If It Works,

Don't Fix It!

What Every Man Should Know BEFORE Having a Vasectomy

by **Kevin Hauber**

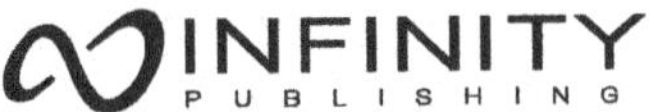

ISBN 978-0-7414-1800-5

Printed in the United States of America

Published January 2013

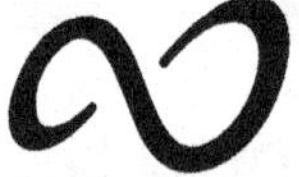

INFINITY PUBLISHING
1094 New DeHaven Street, Suite 100
West Conshohocken, PA 19428-2713
Toll-free (877) BUY BOOK
Local Phone (610) 941-9999
Fax (610) 941-9959
Info@buybooksontheweb.com
www.buybooksontheweb.com

From Kevin's Doctor

"It seems like just yesterday that Kevin came to my office for a general physical and requested a referral to see a specialist. Kevin and his wife Kristen were contemplating contraception options and were interested in finding out more information about vasectomies. At the time Kevin was a healthy, vibrant, and active individual. Sadly, today Kevin suffers from chronic pain due to complications arising from his original vasectomy procedure.

"I think many people living with this kind of pain would have been tempted to give up; but Kevin, with his persevering spirit, began to ask pointed questions and embark on his own research. He did more than become a partner in his health care: Kevin became the captain of his body as he guided the course of his treatment. Unsatisfied with results, he continually sought out alternative and conventional Western models of care and settled into those modalities his body responded to the best and made the most sense for his situation. He maintained contact with providers, began a dialogue with other men who had undergone vasectomy, allowed himself to be guided to experience various modalities, maintained a daily discipline of relaxation techniques, and was judicious with taking his medication/herbal regimens.

"I know many men will benefit from reading this book. It takes us on an odyssey from the initial procedure with the radio booming Aretha Franklin's "Rescue Me" through the trials and tribulations of multiple specialists and numerous invasive procedures and other forms of treatment. We are also exposed to first hand insight of the frustration and cost of dealing with our current medical and insurance systems. Kevin writes from his own experience with great clarity, humor, and a growing respect for the awesome complexity of our human bodies.

"I would like to end my comments by noting that in my ten years of medical practice, I don't think I ever have met an individual who has impressed me with their drive to overcome what must have seemed at times an insurmountable wall more than Kevin. He is truly a shining example of a spirit who has been able to transform tragedy into a bright, shining light by illuminating a subject which has been kept quiet for so very long. This book will undoubtedly help other men seeking contraception and those dealing with complications arising from what Kevin aptly describes as a not-so-simple vasectomy."

Dr. Diane Stern

Contents

Acknowledgements i
A Physician's Forward iii
Introduction iv

Part I. Getting a Fix   1

A Book About What? 2
Chapter One. Bellying Up to the Bar 5
Chapter Two. Holding on for Dear Life 11
Chapter Three. How Is This Thing Put Together, Anyway? 21
Chapter Four. I've Never Seen This Happen Before 34
Chapter Five. On Pins and Needles 36
Chapter Six. I Think I Need a Creative Outlet 45
Chapter Seven. Once Is Not Enough 52
Chapter Eight. I'm Off to See the Wizard 57
Chapter Nine. Here, Eat This Root 61

Part II. Fixing "the Fix" (or Trying To)   65

Chapter Ten. Tied to the Cross 66
Chapter Eleven. I've Got a Lovely Pair of Coconuts 74
Chapter Twelve. All the Kings Horses and All the Kings Men, ... 78
         Couldn't Put Humpty-Dumpty Back Together Again 78
Chapter Thirteen. Life Finds a Way 84

Part III. Good Reasons for Not Getting a Fix in the First Place   88

Chapter Fourteen. How Do You Make a Hormone? 89
Chapter Fifteen. Vasectomies and the Immune System 92
Chapter Sixteen. Invasion of the Antibody Snatchers 102
Chapter Seventeen. Here's a Crazy Idea 105
Chapter Eighteen. Do You Smoke After Sex? 109
Chapter Nineteen. What is This Doing to My Brain? 112
Chapter Twenty. Just Cut It Out! 117
Chapter Twenty-One. Living With Mr. T 120
Chapter Twenty-Two. I'm Sorry; That's Not a Covered Benefit 127
Chapter Twenty-Three. Of All the Nerve 132
Chapter Twenty-Four. Stories, Myths, and Facts 143
Chapter Twenty-Five. Adventures in Inner Space 151

Part IV. Where Do We Go From Here?   155

Chapter Twenty-Six. Extra, Extra! 156
Chapter Twenty-Seven. Show Me Another Way 159
Chapter Twenty-Eight. Testicles On Trial 170
Chapter Twenty-Nine. Doc, It Hurts When I Do This 175
Chapter Thirty. Let There Be Light 186
Chapter Thirty-One. The Challenge 191
Chapter Thirty-Two. How Does This All Add Up? 194
Chapter Thirty-Three. On a Personal Note 200
Chapter Thirty-Four. As If That Wasn't Enough 207
Chapter Thirty-Five. Getting a Firm Grasp on the Obvious: 211
         Relevant Quotations Regarding Post-Vasectomy Pain and Other Side Effects of Vasectomy 211
Bibliography 223
Index 245
Author Contact Information 249

Acknowledgements

There are many individuals who have offered me innumerable blessings throughout the course of my vasectomy and post-vasectomy experience. I would like to recognize all of these individuals by name; however, there are some that preferred not to be mentioned in this text for personal reasons. The loving and caring souls that I can name here are:

My loving wife and children, Kristen, Kate and Kenton; Susan and Erik Amerikaner; Sandy Baer, who helped me extensively in the final preparation of this book for publication and has become a champion of this cause, Dr. Rick Berg my radiologist neighbor and friend who has repeatedly and unflinchingly made numerous images of parts of my body that I never considered photogenic; Sattie Blanton, whose sage advice has been tremendously beneficial to me; Fred Bond, who has put up with a lot from me over the years and has been completely understanding along the way (Of course, I've put up with a lot from him too, but this isn't the time or place to discuss that.). Also, I wish to recognize Carolyn Braddock for her leading edge work with patients who have experienced sexual trauma of various sorts; Dr. Margaret Carmen, whose gentle touch blessed me repeatedly; Judd Clark, who is not only a great swim coach, but has a terrific grasp of the English language and helped me a great deal in the initial editing of this book (Who would have thought?); Jill Cohen for the magic of her touch and unwinding skills and her willingness to share them; Dr. Mark Eckert for his openness and kind sharing of his experience, and for his support of me throughout my experience; Rev. Leona Evans for helping me to remember the greater plan God has for all of us; Dave Farley for the use of several of his cartoons that helped me to smile when needed and hopefully will do the same for you; Rodney Foster of CBS News; Laura Fraser, who was willing to boldly go where no man (or woman) has gone before, quite literally; Dr Jeffrey Freidman, who has been a great source of encouragement and is a very wise and kind man to boot; Scott Freutel for affirming for me that I actually could write a publishable work; Tom and Melanie Fulks for listening and helping me get the word to the right people; Dr. Raymond Gaeta for telling me the truth without sugar coating and helping me to better understand the path I needed to take; Dr. Paul Georgiou, who helped me through a traumatic Emergency Room experience; Christian Giardina, whose hands can break through the impenetrable knots pain can cause; David Goldeen, who has helped me walk the edge I've needed to in my healing process; Connie R. Graves, who can actually make going to a urologist appointment a more enjoyable experience; Linda Griffith, who is just plainly a warm and wonderful person to be around; Dr. Connie Haber, who took on the challenge of my case willingly and "shined the light" on my problem; Dave Hartshorn, who joined me enthusiastically in my shameless efforts to bring the issues discussed in this book into public awareness; and Erwin and LaVerne Hauber (my dad and mom) for supporting me in an unwavering manner through my medical and all other manner of personal crises.

I also recognize Dr. John Hannon, who has helped me to see another way when all else was failing; Jere Hench, who has suffered mightily himself but reached out to me when he found out that I was hurting; Dr. Stephen Hilty, my internist and one of my greatest allies, who willingly ventured into the unknown and repeatedly helped me in ways I never would have expected or imagined; Dr. Gene Hori for saving my bacon numerous times (more literally than I want to think) and for getting me to the right people at the right times; John Hupp, who was willing to share his own experience with me and use his hypnotherapist skills to help comfort and improve my world; Joseph Jastrab, who has been an example and inspiration for me in the personal redefining process I have undergone; Jon Jenkins, whose advice and counsel I have enjoyed for more than 20 years; Dr. Dale Kiker for his incredible willingness to help me as my options narrowed; Kyra Kitts for her wonderful healing energy and love so willingly shared; Archer Koch, my friend and web master/web page designer extraordinaire (If you don't believe me, just check out the www.dontfixit.org web site); Matt Koivista for his steadfast and prayerful support of me; Sandra Lee for her encouragement and savvy media advice; Rev. Richard Levy, whose love and friendship always reminds me of God's unconditional love for all of us; Larry Lima for his commitment to men's work and for the compassion and help he has shown me personally; Cindy Luis, without whose devoted and loving support I would have sunk a long time ago; Dr. Steve Mangar, who counseled me repeatedly and helped me remember the big picture of what I experienced while still wielding an amazingly well-placed needle; Dr. David Marquis for his efforts for my benefit; Dr. Arthur McLean, who is an excellent immunologist; Sharon Mesker, my friend and prayer partner, who is just plainly the most loving person you could ever meet; Patty and Jack Morales for keeping the faith in me, and everyone else for that matter; Michael Moran for helping me sort out the pieces as they fell, and then as they fell again; John Morgan of USA Today for being willing to tell the story; Sheri Nelson, who introduced me to Watsu as a wonderful way to relieve chronic pain; Trish Norman for her insightful and loving touch; Faith Norton, R.N., for helping me to get my research going in the right direction; Mike Owens for the many phone calls back and forth encouraging each other through our respective dilemmas; Gayle Peron, my attorney, who counseled me well and took on a tough case because she knew it was the right thing to do; John and Roz Phillips for their friendship and help in the composition of this book; Dr. Neil Pollock, who has been a saving grace for me and many others, not only for his treatment approaches that he has developed, but by his willingness to bring the issues raised in this book to the attention of the medical community.

In addition, I recognize John Pratt, who researched my legal case tirelessly; Annette Roberts, my mother-in-law and the loving anchor of our family; Dr. Edward Roberts, my father-in-law for being the other sensible anchor of our family; H. J. Roberts, M.D. for blazing the trail of exposing the problems associated with vasectomies and for his endorsement of my work; Margaret and Mark Roberts, who have been willing to put up with me through many situations over the years; Deborah Sampley, D.C. for her helpful guidance; Dr. Mark Schecter for being the peaceful and kind man he is and sharing that with others; Carol Scholl for her support of Kristen and me even when I was quite loopy; Andrew Silva just for being the good friend he is; Kathy Silva, my other prayer partner and friend with a heart as big as the world; Lou and Jeannie Silva (Kathy's parents), whose hearts are equally big; Ralph and Anne Slocum, my long-time friends and supporters (you notice I didn't say old); Diane Smalley, who knows how to place an acupuncture needle in a way that gives me a charge like no other, quite literally.

I cannot forget Bob and Therese Solimeno; Jeff and Rev. Norma Spry for being the loving light they are; Dr. Roger Steele for his help and sense of humor throughout hospital and doctor's office visits; Peter Sterios, who's not only a skilled yoga teacher, but a great friend and human being with a sense of humor almost as twisted as mine, maybe even more; Dr. Diane Stern, who helped me repeatedly throughout the first year of my medical dramas and always reminded me that I was more than my "dis-ease;" Paul Texiera, who led me to find helpful methods of physical therapy; Dave Tuck, who helped me with insights on pharmacy matters; Dr. Marisa Upson whose skills at lymphatic massage and just her presence have helped me immensely; Grace and Mike VanDoren for their support and help in putting this book into better form; my friend Thomas Varner, who helped me practice just hanging out with the depth of what God offers me, even if I don't like much of it; Stacey Warde, who fearlessly wrote about this subject for the New Times and worked with me on the editing of this book; Dave Wardlaw, another long-time friend and supporter; Dr. Philip Werthman, whose technical skills are only exceeded by his compassion and understanding; Owen and Jeannie Weyers for their friendship and loving support; Steve and Lynn Wolter, whose friendship spans the miles; Dr. Jean Yu, who gave me a "charge" every time I saw her; Dr. Lou Zaninovich, who encouraged me in presenting this material and has been a tremendous resource in the field of men's health issues.

Last but certainly not least, I want to recognize Louis Zimmerman, who is an exceptional artist and has the ability to take some sick, twisted ideas I have and turn out even more twisted graphic images.

My gratitude and my blessings go out to all of you.

They say it takes a whole village to raise a child. In my case, it takes a whole village to heal from a vasectomy, and I have been lucky to have been accompanied on the journey by these and so many others.

A Physician's Forward

This book is "one man's story," but it is NOT the story of "one man". It is, in fact, the story of many men. As a doctor with thirty-five years' experience, I can say that unequivocally.

This is not a unique, one-only story. Kevin Hauber's post-vasectomy problem is not a freakish one-off occurrence, not pure coincidence, not "all in his mind".

Sure, he and I both agree that many men have vasectomies and never have any regrets. He was led to believe that those with regrets were very, very rare. But they are out there, and not as rare as he thought, and I agree with his mission to inform and present the "other" side of the vasectomy story.

Vasectomy is a crude surgical insult to the organs directly involved with the greatest and most profound mystery of life: The very propagation of life itself.

Somewhere between forty and two hundred MILLION sperm are produced in every man EVERY SINGLE DAY. A vasectomy blocks the sperm's exit through the vas deferens. But after the surgery, the testicles just keep producing more and more sperm. PRESSURE builds up in EVERY man. Internal ruptures occur.

This amazing body of ours has to adapt, accept the changes, make changes itself to deal with this insult. That it does, and does so well in so many cases is a miracle in itself. That the body fails in some cases to adapt should surely not be surprising.

Read on: Be amazed if you will, but don't be surprised!!

Dr. Lou Zaninovich, M.D.
Male Health Specialist

Introduction
by Dr. Neil Pollock

Kevin's experience with Post-Vasectomy Pain Syndrome, as it is so vividly and meticulously documented in his book, will have a profound effect on the reader whether he is a vasectomy patient with Post-Vasectomy Pain Syndrome, an individual considering vasectomy, or a vasectomy physician.

As one of North America's largest providers of vasectomy, reading Kevin's book and my subsequent discussions with him have provided me with an increased knowledge base to use in helping patients with post-vasectomy pain. As well, I now have an increased sensitivity to better understand these individuals and to help them cope with this very difficult problem. Kevin's work brings up some very important questions that we as vasectomy providers must consider seriously, because it is our ethical obligation and responsibility to our patients to do so.

One key question is: What is a man's true risk of developing chronic pain that may, as in Kevin's case, significantly impair and disable him for a prolonged period? It is important for physician providers to be absolutely sure that when we communicate the risks of such a problem to a patient it is the true risk from our own work, because that is the only statistic that is relevant to the patient coming to see us. For me to be able to tell a patient the true risk of developing chronic disabling pain after a vasectomy done by me, I need to have a system in place by which I have been able to accurately quantify that risk. If I don't, I will inadvertently underestimate that risk for many reasons. For example, the memory of the physician is not infallible; we forget our complication unless we keep accurate written statistics of each and every outcome. Patients who we operate on who develop problems and may see other physicians for treatment never returning to us will also obscure our perceptions of our own complications.

Kevin's book has motivated me to carry out a large scale study of 4,000 of the vasectomy patients who I have operated on over the last four years. My objective is to have as many of the 4,000 as possible telephone-interviewed to carefully document any and all complications including post vasectomy pain that they have experienced that I may or may not be aware of. Once I have these results I will then publish them because I think these results will make a significant contribution to the literature that currently documents vasectomy risks.

Should the results confirm the findings of McMahon's work in his article "Chronic Testicular Pain following Vasectomy" where he reported that 15% of post-vasectomy patients at his institution reported troublesome chronic discomfort, I think it would raise another red flag about vasectomy. On the other hand, should I find that the percentage of individuals experiencing post-vasectomy pain in my patient group is negligible, the procedure of vasectomy may be vindicated to a degree and possibly raise questions as to why some providers have higher rates of serious complication than others. This may lead to us taking a closer look at what procedural aspects of vasectomy may or may not be responsible for these different outcomes.

I do feel it is important in any surgery to cause the most minimal amount of trauma and tissue disruption possible while carrying out the surgical objective. With this in mind there are a number of differences in the approaches of various vasectomy providers that may lead to significant differences in outcomes. I personally subscribe to the following approach which can be viewed on my website at www.pollockclinics.com in the vasectomy video section. I use the No-Scalpel Vasectomy technique as developed by Dr. Lee in Sechuan, China which has been shown to have an eight-fold lower complication rate. I use the open-ended vasectomy technique as described by Silber which involves leaving the testicular end of the vas unblocked with the goal of decreasing post vasectomy congestive pain. I use the No-Needle Anesthesia method for anesthetic delivery which obviates the need for blindly introducing a needle into the scrotum. My approach has allowed for the provision of a virtually bloodless, painless vasectomy done in eight minutes with an extremely low complication rate. We have also seen no vasectomy failures in our last 4,000 surgeries. Of note, the McMahon study that I previously referred to used a completely different technique for performing vasectomy.

So what can a patient do when trying to calculate his true risk of developing complications with a given vasectomy provider, if he may not be getting a true estimate of risks from the provider? There is no question that experience is a key determinant of outcomes. Look for a provider with experience in the area of vasectomy, not in the area of general urology or general surgery. Doctors like myself, dedicated to performing vasectomy as the focus of their surgical practice, may perform 1,500 or more vasectomies annually. This level of experience is quite different than the experience of someone performing 20 or even 200 vasectomies annually. Physicians may be slightly more accurate in estimating the numbers of surgeries that they do rather than recalling post-surgical complications. Secondly, seeking a provider who understands and uses the same technique that I have described may also help to lower post-surgical morbidity and possibly short and long-term complications.

For those individuals who have developed post-vasectomy pain and are now considering what they should do, I can only say that seeking the care of an experienced physician who has a good understanding of post-vasectomy pain and treatment options is critical. Let me state plainly that these individuals are not easy to find. The most common experience patients may have is to see a provider who denies the existence of their problem or who acknowledges it but because of his own frustration in treating it makes the patient feel like a nuisance or encourages them to have another surgery that often ends up putting the patient in a worse situation than before.

On my website I outline a number of potential causes of post-vasectomy pain and potential treatment options. However, before considering treatment options that are invasive, i.e. surgical, I can only say that I advise my own patients not to consider such things for up to three years post-vasectomy, because very often time heals all. In addition, it must be understood by the patient and the medical provider that post-vasectomy pain symptoms may manifest in a variety of ways and at differing lengths of time following the procedure. These factors must be considered in the process of making a diagnosis and recommending any course of treatment. There is no "one size fits all" approach to the treatment of this problem.

Dr.Neil Pollock

Dr. Pollock is a vasectomy surgeon in Vancouver, B. C., with a special interest in the diagnosis and treatment of Post-Vasectomy Pain Syndrome. He can be reached by email at drneil@netrover.com. Dr. Pollock's website can be found at www.pollockclinics.com. This introduction is in no way intended to be medical advice to any individual. It is simply a general discussion of Dr. Pollock's experience with post-vasectomy pain and reflections on Kevin Hauber's book. Individuals with any medical problems should seek out the advice of a qualified medical practitioner.

Part I

Getting a Fix

If It Works, Don't Fix It-
What Every Man Should Know **Before** Having a Vasectomy

By Kevin Hauber

A Book About What?

I know what you are thinking. A book about vasectomies? Why would anyone possibly want to write that? Why spend the time and effort to write (or read for that matter) a book about a widely accepted medical procedure on a perfectly unmentionable part of the body that everyone would just as soon not discuss anyway? I'm sure you have asked these types of questions of yourself by now. But it is precisely because of the fact that this surgery is so widely performed and the results are discussed so little that this needed to be written.

A famous playwright was once asked about where he got his inspiration for what he wrote. "Whatever it is that wakes you up at four in the morning," he replied, "That is what you must write about." I have taken this idea to heart. Well, not exactly to heart, but close. I cannot count how many sleepless nights this subject of vasectomy has caused me. In this regard, I now know that I am not alone, as you will see.

This book is an outgrowth of my own personal experience with a vasectomy, or in my case, vasectomies, and what can go wrong. Some might claim that mine is an extreme example, despite the fact that a good deal of evidence shows otherwise. My experience turned into what has truly been the most significant medical situation I have ever faced, and one that has struck fear in the hearts (and other places) of every man I have described it to. Hopefully, you can benefit from this knowledge, which I gained the hard way.

This is a subject that is uncomfortable for most people. The discussion will be in open and frank terms. A frank discussion is necessary because of the great deal of information concerning vasectomies that needs to be shared with men and women before the procedure is done. This information is most commonly not known by the patient or disclosed by the doctor. This lack of information, or in some cases, actual misinformation, does not allow an informed choice about what is often a permanent change in a man's bodily function. Serious ramifications can result. I discuss these facts in plain language.

The more we know about what works well for our bodies, and what doesn't work well, the better off we will all be in this life. If open discussion about bodies and some of their most basic functions is more than you can handle right now, you may want to put this down and go read something else. However, if you are a man or woman who is concerned about reproductive health, and, in fact, your health in general, or care about some one who is, keep reading. I am not a writer by trade, nor am I a doctor, but spend my work-a-day life as a mortgage loan officer. This is not a profession noted for its adept skills at handling medical issues or sarcastic humor, not necessarily in that order. However, I've found great motivation to share the information contained here. I won't give any medical advice, but will share my medical experience and the research of many doctors with you.

Will Rogers said, "There are three kinds of men: The one that learns by reading; the few who learn by observation; and the rest of them who have to pee on the electric fence for themselves." Unfortunately, when it came to vasectomy, I had to learn by the last method, which is a surprisingly accurate analogy for the sensations I experienced afterwards. Maybe, by reading this, you won't have to do the same.

Part I of the book discusses the circumstances that can lead up to considering a vasectomy, what you are likely to be told beforehand, and what you might experience during and after the procedure. I will tell about this through my experience and the experience of others. There is also be a candid discussion of some of the anatomy involved and why reactions can occur.

Part II deals with what is often involved in the undoing of the effects of vasectomy, and the types of medical procedures needed to do so. As you might be able to tell, there is a progressive intensification of subject material here.

Part III continues and broadens the discussion of the long-term effects of vasectomies. Based upon my experience and the research presented, I draw some very specific conclusions about the overall viability of vasectomies as a form of permanent birth control.

Part IV discusses the various alternatives available and the need for accurate information to be given about this subject. Hang in there. By the end you will understand enough to make up your own mind. Hopefully, you will know the reason why I was compelled to tell this story and share the evidence.

My personal journey started as an attempt to permanently resolve the issue of contraception for my wife and myself with what I thought was a well-researched and well-advised solution. Along the way, I encountered complications that have implications for millions of other men as well as myself. I learned what kind of truly painful consequences a vasectomy can result in, and what drastic measures are often proposed for the resolution of that pain.

I learned what significant autoimmune responses are all about and why three out of four men who have vasectomies experience this type of reaction. I also learned a great deal about the long-term health consequences of such reactions. In the process, I discovered a great deal about the anatomical and hormonal changes that occur after a vasectomy, and how these changes can affect your health. I also learned how little medical science knows at this time about how to treat and resolve such conditions, and why much of this evidence has been undisclosed in many cases.

It became abundantly clear that I would need to judiciously guard my own health and act on my inner guidance in this process, while critically evaluating the medical advice I was being given. In short, what started out as an effort to resolve a problem that was presented to me as uniquely mine, became something with far-reaching implications.

In some cases I have changed the names of those involved to protect the injured. It may read like a script from a bad Mel Brooks movie, but alas, it is true. Or, this may be regarded as more of a dark comedy, which is all the rage these days anyway. Fortunately, most of the people who read this don't know me personally, and for those who do, well, it will give them something to smile knowingly about the next time they see me.

I want to acknowledge the love and support of my wife, Kristen, and my two children, Kate and Kenton, who have loved me without fail throughout my situation, even at times when I was not acting in a very lovable manner. I have also been blessed with encountering many caring and competent medical providers and other healing professionals along the way who have given me wonderful assistance and guidance.

In addition, I credit my somewhat twisted and frank sense of humor for helping me through my situation. Humor is an incredible coping device, as I'm sure you'll see in this case. At times, humor was the only coping device I had left. So many possible titles came to mind for this work: Scrotal Scribbles, The Testicular Testament, and Great Balls of Fire were all contenders. However, I finally settled on "If It Works, Don't Fix It" because that idea embodies the message of what I experienced, and what I learned along the way.

I found a surprising number of sources on this subject while writing this book. Most references were written in a rather sterile (pardon the pun) medical style that relays a good number of statistics and other technical information. I've always felt that, while interesting, statistical information doesn't convey the full human experience. For that reason, you will find the information presented here in the context of the very human stories of myself and others. Hopefully, in this way I can share the true impact of what is being discussed.

However, if you are the kind of person who likes to read the last chapter of a book first to see how it comes out, or you are a man who has already had a vasectomy and want to skip the story line stuff because you think you know it all, start reading at the chapter titled "How Do You Make a Hormone" and go from there. If you are a real bottom line, Reader's Digest version-type of person, look to the chapter titled "Stories, Myths, and Facts" and you will find a good summary of what the experience entails and what results can occur based on documented medical facts, not claims for advertising purposes.

If you are experiencing chronic pain or other post-vasectomy problems, you may want to look at the chapter titled "Doc, It Hurts When I Do This" initially and then rejoin the story line to expand your understanding. The last chapter contains numerous quotes from medical journals on the subject of vasectomy and the problems that can and do ensue for your reference.

It would be quite easy to become self-conscious about this subject. Believe me, this is an issue I have confronted throughout the entire experience. To address the feeling, I'll share a piece of wisdom that a friend several years my senior shared with me:

"When I was in my teens and 20s, what everyone thought of me was all-important.

"In, my 30s and 40s, I didn't care much about what everyone thought of me.

"By the time I reached my 50s and 60s, I realized that others weren't thinking about me much at all, but were more interested in their own lives."

I'm not in my 50s or 60s yet, but the wisdom presented here makes sense. It is my hope that, in sharing the stories and research contained in this book, you will gain a greater appreciation and understanding for the amazing and pervasive creative process going on inside your body. I know I have.

I hope also that the respect you may gain for this powerful natural gift will endure long after you forget my name and many of the details of the story, and that it might help you in making some very important core choices in your life. And please, share this information with others whose health you care about.

Chapter One

Bellying Up to the Bar

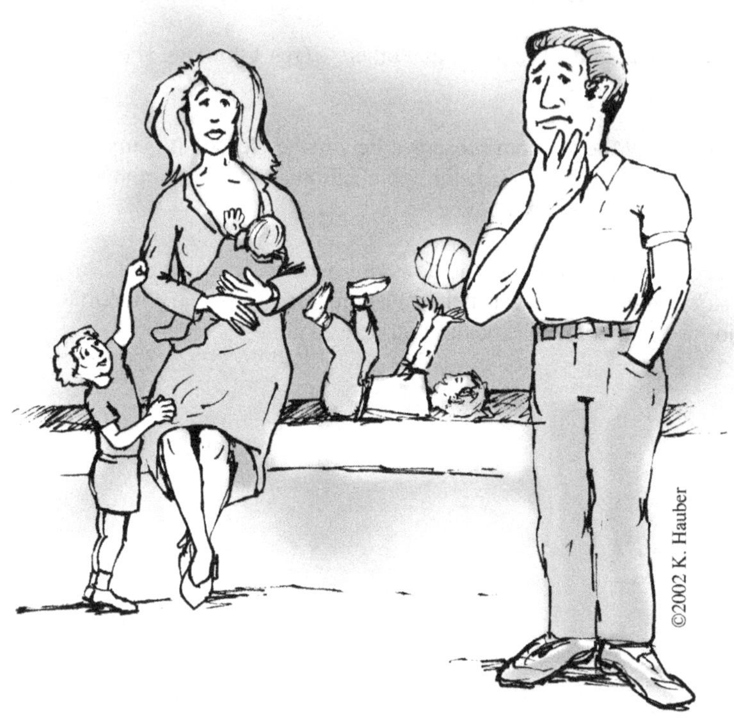

"Since the first human vasectomy was performed by Reginald Harrison in 1893, it has had the uncanny knack of gathering enthusiastic support from the fringes of the medical profession and the public. Both the use and study of vasectomy have been marred by the intrusion of many of the passionate social issues that have wracked the twentieth century. It has been dogged too by the intrusion of man's deepest fears and irrational buried yearnings. For not only does vasectomy, by physical and functional propinquity, keep close companionship with the dark art of castration, but it has been used to cast out the devils of insanity, to chase the Faustian legend of eternal youth, to hasten the coming Neitszche's Superman, and, latterly, to save the world from ecodoom" (Wolfers, 1973)

That's a hard act to follow, but let me try in my own simple way. A vasectomy is not something most people talk or think about a lot, unless they happen to be a urologist, of course, or someone who has had complications from his vasectomy. For many men, in fact, it is often treated as a relatively minor decision, and an easy procedure. Guys will talk about having gotten their "license to love" almost as if it were a war medal. Depending on which statistic you believe, up to a million men per year in the United States apply for that license. Some estimates are only about half that number. However, "It has been estimated that approximately 500,000 men undergo vasectomy for elective sterilization in the United States annually. This number is most likely an underestimate, since there are many unreported cases" (Kessler, 1982).

"The use of vasectomy is growing and bypasses the frequency of female sterilization in some parts of the industrialized world…. As a couple ages, their likelihood of choosing some form of permanent sterilization increases" (Sandlow, et. al., 2001). Vasectomy is the most common male surgery performed, second only to circumcision, and has been done with regularity for many decades now. "Vasectomy was first preformed on humans in 1893 and was originally used mainly to prevent epididymitis following prostate operations" (Kaufman, et. al., 1996). Although the procedure has been performed with increasing frequency since around the turn of the century, the popularity of vasectomies as a means of birth control really took off in the sixties and seventies, as the age of "free love" burst on the scene. Millions more are done each year if you look outside the United States, especially in developing countries such as China and India, where there have been forced sterilization programs or "incentive" programs in place as a means of population control.

Forced sterilization programs have a fascinating social history, and not just among a few religious orders. From 1933 on, over a million men were sterilized by order of the Nazi government in Germany because they were deemed unfit to procreate. Many of these "unfit" persons were, not surprisingly, Jewish, as this "Prevention of Hereditary Disease in Posterity" law attempted to affect ethnic cleansing on the population (Carruthers, 1997). "No one knows how many sterilizations were performed in Germany during Nazi rule. Estimates range from 200,000 to 2,000,000. About half of these were vasectomies" (Wolfers, 1973).

Politics can get involved in all this snipping, too. A series of forced sterilization programs in India in the 1960's and 1970's are credited as having had a large effect on the outcome of the election that removed Indira Ghandi from power (Bower, 1995). Sterilization programs in India have persisted since, relying more on persuasion and various incentives, like free radios and cash payments, to entice patients. In India, two studies showed that, "43 percent and 36 percent [respectively] of the men reported that the money was the 'sole motivating factor'" (Wolfers, 1973). Other countries, such as the Philippines, still engage in mass sterilization campaigns, particularly in rural areas.

Forced sterilization of men has been practiced regularly in the United States also. "In 1922, 31 states had statutes permitting involuntary sterilization of 'defective individuals'" (Carruthers, 1997). What kind of defects might we be speaking of here? Some convicts are forced to be sterilized as a condition of parole or even while in prison. Up to the 1970's, welfare recipients in some states were required to be sterilized if they had two or more children. This quote from Chicago's Chief Justice Harry Olson may give you an idea of the rational and legal arguments that went into these decisions: "By eugenic measures, …our burden of taxes can be reduced by reducing the number of degenerates, delinquents, and defectives supported in public institutions" (Wolfers, 1973).

In the early 1900's, one particularly zealous doctor attempting to rid the world of social evils at the Jefferson Reformatory in Indiana, "compulsorily vasectomized 280 men because they had defects of character such as 'selfishness, ingratitude, inconstancy, egotism, and inability to resist any impulse or desire' or masturbated excessively" (Carruthers, 1997). Obviously, you would hate to have met this doctor when either of you was having a bad day.

The list of reasons to forcibly sterilize people expanded at a lightning pace. "By 1939, sterilization had been recommended for leprosy, tuberculosis, epilepsy, alcoholism, insanity, sexual deviation, moral turpitude, mental defect, criminal conviction, Huntington's Chorea, 'hereditary' deafness and blindness, severe physical deformity, neurasthenia, syphilis, rape, drug-taking, carnal knowledge and, ultimately, chicken stealing!"(Wolfers, 1973).

Despite its use as a means of social control, most men alive today who have undergone vasectomy have done so of their own free will, sort of. This is not to say that there aren't other coercing influences, which we will discuss in detail later.

It is commonly proposed that sterilizing a man by a vasectomy is simpler and safer as a means of permanent birth control than his female partner having her "tubes tied." Statements in various forms of public media often convey the idea that vasectomies are practically foolproof. According to the U. S. Department of Health and Human Services, around 50 million men have had vasectomies, equaling about five percent of all married couples of reproductive age (National Institute of Health, 1996). Other recent estimates run as high as 70 to 100 million total vasectomies performed (Weiske, 2001). However you look at it, that's a lot of snipping going on. Looked at another way, about one of every six men over the age of 35 in the United States has had a vasectomy. The prevalence increases with education and income (National Institute of Health, 1996).

According to the Journal of Urology, complication rates for vasectomies run 3% or less. Remember that number, less than 3%. Is this really the case? What constitutes a "complication" anyway, and who gives and compiles this data? Let me share some facts and a few stories with you, and let you judge for yourself.

In one study, the mean average number of children in the family was 2.4 when the father sought a vasectomy (Sandlow, et. al., 2001). In my experience, 2.4 or more children can more than fill an ox cart with the volume of stuff babies require to be hauled around with them. Simply put, most vasectomy patients are "typically in their thirties, of high socioeconomic status, white, with some religious affiliation, married, and [have] approximately two to three children" (Sandlow, et. al., 2001).

Modern life has a curious collection of pressures and expectations associated with the maturation process. On a physical level, as you enter adolescence, there is that rush of desire to perfect your procreating skills without actually procreating. This process has gotten countless folks into many unforeseen problems, and is the subject of many other dissertations by everyone from parents, to ministers, to politicians. I shall not enter this discussion. I merely observe these varied influences and opinions all exist.

Next there is the urge and pressure to choose a mate and actually make children. At this point the anxiety of the expectations surrounding this process is tremendous, not least among them the "So, when are you going to give me a grandchild" syndrome. This kind of pressure, along with any physical or genetic factors, makes the process of conceiving quite difficult for many couples.

There are many who struggle through the attempt at the American Dream of family, career, home (with the unthinkably large mortgage that loan officers like me will happily provide), and 2.5 children in the back of the SUV. At some point, we realize that our dance card is quite full, and that continuing to contribute to the population increase is not only a social and environmental issue but is wearing us out.

Here's how the conversation usually goes:

Husband: "Honey, we're so lucky to have such a beautiful new baby."

Wife: "I know, but I didn't realize how much work two (four, eight, twelve) children would be."

Husband: "So, how did your appointment with the doctor go today?"

Wife: "The doctor says everything is fine, but we may want to consider some form of permanent birth control if we don't want any more children. You know the risks associated with pregnancy go up quite a bit as a woman ages, along with the risk of blood clots and stroke if I stay on the pill."

Husband: "I understand. What would you like to do about it?"

Silence. Probably a long silence with a glare attached. A pregnant pause, if you will.

Wife: "I figure that since I'm the one who carried these kids around for nine months each, went through the 36 (98, 412) hours of labor and pushed them out, now it's your turn!"

Silence again: Probably an even longer silence.

Husband: "(Gulp) OK honey, I'll look into it."

Obviously, my wife and I had a discussion similar to the one above. A friend of mine who is a few years older told me once that when a guy has fathered all the kids he and his wife want, his biological usefulness has just expired and he had better have other redeeming qualities. Besides, as a "modern father" I had witnessed and participated in the birthing process with my wife twice, which gave me a tremendous respect for womankind in general and my wife in particular. Any man who still thinks that women are the weaker of the sexes has obviously not been a part of the birthing process. Deep in my heart I know this to be true. In this light, the prospect of a little snip, snip didn't seem like too much of a sacrifice.

So, having a vasectomy almost becomes a rite of passage into the "now I need to support what I've created" stage of life. One male friend of ours put it quite delicately, "I've fired two live rounds and now the rest are going to be blanks!" A lot of people have fun with the process, and not necessarily just the men. One friend of mine had his vasectomy and his wife threw him a party, complete with a weenie roast.

Another acquaintance told me that during the procedure, he and the doctor were rocking out to the Beatles and he felt quite comfortable and safe throughout the entire process. He must have had better drugs than I did, but I don't doubt the story.

For most guys, it's just a great way to extract a couple days of sympathy, and catch up on some TV sports before those "Get back on the horse and ride!" messages come. There was even a TV commercial for a sports channel picturing a guy looking over his feet in a hospital bed at a nurse who is smiling at him and picking up some instruments. The caption comes on saying, "Vasectomy?" and going on to give information about how to order the sports channel. It would appear that the marketing people for this channel knew their demographic pretty well. It would also appear that the guys who watch that channel are into several kinds of sport.

Some people make a real party out of this life event. In Thailand in 1990, the "King's Birthday Vasectomy Festival" was held during which a reported 1203 vasectomies were performed by 50 doctors throughout the course of one day (Nirpathpongporn, et. al., 1990). There was even a pop radio song released commemorating the event. This is an example of someone who just isn't content with blowing out the candles. It's funny, but I remember stories as a kid where the king and queen used to throw a ball in celebration of some major event. This added a whole new twist to that form of entertainment.

Some men turn a vasectomy into a form of recreation. In France, vasectomies are illegal due to an old Napoleonic law against "self mutilation." The British recognized this as an opportunity to increase tourism and draw some of the amour conscious Frenchmen across the Channel for a couple of days by arranging tour packages that include the vasectomy, the transportation, and the lodging (Mayor, 2000). I think this should be called the "Trip and Snip," but I don't know how that would translate into French. The first man to take advantage of this package commented "It's just like going to the dentist except in a slightly different place." This brought about observations that he might not know his balls from a hole in his head.

Despite all the jokes that can be made about undue influence and coercion, most men have made up their minds that they are done fathering children by the time they seek a vasectomy. It must have something to do with pulling around an increasingly heavy ox cart all the time. Sandlow, et. al., (2001) found that 85% of prospective vasectomy patients had a high level of certainty about their decision to seek sterilization, and that in 91% of cases the wife, girlfriend or partner had been involved in the decision making process. Ninety percent of the partners had been highly in favor of the decision to seek a vasectomy (that's an easy one, isn't it?).

All kidding aside, I believe that most men who choose to have a vasectomy do so because they feel it is the best and simplest thing to do for themselves and their families in this rather important procreative aspect of life. "Men want to be partners in family planning and will access services if available. Current political and social policies are demanding more personal responsibility for the outcome of unintended pregnancies" (Fortunati, et. al., 2001).

I know my motivation in seeking a vasectomy included concerns for my wife's health. I was concerned about what could happen if she were to become pregnant again as she entered her late 30's given the dramas of her prior pregnancies, and I'm sure this concern is common.

There have been reports of some men, even teenagers, seeking vasectomies to allow for uninhibited sexual promiscuity, but I sense that this is quite exceptional, especially in the era of serious sexually transmitted diseases that even a vasectomy won't stop. Besides, research shows that men who seek vasectomy at a young age often regret the decision later on.

What are some concerns of the typical vasectomy candidate? Sandlow, et. al., (2001) determined that men who seek a vasectomy experienced "anxiety about vasectomy surgery [that] was mostly driven by fear about pain and fear of the unknown." Concern about pain during and after the procedure was expressed by 27% of the subjects in this study, while 23% expressed concern about unknown factors. Other concerns expressed included fear of the surgery itself, complications from the surgery, general anxiety, "being cut on," side effects, lack of information, doctors in general, and that someone will make a mistake. These all seem like legitimate concerns to me. Surprisingly, only 5% of subjects expressed concerns about the finality of the procedure, indicating a high degree of conviction about the need for what the overwhelming majority of the men were doing, but anxiety about how they needed to get there. It was also noted that vasectomy "subjects are better problem solvers and have a higher self-concept than people in general." I like that characterization.

"The great majority of men who seek vasectomy have been married for ten years or more and have a stable relationship. Some reasons for a vasectomy include: having all the children the couple wants; not wanting or able to use other methods of contraception; a health problem in the woman that makes pregnancy unsafe; a genetic disorder; or a desire to enjoy sex without fear of unwanted pregnancy" (Simon, et. al., 1998). These are all perfectly viable reasons.

The pressure to seek sterilization is often motivated by medical, social and other sources as well. It is common for a woman's OB-GYN to suggest that her husband/partner consider a vasectomy as a safer form of permanent birth control than the alternative of tubal ligation because of what is commonly perceived to be a greater surgical risk involved in the procedure for a woman.

Doctors aren't the only sources advocating vasectomies. Sterilization has many social components to it and is an element of many a person's and organization's agenda. Witness this ad by Planned Parenthood in a 1999 issue of Hope Dance magazine, a popular newspaper on the Central Coast of California:

The implication here is clear. If you are the partner of a woman and you both desire not to create any (more) children, then the responsible thing to do is to get a vasectomy. You shouldn't make it the woman's responsibility. Let me be quite clear, I have nothing against Planned Parenthood, and in fact support many of the good works that they do in the name of community service. But, regardless of how you feel about such messages and agendas, they influence the decisions men make about their bodies.

Like so many other issues, it is hard to get a neutral (or is that neutered?) opinion when it comes to the issue of sterilization. "Vasectomy is a highly emotional issue to several groups in the community with (real or imaginary) conflicting interests. On the one hand, one can appreciate the zeal it has aroused in family planning circles as a safe, simple, and reliable form of permanent contraception. On the other hand, it involves issues of the most fundamental nature to psychoanalysis. And still again, it is the first attempt to engage the male in biological (as opposed to physical) forms of contraception which may involve pain and risk. The polarization of this research into camps of those in favor and those against is therefore not surprising. It has led to animated criticisms of one by the other." (Wolfers, 1970).

Controversy abounds over the potential health hazards associated with vasectomy and other forms of surgical sterilization, with all of the usual politicizing and publicity spinning that humans are inclined to do to defend and promote their particular world view. Wolfers (1970) offers a further caution in this regard to the promoters of sterilization, noting that, "a contraceptive method with harmful side effects released on large sections of a population will ultimately do more to retard than advance the cause of family planning." But what could possibly be the "harmful side effects" of vasectomy? Read on!

The information you will usually see about vasectomies will inevitably contain the word "simple." This may be true, at least from a surgical standpoint, if not from a functional view. Of all the choices a man can make that involve having his body cut to change something, a vasectomy is one of the fastest procedures that can be experienced. Having a mole removed could take longer, albeit with substantially different implications.

However, when things go wrong, they tend to really get a guy's attention. What could possibly go wrong with such a simple procedure? Hold onto your, er…, hats guys, and let me tell you. You may find that this ability to express your "free love" can have a really high price.

I first contemplated having a vasectomy about a year after the birth of our second child. My wife had experienced enough difficulties related to her pregnancies that we decided to stop at two. Besides, we were running out of room, what with the volume of stuff that such tiny beings seem to generate.

Kristen and I watched the requisite video and had the consultation with the urologist. During this visit, I asked a simple question, "The body continues to make sperm after a vasectomy doesn't it?"

"Yes," he replied.

"So what happens to all those cells? There are a lot of them after all, aren't there?" I inquired further.

The doctor hesitated as if scanning for an answer that would satisfy the concern. "They are just reabsorbed into the body" he replied.

Really? "What about the media stories of vasectomy causing prostate cancer?" I inquired.

"Oh, those have all been disproven," he assured me.

Hmmm, I didn't have complete faith in this response. This seemed like an awful lot of cells to "just reabsorb," but not knowing any better, I agreed to proceed anyway.

In the interim between the consultation and the planned surgery date, a friend of mine had his vasectomy. In his words, he swelled up like he had a third testicle for several weeks afterwards. Yikes!

Then a co-worker of mine had his vasectomy and ended up with what he termed "large painful melons" for days afterwards. Yet another coworker of mine told me of how he developed painful cysts in his scrotum that had to be removed surgically after his vasectomy. Ouch, ouch, ouch!

Another friend went into what seemed like a prolonged depression after his vasectomy, questioning his continued usefulness, which mystified me. Less than a three-percent complication rate? I didn't think I could know that many guys and still be hearing about all this. My wife and I decided to put the whole idea on hold for a while.

Several years later, I read an article in *Men's Health* magazine about "no-scalpel" vasectomies and how the incidence of complications was drastically reduced. The idea of surgery without large knives intrigued me, especially given the location of the prospective cuts. I searched the Internet, and found a web site with a directory of doctors who did the no-scalpel procedure, the closest of whom was about two hundred miles away. This seemed like a potentially long and unpleasant ride given what I was considering having done. So I waited and watched.

One day, I asked my wife's OB-GYN what the difference was between a procedure, a "minor" surgery, and a major surgery. He said that there was no well defined difference, but concluded, "It's never a minor surgery if it's on me!"

Chapter Two

Holding on for Dear Life

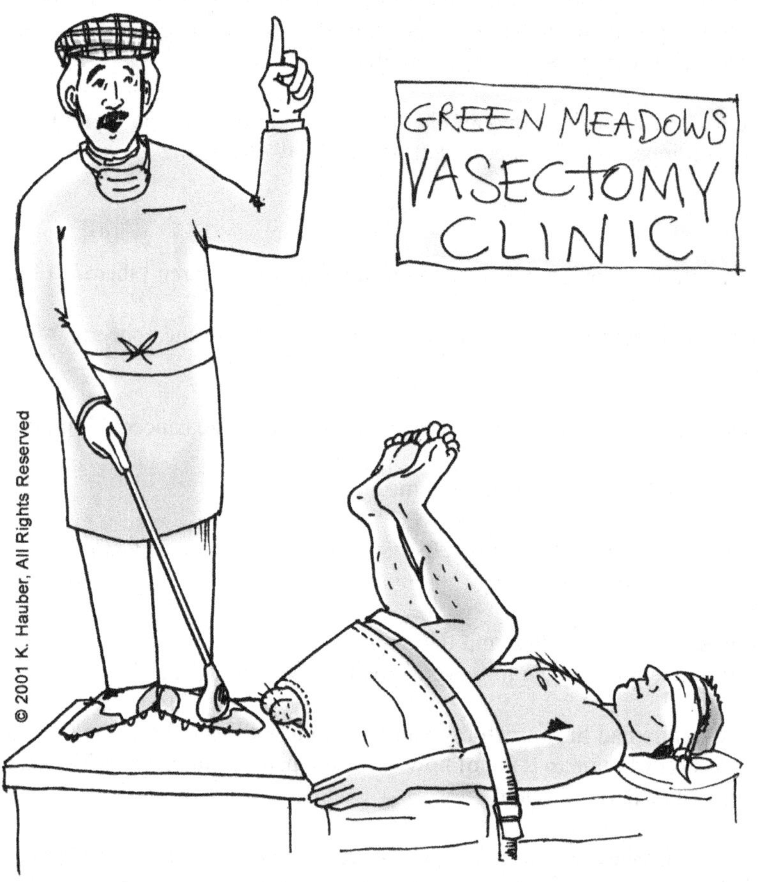

*Now, I need you to hold still. You might feel a
little pressure, but it's only one quick slice.*

The nightmare or the reality?
(I know it's "guy" humor and a little rough, but this is what it can feel like.)

I have avoided doctor's offices most of my adult life. I have nothing against doctors and their work in general as long as they're working on someone else's body. My attitude has always been that with bodies and cars, good preventative maintenance is far better and cheaper than repairs when you have a breakdown. For me this meant exercise, eating well, and passing by hospital zones as quickly as possible.

After years of "loving encouragement" from my wife, I finally went to see a doctor who was a friend of ours from church, scheduled a physical which I hadn't done in about twenty years, and asked for a referral to a urologist to discuss a vasectomy, all in the name of good self care. My physical (including a testicular exam, which was a new experience for me) pronounced me in great health. My doctor told me that even though I was in great health, I should make a regular practice of a testicular self-exam and a breast self-exam checking for lumps.

Really? Breast cancer in men? That was news. The stuff you learn as you go along is amazing, isn't it?

According to my doctor my workout and diet habits were good, because I had a "heartbeat like a giant sea turtle, and they live for two or three hundred years." I wondered what I would do with all that extra time. I don't consider myself a health nut, just a nut who tries to eat well and work out regularly. This was all very reassuring, and I wondered why I had resisted any involvement with the medical model for so many years. My answer was soon to come.

Getting a vasectomy seemed like the perfect move at the time. My wife, my kids and I were all healthy. I was having my best year ever in my business. In short, I was at the top of my game. A little family planning insurance seemed in order. Besides, I had done some research on the Internet about vasectomies and knew what to ask for in the procedure with the least complications. Sure! Do you sense the impending disaster yet?

I was referred to a urologist who was supposed to be the best guy in town. I had another consultation with this new urologist, signed all the necessary consent forms, and received the perfunctory pamphlets on vasectomies. I mentioned the fact that several of my friends had some dramatic results after their vasectomies, then I asked, "I'll be getting a no-scalpel vasectomy for which the incidences of complications is lower, right?" Right, I was assured once you start using that method, you never go back to the old way. Once will be enough for me, thank you. He also assured me that this was a far better method of permanent contraception than removal of the testicles, a fact which I had a hard time arguing with. We scheduled the procedure to be done after an upcoming vacation and parted company. The doctor was a nice guy and he made it very easy, and very simple. The signs were good so far.

Most guys will try to have a vasectomy done on a Friday, rest up over a weekend, catch a few games on the tube, and then head back to work on Monday. I figured that I would give myself an extra bonus and scheduled to have mine on a Thursday afternoon and take the extra day off, sort of my own version of a weekend special. I knew this would be more than enough healing time to get back in the swing of things.

The pre-surgical instructions specified that, among other things, I shave down. Being a neophyte at this and certainly not trusting the job to anyone else, I can now offer this piece of advice: Guys, should you ever find yourself in a similar circumstance, do not use an electric razor. It might seem simpler and less hazardous, as I thought, but you will be reenacting the war dance scene from Custer's Last Stand in no time, take my word.

Regardless of how you perform this shaving exercise, it feels like risky business. Don't think that you can leave this job to the nurse when you get to the doctor's office either. In all likelihood, the nurse will be in a hurry and annoyed that you didn't shave yourself. This is not the frame of mind you want someone in when they are pulling a razor across your scrotum. Just get your hand to stop shaking long enough to do the job yourself and make a fashion statement.

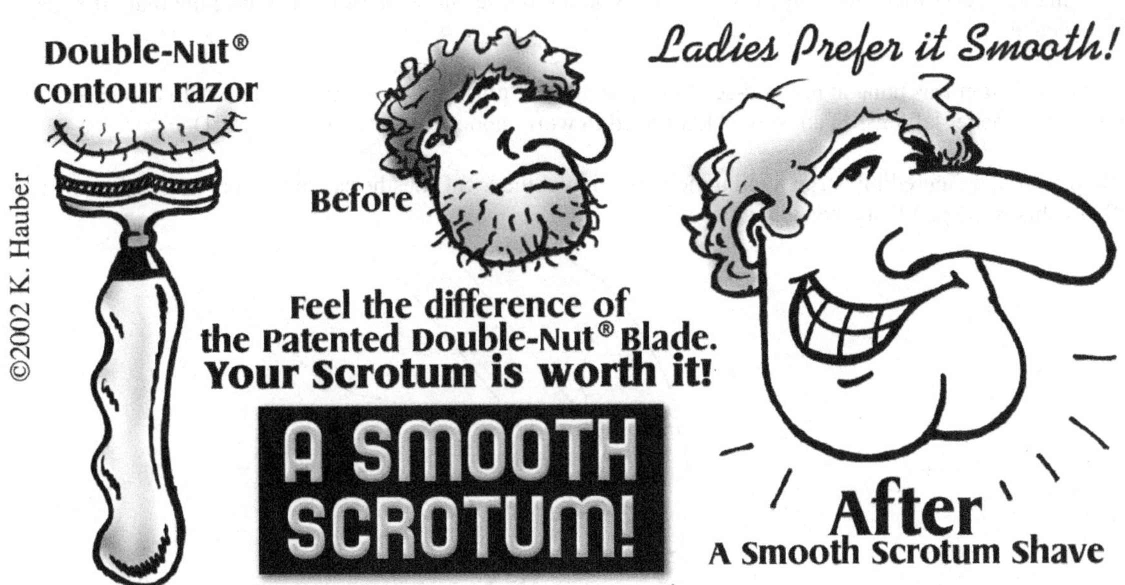

A friend of mine who is still in college claims that among the younger set, scrotal shaving has become quite popular and that "chicks dig it." Just goes to show that beauty is in the eyes (or hands) of the beholder. For me, the shaving experience wasn't so bad, but afterwards when that three-day scrotal beard started to grow back it felt like a cross between cactus apples and a Chia Pet between my thighs.

Cleanly shaven in new and invigorating ways, I operated in a complete state of denial about any anxiety I felt on the day of the surgery.

As we drove to the doctor's office, my wife asked "Are you sure you want to go through with this?"

"Sure, honey," I squeaked (OK, we can talk about denial as a coping device at another time).

Upon walking into the room where the procedure was to be done, I noticed that the radio was playing the local oldies station.

"Would you like some music?" the nurse asked.

At that moment, as if on cue, Aretha Franklin came on the radio belting out "Rescue Me!" I should have paid attention to the sign.

"I think silence will be good, thank you," I replied.

I was directed to undress, climb up on the table and cover myself with what amounted to a large paper napkin, as if that made any difference. The nurse put a bunch of goo on a grounding plate from the cauterizing machine and slipped it under my tailbone.

"I've never been arc-welded before," I observed and got a little smile from her.

Enter the doctor. "Are you nervous about this?" he asked.

"Given what we're about to do here, I think I'm as calm as I can be," was as honest a response as I could give.

This must not have been too reassuring, because he looked at me again and asked, "Would you like a Valium?"

It was almost like being in a restaurant, "Hi, I'll be your surgeon today. Would you like something narcotic from the bar?"

"No thanks, never touch the stuff, just give me a bullet to bite and go ahead." He gave me that "It's your funeral" look and proceeded.

A small curtain was hung at my mid-section, so as not to "give away any trade secrets." In this case, I think some things are probably better left unseen anyway. Don't need to worry about competition from me, Doc.

He prepared an incredibly large looking needle to inject the local anesthesia, and before putting it into my scrotum warned, "Now this is the part that tends to hurt a lot."

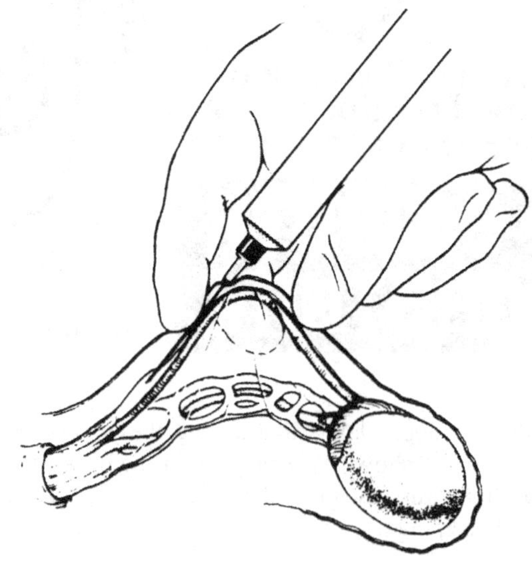

He was right. At that moment I found there was a distinct lack of grab handles on the table. I mentioned this to the doctor, and he relayed how when he was in residency at the VA hospital they had a great grab bar for when he used to do prostate tissue samples. He described how a device is inserted through the rectum and plunged repeatedly into the inside of the prostate to remove the samples, but I didn't have to worry about something like that until I was a few years older. There's something to look forward to!

The conversation actually improved from there, and as the local took effect, the faint cutting and tugging sensations bothered me less and less. I had the somewhat surreal experience of carrying on a perfectly pleasant conversation with a man operating on my loins. How many vasectomies had he done? Over a thousand now in all likelihood, he claimed. What did he do for the thousandth; get a band, order a buffet? No, but that wasn't a bad idea.

There was only one point when he connected with something that made me feel like he was trying to pull out my tonsils through my scrotum, as my whole body convulsed.

"You felt that?" he looked up and asked.

Was he kidding? "I felt that all the way up in my chest," I explained. What was he using to do the procedure, a cattle prod?

The promised twenty minutes turned into 35 or so, but I made it through the rest of the eye-bulging and toe curling stuff in fine form. Later, the doctor would characterize the procedure as uneventful. I suppose that depends on which end of the tugging and snipping you are. Not necessarily from my perspective, but from his, maybe if you've snipped one vas, you've snipped 'em all. After all, I lived through it, right? I thanked the doctor and the nurse expecting (hoping) to not ever see them again in this type of setting, and went home.

You never really know how bad the roads are in your hometown until you are on your way home from a vasectomy. You get to experience every rut and pothole at a new level of your physical being. After experiencing more road construction zones than I'd seen in years, we arrived home. I made several bowlegged strides to get upstairs and I climbed into bed, assuming a somewhat meditative pose perched on a package of frozen peas my wife had the foresight to pick up. Bet you'll never look at frozen vegetables the same now, will you?

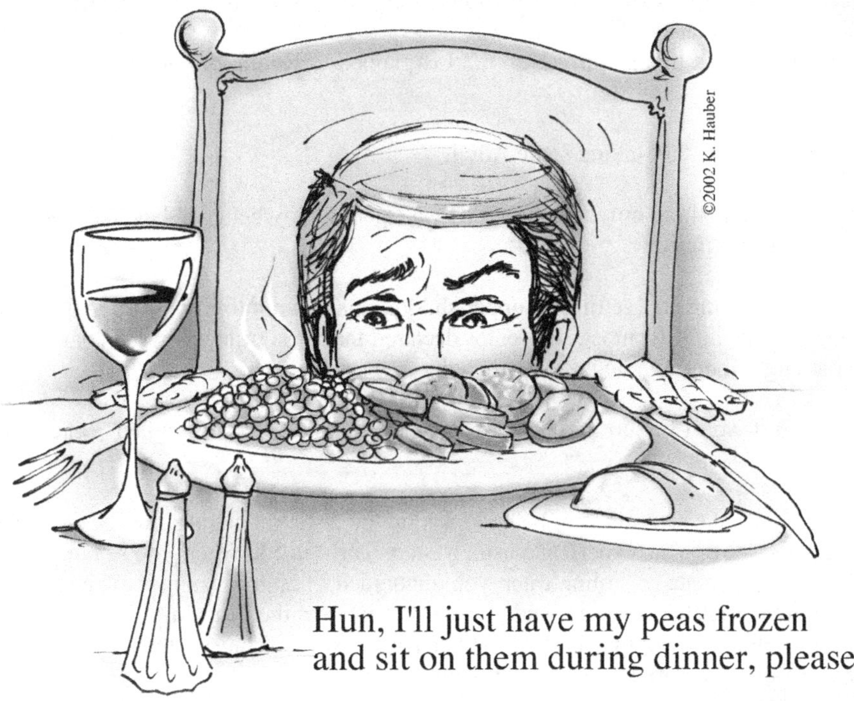

Hun, I'll just have my peas frozen
and sit on them during dinner, please.

I decided to do a little reading and unwind. I picked up Wayne Dyer's "You'll See It When You Believe It" seeking some good inspiration. When I read a book like this, I have a habit of thinking to myself "OK God, what message do you have for me today?" I did so and opened the book, straight to the chapter on "Detachment."

I called to my wife "This is great, I'm sitting here on a package of frozen peas fresh out of a vasectomy, and I'm getting a message from God via Wayne Dyer about detachment." Little did I know how prophetic this was and how detached I would learn to become in what was ahead.

A message like this was just too good not to share, so I fired off an email to several friends, which started several weeks of electronic banter. One friend's response asked if our male dog, who had been neutered recently, was giving me much sympathy. I replied that he would come up and give me a compassionate, soulful-eyed look, and then walk across my groin. Man's best friend, hah!

As an aside, Wayne Dyer was actually speaking locally a week later. A friend was organizing the event, and she called me the night before, asking if I would like to join her in taking Dr. Dyer to lunch before the presentation. Sure, I agreed quickly.

"But you've got to tell him the vasectomy story" she insisted.

Why not? I'll probably never see the guy again, so I might as well make a lasting impression.

Back to the story. I rested the remainder of the day of the surgery, being waited on, which lasted until the next morning when I had to start getting things for myself again. All good things come to an end too soon, don't they?

I didn't concern myself too much with the stinging and twinges I felt as I moved about, assuming this all to be normal post-operative stuff. But the stinging and twinges increased over the following two days, even though I took it easy. I didn't want to use the codeine prescription the urologist had given me, but dang, this was really starting to hurt more and more.

By the fourth day following the procedure, in addition to the stinging, tearing and shooting pains, it felt as if my testicles were ready to explode. That was a Sunday, so I went to church per my usual habit, and it was very uncomfortable to sit through the service which, by the way, had nothing to do with what the minister was saying. I tried going back to work on the fifth day and made it about a half an hour before going home and calling the doctor's office.

"Not meaning to be a wimp, but this is hurting a lot," I explained to Robin, the nurse who had assisted with the surgery.

"You need drugs," she implored, "try taking some Advil.

The next day brought the same thing only worse. "This isn't getting any better" I begged of Robin and she made an appointment for me to see the doctor that day.

By now I was aching all the time and getting whopper shooting pains up into my groin. After examining me and being sure to mash in all the spots that hurt the most, the doctor declared that, yes, in fact, I was in pain and needed bigger, stronger drugs. Prescription-strength Ibuprofen ought to do the job.

"Try a week's course so it won't be too hard on your stomach, and wear some tighter jockey shorts" he stated. Anything, just help me end this!

Every man knows and dreads the sensations of being kicked in the testicles: aching, nausea, doubling-up type pain, and muscle guarding. You get the idea. This experience usually starts early in life when you're not watching where you are walking, or have some sadistic playmate or sibling catch you unguarded. I am no stranger to pain, having experienced several surgeries earlier in life, numerous back injuries and muscle spasms over the years, along with the normal less-than-pleasant parts of participation in athletics and martial arts. What I was experiencing by then was a new level of agony beyond anything I had ever experienced before in such an unrelenting way.

What was this like? Well, let me answer that inevitable question frankly. This is going to be one of those explicit parts, so if you can't handle it, close your eyes and skip a few paragraphs.

As a man, imagine that your testicles ache all the time, regardless of what you do. I know this is an unpleasant thought, but stay with me anyway. The aching increases in a wave-like manner every few hours or days when you are a little more active, or, alternately, for no apparent reason at all. That aching spreads to your groin, stomach, low back, and inner thighs to the point that all you want to do is curl up in the fetal position with a pillow between your knees. At some points you will want to run away from the pain. If you were to try this, you would find that the pain becomes worse, as movement aggravates the problem.

If you are a man, notice the sensations in your testicles for a moment. I'm not saying grab and tug, but just notice their presence. Notice when you sit or stand or walk that there is a slight pressure created on the back of your testicles from your legs or the seat. Notice how even wearing briefs creates the slightest bit of pressure with the support that is afforded. No big deal, right?

Now what if every time that slight bit of pressure is created, your testicles ached even more than I previously described, and you experienced stabbing and stinging pains up into your groin and stomach. What if a little bladder or bowel pressure was added to your groin and the stinging and tearing sensations increased? This pain wakes you up with this in the middle of the night and you can't go back to sleep as a result. You try to modify the way you sleep, sit, or walk to minimize the pressure and the pain that resulted. Imagine how your posture, appetite and digestion might be affected.

These are the sensations I experienced. This led to constant nausea as if I had been kicked in the groin. If you still don't comprehend what this is like after, try what I call the Vice-Grip Empathy Test. Chronic testicular pain (CTP) is usually defined as testicular pain lasting longer than three months that interferes with a man's daily activities (Heidenreich, et. al., 2002). So try this experiment: Just take a pair of Vise-Grip pliers and snap them quickly on your testicles or the testicles of a man near you. Then watch the writhing begin. You won't need too much empathy to get the idea after this. Leave the pliers in place for, say, three months or so and take note of what is left of the man when you return.

That is a pretty succinct description, which is all the more I hope you ever experience. Doesn't sound like a lot of fun, huh? It isn't, let me assure you.

What does chronic testicular pain feel like?

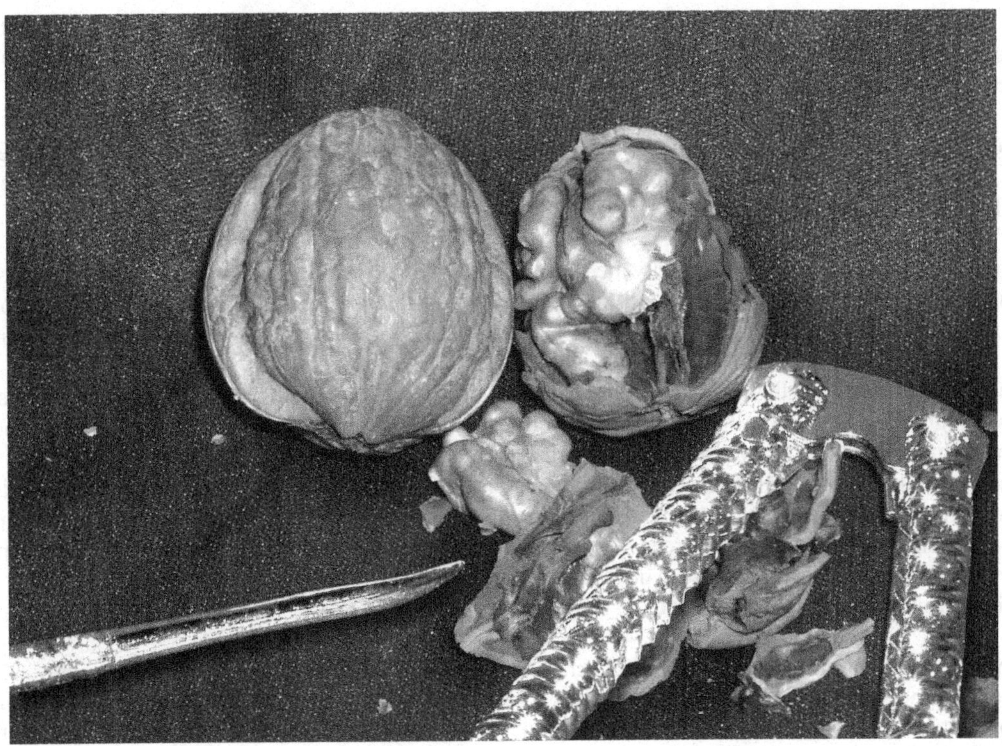

Does this give you any idea?

My habit in life has been not to share or demonstrate any distress I might be experiencing. It's kind of a guy thing in that respect, and besides, I really disliked going to doctors. My coworkers had once given me an accolade titled the "Never Let 'Em See You Sweat" award noting this iceman-like quality. But this vasectomy experience was beginning to push my control buttons in a big way.

Back at the ranch, I limped in to see my urologist again later that week walking like I was John Wayne after a long trail ride. Why wasn't this getting any better?

"You may have some connective tissue damage or something else going on" my urologist told me, "but let's get an ultrasound to take a look."

So I shuffled over to the hospital to have ultrasound images made of my sore testicles. This was yet another new experience.

No man has ever been truly humbled until he has had a testicular ultrasound (a.k.a. man-o-gram) done by a demure young female technician as she pushes a cold piece of sounding equipment into his aching privates. The hospital policy necessitated a male chaperone be present for this undertaking so that "she wouldn't take advantage of me."

"Don't worry," I reassured, "I'm not in a very receptive mood to overtures at this point."

The pictures showed nothing that wouldn't have been expected a week or two after surgery. This purportedly mystified the doctor and his partner as to why I was in so much pain. Was it possible that I had a hernia? Not possible, according to the doctors. Try to ride it out and take it easy was the best advice they could give.

By this time it was a week or so after the surgery, and I wasn't resting, working, or doing anything but lying around and moaning a lot. I was on the couch in my den with one of those frozen pea packs on my groin.

My wife walked by and quipped, "I'm so tired of seeing you with your pants off!"

This was supposed to make me feel better? "Believe me, honey, I'm pretty tired of this too."

The following Saturday morning marked a week and a half after the procedure, and by about 8 AM I was rolling around on the floor trying to find some position of comfort. My wife took that "I've seen enough of this B.S." approach and called the doctor, getting the answering service.

My urologist wasn't on call, but his partner who had also examined me that week without any revelations called back and in a very terse manner insisted, "There is nothing more that I can do for you. Now I want to get back to breakfast with my family."

My wife was incensed. He was lucky he wasn't nearby or he would have been wearing that breakfast he so eagerly anticipated. If you knew my wife, you'd know that I'm not kidding. She has even less patience for that kind of arrogance than I do. I secretly appreciated the mother lioness approach to taking care of me that came so naturally to her.

I found it hard to believe that a doctor would ignore concern over pain being expressed by a patient, and assumed I must have just caught the doctor on call on a bad day. In discussions with my attorney sometime later I found out that this is a common attitude taken by urologists toward their vasectomy patients. She had just finished litigating another vasectomy case and had found out this and some other curious facts in the process, which I will bring out in more detail later. As time went on, I talked to other men who had encountered severe pain following their vasectomies, and the reality of this attitude as being common was reinforced. Please understand, this observation is not a blanket condemnation of all doctors. However, it is a criticism of those who adopt an attitude of the sort exemplified here and leave their patients flapping in the breeze; painfully so, I might add.

No man in his right mind likes to have his genitals cut on, and many underestimate the pain they will experience. In fact, "A focus group sponsored by the Association for Voluntary Surgical Contraception found that men who had undergone conventional vasectomy experienced more pain and discomfort during and after the procedure than they had been led to expect by the operating surgeon" (Li, et. al., 1991).

"Pain isn't taken seriously as a problem, Dr. [Allan] Basbaum says. It is now required of all physicians in California to take pain management classes. But this isn't enough" (Infinite Mind: Pain). So the response of some less-empathic doctors, unfortunately, becomes one of placating the patient, trying to get him to take more pain medication, or just plain blowing off the patient's concerns and telling him to tough it out.

The latter appeared to be the approach of the particular doctor we called on that Saturday morning when the aforementioned rolling around on the floor was occurring. He was the one I had consulted with about getting a vasectomy the first time, and now I knew why I didn't follow through. This harsh attitude was exemplified well by Dr. Boris Klopukh in an interview with ABC News on March 12, 2001: "I do a lot of vasectomies and the No. 1 concern is fear of pain…. Men are wusses for the most part." Maybe Dr. Klopukh needs that Vice-Grip Empathy Test for about three months to show he isn't a wuss, huh?

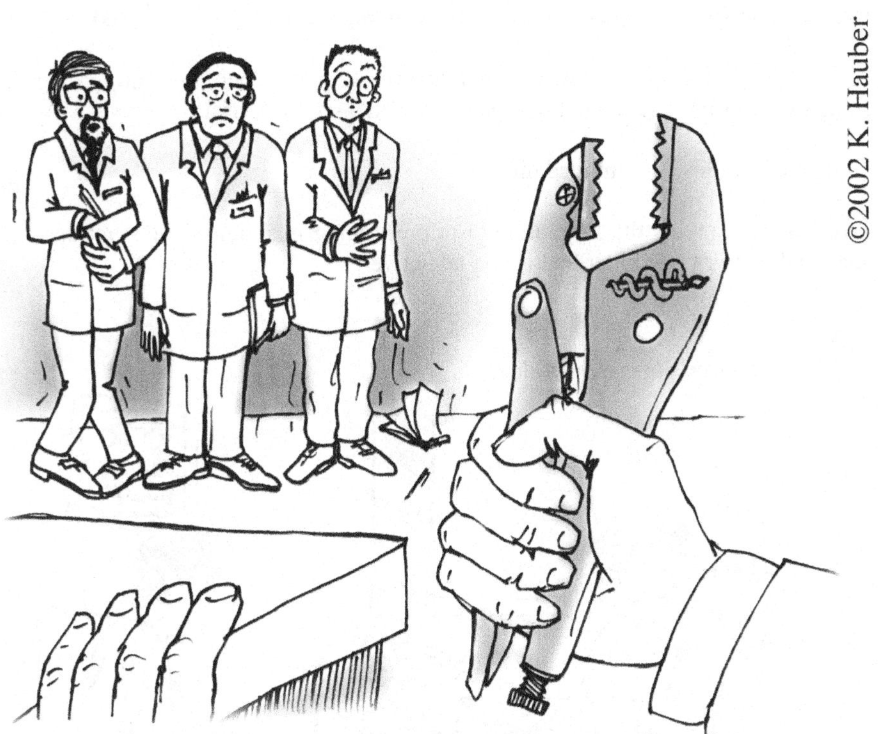

OK, gentlemen, line up and place your testicles on the
table for the Vice-Grip Vasectomy Empathy Test…

The perception that men are "wusses" when it comes to pain needs to be questioned. Remember, men have been the ones who have gone out and started wars for thousands of years only to come back hacked up and maimed, or not come back at all. Evidently, in the process of this or whatever other natural selection has occurred, men have developed a significant tolerance for pain.

"Women experience pain more than men. Their thresholds for pain are lower," according to Dr. Louann Brizendine of UC San Francisco (Infinite Mind, 2003). Please note that it is actually a woman saying that women's pain thresholds are lower, not one of us male chauvinists. Maybe this helps to make women smarter than men and keeps them from doing many of the stupid things we do that hurt us. I can only speculate.

Another common assumption is that people will usually exaggerate about the pain they are experiencing to get attention, make some one feel guilty, or just because they are "wusses" as previously mentioned.. Not true, according to recent scientific research measuring brain responses to pain stimulus. "Self-reports of pain, the validity of which have been questioned by experts, have been shown to be accurate" (Mullich, 2003). Pain responses vary between individuals, but, patient's perceptions regarding the severity of their pain have been validated (Coghill, et. al., 2003). So, my dear doctors, if your patients say it hurts when you cut on their genitals, please believe them!

Needless to say, this situation was a lot more than I had expected. By the time three weeks had passed and the same symptoms were still present, I went back to the doctor yet again.

"Why do I feel like I've been kicked in the balls all the time?" I asked expectantly.

He explained that I was experiencing the kind of response that a cowboy gets when he falls off his horse and gets kicked in the groin. That was a special image, but not being into rodeo and not being very reassured by this I waited for him to continue.

"We don't know why this happens sometimes," he went on, "but apparently you are experiencing chronic testicular pain."

We were in agreement so far, at least in so far as the chronic pain part was concerned.

He continued, "This is a condition known as neuralgia (nerve pain) where the pain sensing nerves get stuck on and won't let up. I'm going to prescribe several medications for you on a six week trial."

"But I don't do medications," I reminded him.

"Don't worry," he reassured, "the Imipramine I'm prescribing is an anti-depressant that should help to ease the nerve responses, and the Ultram is a painkiller that is non-addictive."

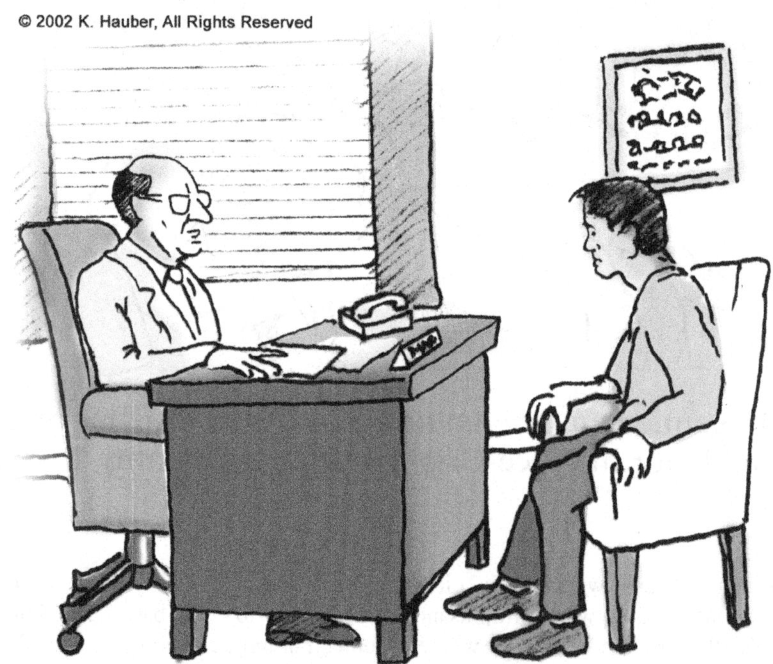

I'm going to prescribe some ⟨scribble⟩ and some ⟨scribble⟩ for you , OK?

I remained quite skeptical and required a lot of reassurance and explanation. Long-term nerve medication and painkillers? I didn't like the sound of that at all. After a good deal of discussion, and because I didn't know what else to do, I agreed.

"How many days should I expect this to go on?" I inquired expectantly.

"Hang in there, this could take months. Try these medications for six weeks and let's see how it goes," he responded. If this was his version of a pep talk, it left a lot to be desired.

What!? I came to him for a "simple" vasectomy, had been in extreme pain ever since, and now he was telling me that I needed to be on anti-depressants and pain killers for what might be months? I suppressed the choke response I felt welling up and the desire to blurt out the previous sentence, realizing my potential need for long-term care and the low likelihood that I would get it in prison.

During this time I attended a lecture by Dr. Deepak Chopra, who is not only trained in Western Medicine, but is an author, advocate and practitioner of holistic medical practices. I will never forget one of the comments he made. He said, "If you don't think that your body is important to you, just see what happens when you get sick." I was truly experiencing the full impact of that notion in a way I never thought possible.

Like many guys I never gave too much consideration to learning about the most personal portions of my anatomy as long as everything worked fine. I had acquired only a few basics from health class and a lot of myths along the way, and was perfectly content to protect my equipment and bring it along for the ride.

What I found now was that chronic testicular pain is really no big deal. No big deal that is, unless it happens to you! Then it will truly consume you and you will have difficulty focusing on anything else. If this type of pain does ever happen to befall you, I can guarantee the months that follow will be the longest of your life and you will be motivated to learn everything you can about your body in an effort to find a way out of your troubled situation. This was where I found myself.

Chapter Three

How Is This Thing Put Together, Anyway?

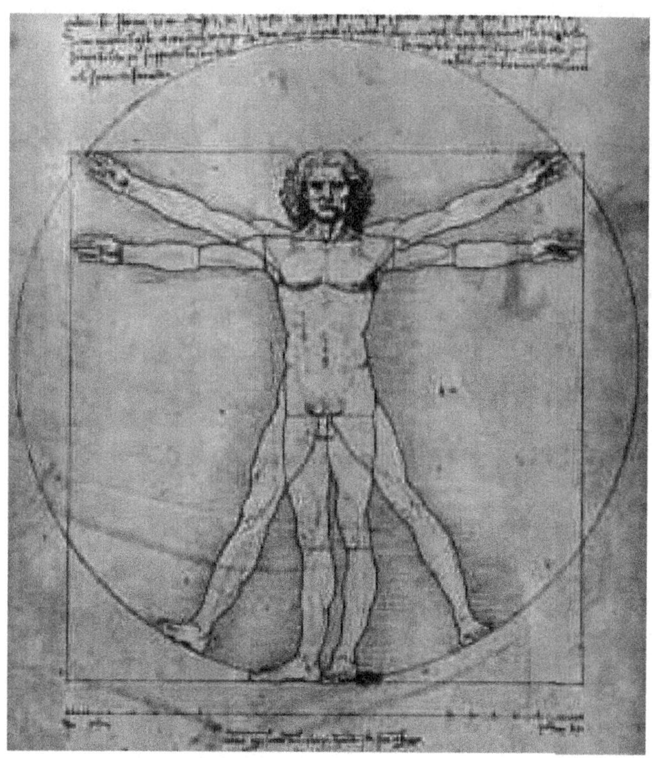

Modern medicine can do some pretty amazing things. If something is wrong with our bodies, there are an incredible number of ways to cut the problem out, repair the damage, or medicate us in an attempt to help our bodies to heal. Anyone who will deny this needs only to reflect on the diseases and injuries that spelled almost certain death in our grandparents' and great-grandparents' generations that are now nearly unheard of.

Public awareness of what it takes to maintain good health has increased also. The exponential rising costs of medical and pharmaceutical technology is another matter altogether, as is access to that technology, but the fact remains that the technology and knowledge needed to cure many of our collective ailments are more widely available.

Any form of surgical sterilization, for men or women, is an entirely different matter if you think about it. You take a perfectly operable and most basic function of the body, i.e. the reproductive process, and deliberately disable it. We are told that doing so has no negative long-term effects on the body by those who supposedly know best, and that we can interrupt nature at will, and enjoy the contraceptive benefits we might derive in the process.

However, in regards to vasectomy, you might ask yourself; if retaining sperm in the body is such a great idea, why did nature give us such a pleasurable incentive to get it out? It has only really been since mortality rates have fallen in the past few decades that contraception for the masses has become more of an issue with worldwide exponential population growth. Having many children used to be a form of social security and indeed a survival mechanism during many eras.

Okay, it's disclaimer time. If frank discussion about male anatomy with diagrams and pictures is somehow offensive or irrelevant to you, I suggest you skip to the next chapter. On the other hand, if knowing a little more about the parts we have been blessed with and how they work would be beneficial to you (I had no choice), read on.

Most men are quite interested in taking good care of their equipment. A guy can be a real pig in many aspects of his life, but will be quite fastidious in tending to his genitals. This was demonstrably true in many of the guys I knew in college, at least in terms of their genital "exercise" programs if their claims had any truth to them. I don't need to mention names, you know who you are.

All that aside, there are numerous unsavory reasons that a man might have to see a urologist. Probably number one on the anxiety hit parade is testicular cancer, which is the most prevalent cancer in men between the ages of 15 and 35. The incidence of testicular cancer is on the rise (Clore, 1993). This situation was brought into the spotlight recently when comedian Tom Green was diagnosed as having testicular cancer at age 28, and publicly shared his experience in the process.

Tom was quoted as saying, "I want to raise awareness among young guys who don't ordinarily think about cancer. Check yourself every day (Green, 2000)." We've come a long way from "Stop that or you'll go blind" haven't we? Tom even established an information source, called Tom Green's Nuts Cancer Fund, headquartered in the city where the biggest nuts naturally end up, Los Angeles.

Another less comical but very inspiring story on this subject can be found in the saga of champion cyclist Lance Armstrong. When Lance won the grueling 2000 Tour de France competition (his second victory for that event), he warmed hearts around the world by lifting and smiling at his infant son in celebration while on the podium. It was a very poignant moment.

What makes this even more inspiring is that four years before, at age 25, Lance was diagnosed with advanced testicular cancer. His cancer had spread extensively, necessitating the removal of his right testicle and spermatic cord by cutting through his groin and pulling them out. His cancer had also spread to his lungs and brain requiring the removal of several of those tumors. This was followed by an aggressive course of chemotherapy.

Not only did Lance beat his cancer, father a child by in vitro fertilization and come back as a champion cyclist once again, he wrote a book about the experience titled It's Not About the Bike. He also created the Cycle of Hope Foundation to help raise awareness about the issue of testicular cancer. My hat is off to both Lance and Tom for their courage in sharing their experiences in an effort to help lessen the suffering of others. These are great examples of the strength and tenacity of the human spirit, and an inspiration for us all.

As with Lance, unfortunately, medical treatment for testicular cancer hasn't advanced beyond removal of the offending organ(s) in many cases, often followed by radiation, and/or chemotherapy which can cause a host of other problems, such as sterility, and a lot of misery. One has to weigh this against the possibility of death due to spread of the cancer, but, nonetheless, this is a traumatic experience. Here is one of those hard-to-look-at pictures of what a cancerous testicle and spermatic cord can look like:

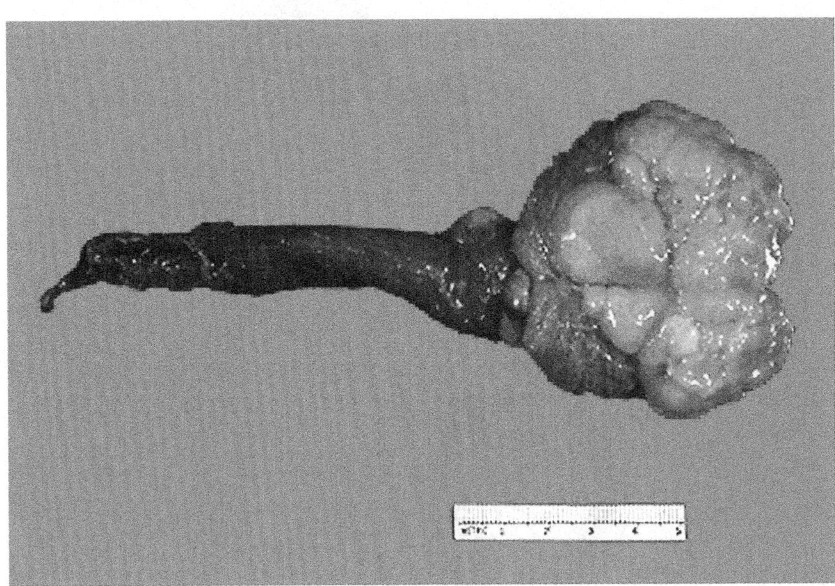

In addition to cancer, cysts of several types can form in the scrotum for a variety of reasons, which are often quite unpleasant and painful. Hernias can extend into the scrotum and require surgical resolution. Then there are varicoceles, which are essentially varicose veins that form in your privates and often lead to infertility. Estimates are that from 15% to 20% of the male population is affected by the presence of varicoceles, making this the most commonly diagnosed cause of male infertility, most often occurring on the left side (Kim, et. al., 1999). Increased pressure inside the spermatic veins leads to a phenomenon known as the "nutcracker effect" (no kidding!) causing varicoceles to form. Reduced testosterone levels and testicular atrophy (shrinking of the testicle) can also result from varicoceles, as can pain, and surgery is often recommended to correct the condition (Brandell, et. al., 1999). In short, varicoceles lead to progressive testicular damage over time. These diagrams shows what a varicocele can look like from the inside and the outside, with the deformation of veins often showing through the scrotal skin:

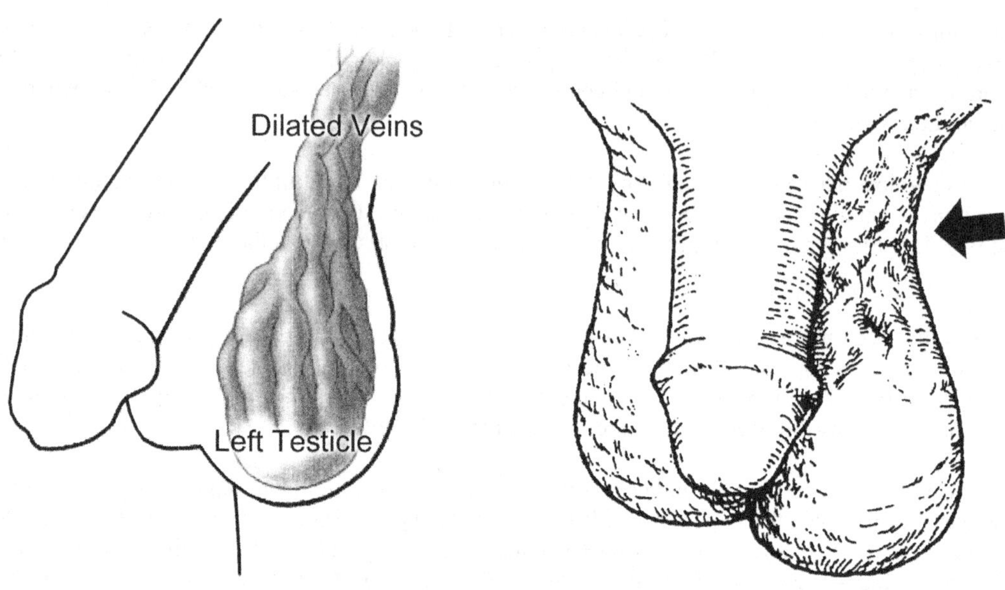

A hydrocele is a fairly common malady affecting the testicles. A hydrocele is essentially a fluid sack that forms between the testicle and scrotum, which can become quite large and require surgery to drain. Here's a diagram to give you an idea of what a hydrocele can look like (Note the fluid sack to the left of the testicle. Also note the absence of scrotal skin in this diagram):

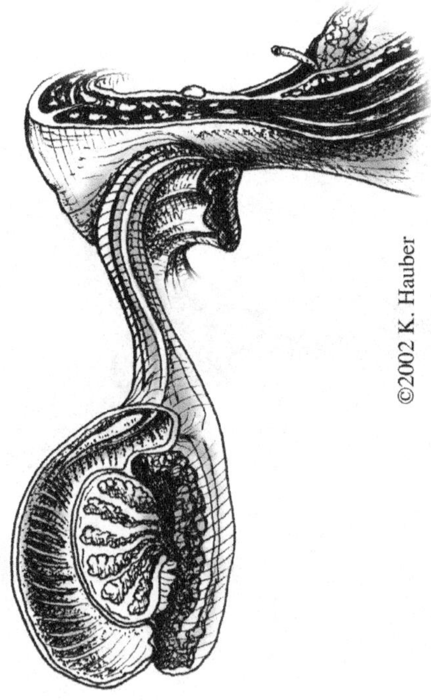

In terms of appearance, most often a hydrocele will typically cause one side of the scrotum to enlarge substantially compared to the other side. Testicular atrophy (shrinking of the testicle) can result from this process also, even though the affected side may appear larger because of the hydrocele. A moderate example of what this might look like is shown here:

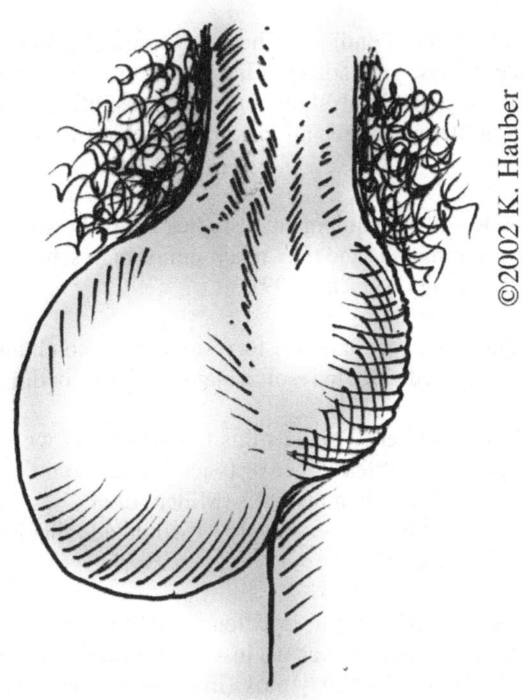

Hydroceles can become alarmingly large. As you can see from the diagram below, the hydrocele can easily exceed the size and volume of the testicle itself, which can cause a good deal of distress and discomfort:

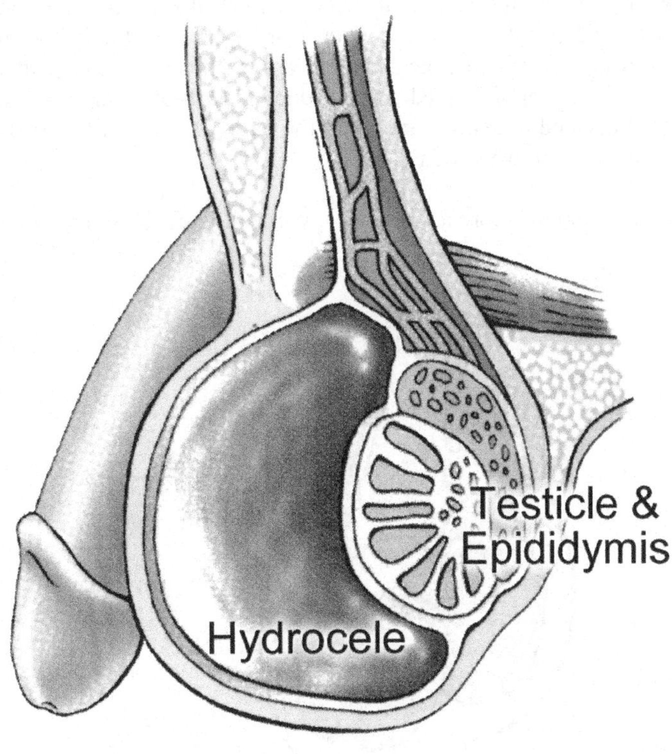

A friend of mine developed a hydrocele following his vasectomy. He says that one of his testicles is now three times the size of the other, but fears the types of lancing and dicing that doctors have recommended for resolution. I've never asked him to show me, so I have to take him at his word. Besides, if a guy is willing to talk to a doctor about his testicles, my experience says it must be something substantial.

Add testicular torsion (a very painful condition where the testicle and cord twists within the scrotum) which is particularly common among adolescent boys, prostatitis (inflammation of the prostate gland), prostate cancer, Peyronie's Disease (excessive curvature of the penis), erectile dysfunction, and a host of other maladies and you have enough to keep the urology profession in business for a lifetime. Keep all this in mind, since these various maladies become more relevant as the story unfolds.

Then there's the issue of abuse of the equipment. Studies have shown that one out of ten males has been the recipient of a heavy-duty kick to the groin by the time they reach junior high school. One out of four of these boys sustain injuries requiring medical attention as a result (Pollack, 1999).

Understandably, most men and boys are anxious to resolve such conditions, even if they are reluctant to seek medical attention. What needs to be done medically to resolve many of these conditions is often an unpleasant reality.

We can look to comedian Dennis Miller to give us this timeless bit of wisdom on the subject: "You know, if you have a son, he is going to kick you in the balls at least once or twice a year, if you're lucky. They claim it's an accident. I don't think so. There are piñatas that get hit less than my balls (Miller, 1998)." As another father of a son, I have to agree, they know just where and how to hurt you, quite unconsciously. I would add that having sensitive balls after a vasectomy increases the odds of that painful shot by a factor of ten.

So what would keep a doctor from doing a vasectomy to begin with? Obviously, if there were something physically wrong or if there was some deformity, such as we just discussed, the surgery would be brought into question. A history of testicular injury or frequent bouts of epididymitis (infections or congestion of the epididymis portion of the testicles) or other disorders may also serve as contraindications. Contraindication is a fancy word meaning it's not a good idea to do some kind of treatment. A few doctors will screen for a family history of prostate cancer; an issue which will be discussed in more detail later. Beyond these factors, most often there is not any substantial screening performed.

In my case, there wasn't even a physical exam or a look-see by the urologist before the day of surgery, which I found to be a very casual approach (from the doctor) to what seemed like a major decision, for me at least. I get the impression that often urologists will just tend to take your word that everything is working fine and sharpen their instruments. Apparently, it is also difficult to predict whether a particular patient will have complications from the vasectomy because of the numerous factors involved. Many doctors just don't, or can't, or won't, take the extra time. Because of what I experienced, I decided to learn more about the parts of my anatomy that now agonized me, other than knowing what had previously felt good and what didn't.

When you go in for a consultation before a vasectomy, you will likely be shown a simple diagram like this one:

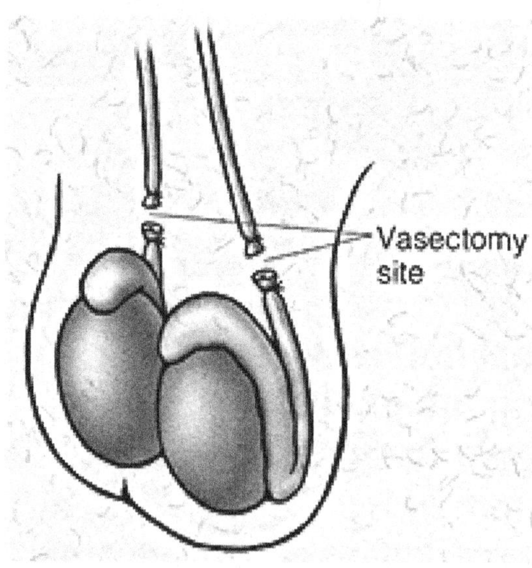

Or, at best, you might be shown a diagram like this:

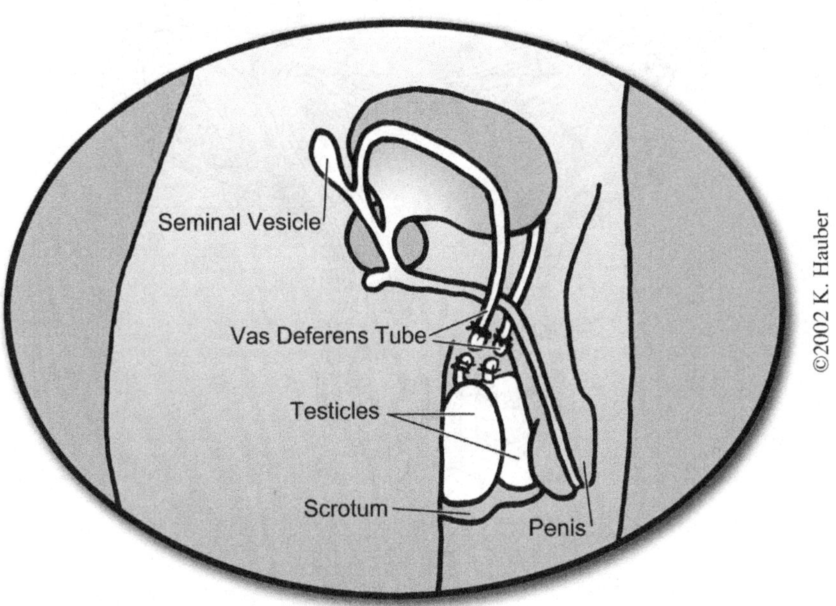

Pretty simple stuff, right? Just a couple of tubes, a little skin to cut through, and a few good Boy Scout knots to tie. Again, not exactly. Actually, there is a lot more going on in this area than the simpler diagrams might indicate, as the diagram below shows:

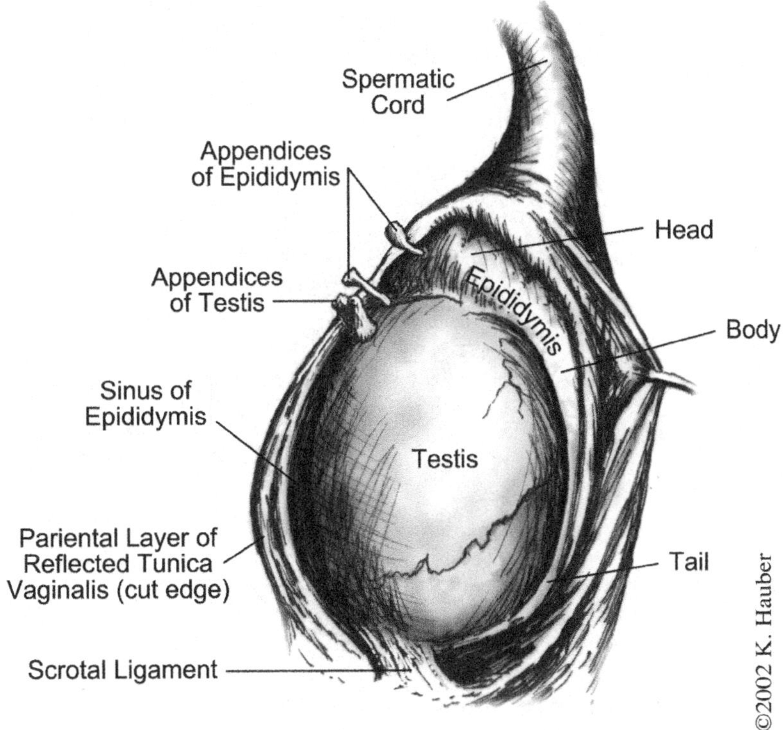

A more detailed sectional diagram of the entire region of the body like you might see in an anatomy book is shown here:

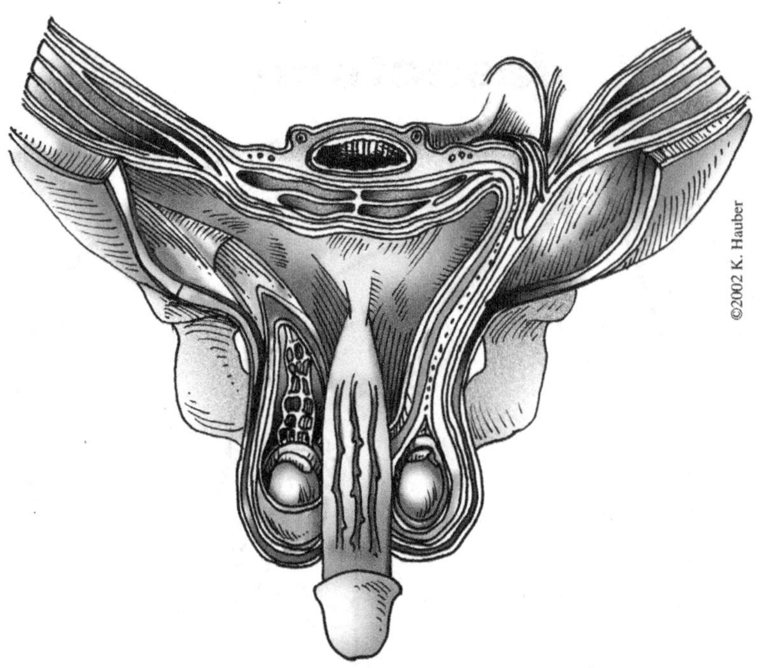

A sectional diagram of the testicle itself looks like this:

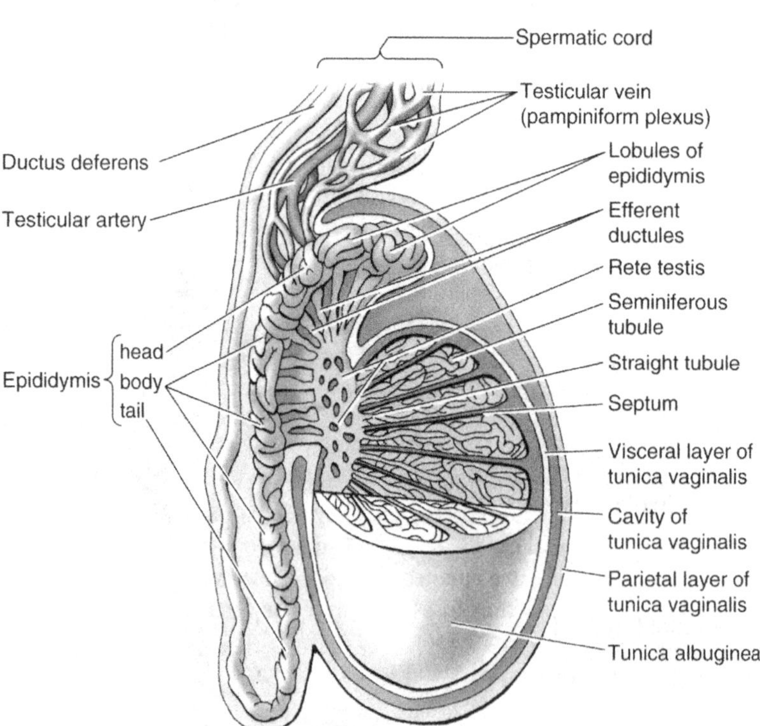

As you can see, there are many layers of tissues, muscle, blood vessels, nerves, etc. One doctor characterized the structures of the testicles this way: "They are very complex organs, with rich nerve, blood and lymphatic supply. Also, they are under intricate hormonal and temperature control to regulate sperm and testosterone production (Carruthers, 2000)."

In terms of function, the pituitary gland produces luteinizing and follicle-stimulating hormones (LH and FSH), among others, which stimulate the testicle to produce testosterone and sperm at the rate of about 50,000 cells per minute (National Institute of Health, 1996). The immature sperm cells move into the epididymis, which lies along the back of the testicle. The epididymis is a delicate coiled structure that would stretch out to somewhere between 16 and 20 feet long.

The epididymis has been described as "friable," which, in this case, means easily broken. Based on the sensations that can emanate from this area when impacted, I would have to agree. The sperm cells travel through the epididymis for about three weeks and in the process become more "motile," which simply means they mature and can move about more vigorously and attack unsuspecting eggs.

The scrotum is actually composed of several layers of tissue. The vas deferens is the thin tube that carries the sperm from the epididymis to the prostate gland. When a man is adequately stimulated to approach ejaculation, the smooth muscle layer of the vas deferens contracts vigorously forcing the sperm upstream. Doctors have observed this smooth muscle layer to be a strong and highly developed muscle even if it's relatively small. This, I'm sure, is the result of countless generations of evolution, not to mention the regular workout most guys enjoy giving this muscle from about age 12 on.

The testicles themselves don't just hang out but are suspended by structures called the spermatic cords, which are composed of the Cremaster muscle, blood vessels, nerves, and lymph vessels that run from the testicles up through the inguinal area of the groin. Up to the point that I learned this by finding out how much they could hurt, I would have thought that "spermatic cords" was just a kinky name for a very horny rock band ("Hey dude, what did you do last night?" "Man, it was great. I went to this concert. The Spermatic Chords opened for Pearl Jam. They rock!").

What's normal size for the boys from down under? "A testicle less than 3.5 cm long is considered small" (Junnila, et. al., 1998). Break out your calipers, guys. No one seems to comment on what is too large, despite all of the euphemisms to that effect, but I'm guessing that walking comfortably would likely become an issue at some point as size increases. I get the image of a human version of a grandfather clock. There is actually a device that has been developed for measuring testicle size in milliliters called an "Orchidometer", which essentially tries to estimate testicular volume. This can be especially helpful if you're experiencing swollen or shrinking testicles for any reason and need to track the healing process:

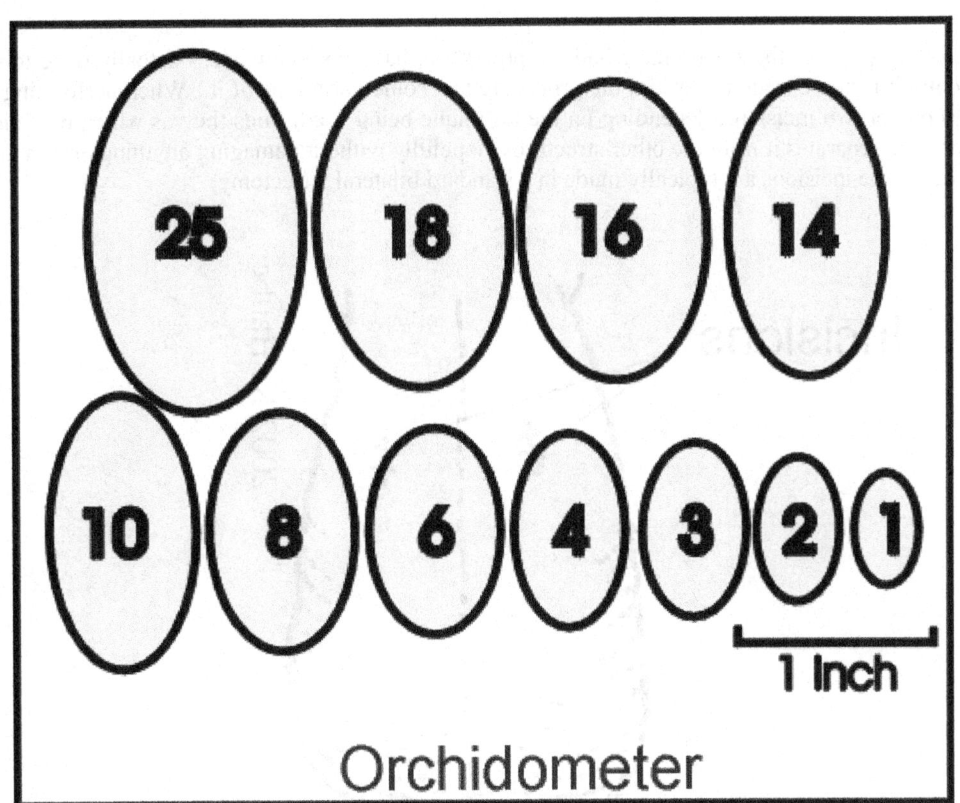

For whatever anatomical reason the Creator had, the left cord is normally longer than the right cord (Gray, 1995), leading to the infamous "one hung low" syndrome for about 80% of males, as shown here in this frontal view:

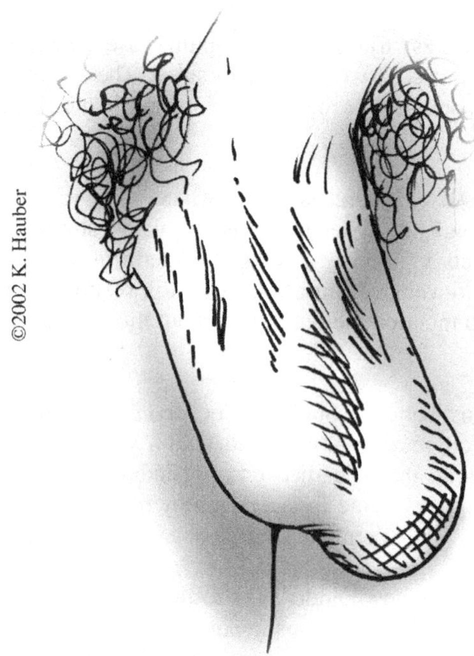

Maybe this is intended to avoid the click-clack effect as we walk down the street. Regardless, at least now you know there isn't something wrong with you guys. The scrotum and testicles will normally contract automatically on cold days, or when a man is ready to ejaculate, when he is in pain, or whenever he gets within ten feet of a doctor. With the amount of time I was spending around doctors being probed indelicately, I practically had to massage mine down from my throat.

Since most guys, even those who have had the procedure, have no idea what is actually done to their equipment during a vasectomy, it is appropriate to discuss the procedure and some variations of it. When performing the vasectomy, the doctor makes one or two incisions, depending on the technique being used, finds the vas which runs along the back of the spermatic cord and separates it from the other structures, hopefully without damaging anything else in the process. This diagram shows where the incisions are typically made in a standard bilateral vasectomy:

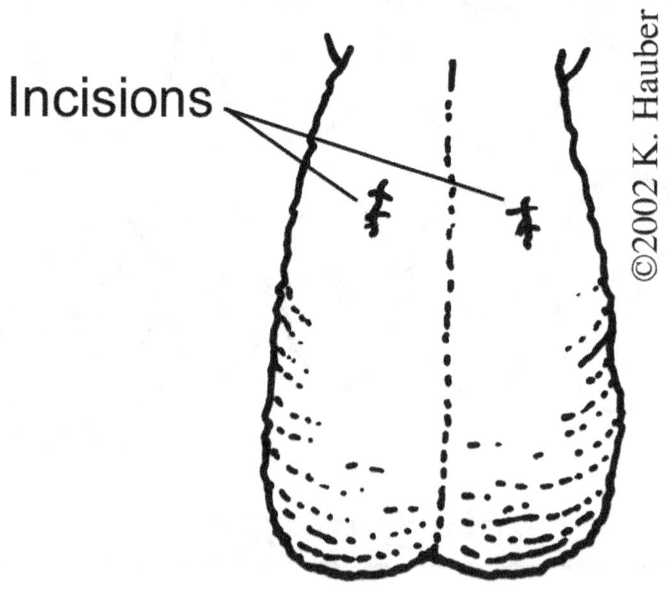

The doctor then cuts, ties and/or cauterizes the ends to stop the flow of sperm. The ends are tucked back into the scrotum and everything is closed up with whatever number of stitches is needed on each side. There are two typical variations of this procedure that are most commonly done. The method historically used in the West has been to make two incisions, one on each side of the scrotum, accessing the vas in this manner.

Standard Bilateral Vasectomy

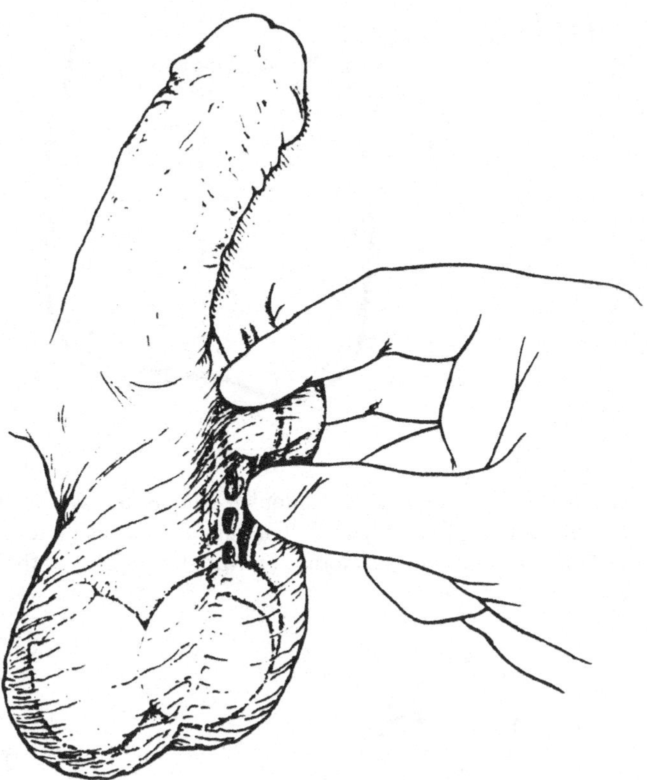

The doctor locates and injects the vas (ouch) as shown previously. Then, presumably when the patient is numb, cuts are made on each side. The doctor then uses a "mosquito forceps" to find the vas and lift it out of the scrotum. This is where the cutting, tying, electro-cautery, and prayer come in:

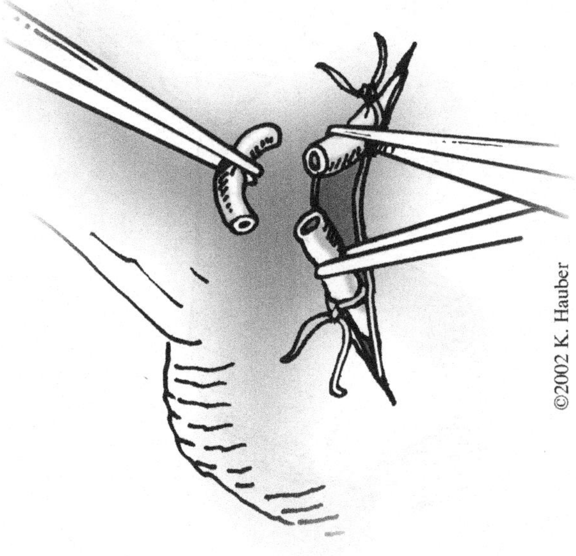

Another method, developed in China in 1974, and introduced into the United States in 1988, is called the No-Scalpel Vasectomy, wherein there is only single midline puncture of the scrotum:

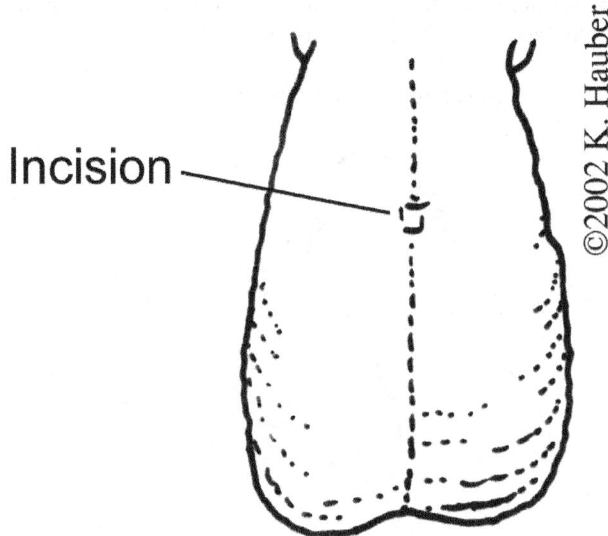

In the no-scalpel method, the vas deferens is manipulated under the skin to the center of the scrotum, and (don't get nauseous on me now) then vas is placed in a "special clamping device" as my doctor phrased it. I had been told once that they used to use a "special clamping device" as a form of torture for heretics in the Tower of London, but I thought that went out of fashion years ago.

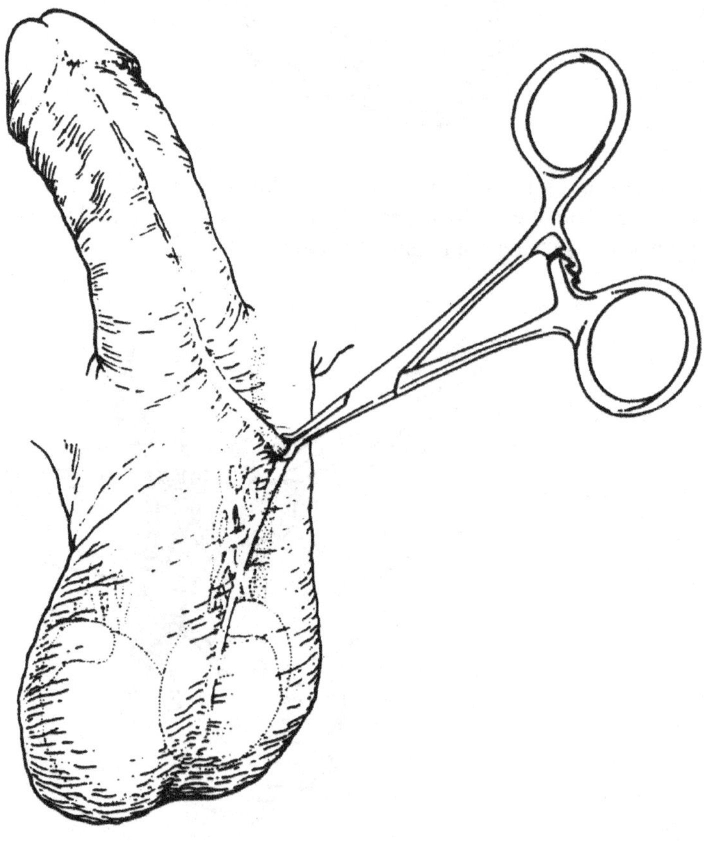

Evidently not. It was strange how none of the literature I had read on vasectomies up to the point of my procedure referenced this particular fact.

The doctor then takes aim and makes a single puncture wound, accessing both of the vas deferens through the same puncture, pulling each out long enough to do the required "ectomy" part of the procedure, severing the vas.

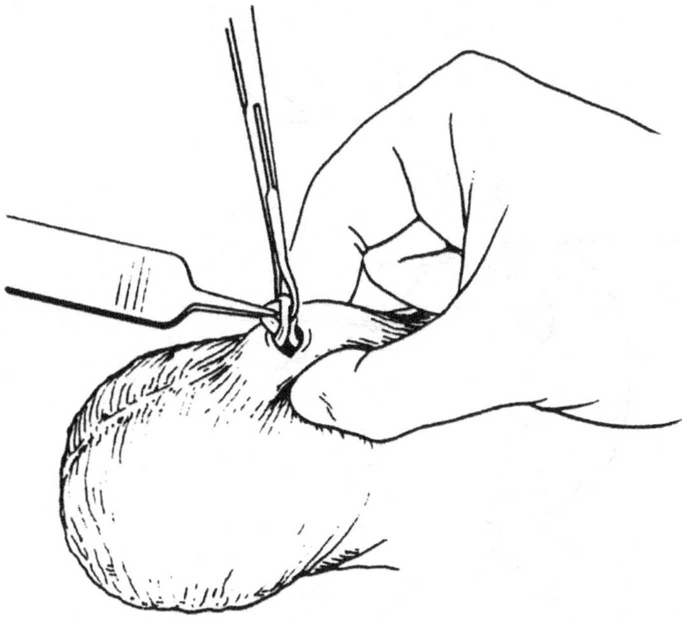

When the snipping, cauterizing, and tying are done to the doctor's satisfaction, the vas is replaced in the scrotum, and the wound closed without a stitch. That's the plan at least.

If you think my description of the procedure has holes in it (sorry), and would like a more complete understanding you can get a narrative with full color pictures and video snips- I mean clips- available at www.beavercleaver.net. It seems as if another guy named Kevin, this one is Kevin B. Cleaver if you can believe that, had his vasectomy done a few months before mine and decided to immortalize the experience on the Internet. If that isn't enough, another guy did the same thing at www.myvasectomy.com to share his intimate modifications with the world.

The advertised advantage of the no-scalpel technique is a (claimed) lower incidence of post-surgical complications such as infection or excessive swelling and bleeding. Who wouldn't want to lessen those possibilities? Many doctors think this is a good idea, and will exclusively use the no-scalpel technique.

A study published in the Journal of Urology in 1999 concluded that "The no-scalpel approach is an important advance in the surgical approach to vasectomy, and offers fewer side effects and greater comfort [really?] compared to the standard incision technique, without compromising efficacy." The study examined the results of vasectomies done at eight locations in five countries. "In the no-scalpel group operating time was significantly shorter, and complications and pain were less frequent than in the standard incision group. The no-scalpel group resumed intercourse sooner, probably as a result of less pain following the procedure (Sokal, 1999)."

A less common variation on the vasectomy is performed by cutting into the inguinal area of the groin on both sides and accessing each vas in its path along the spermatic cord. This is often done in conjunction with a hernia repair if that is deemed necessary.

Regardless of the variation on the vasectomy procedure that is used, the doctor will typically use some form of cauterization (burning) on the vas and the other cut tissues. This usually occurs without a hitch, but not always. I found out just what could result from overkill in the cauterization department. It seems as if the cauterizing issue is kind of like Goldilocks (Goldiballs?) and the three bears: "My cauterizing is too hot!" "My cauterizing is too cold!" "My cauterizing is just right!"

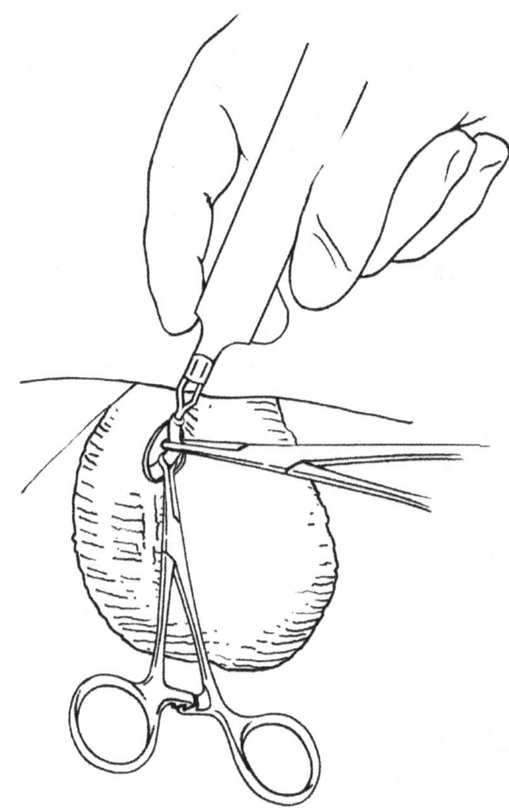

Inadequate cauterization can be a problem too. A problem case with which I became familiar occurred when a friend of a friend was having his vasectomy done and the cauterizing equipment broke in the middle of the surgery. Surgeons often use the cauterizing equipment to avoid excessive bleeding, especially in areas with intense numbers of blood vessels, such as the scrotum. The results weren't pretty. Much of the closing had to be done by hand stitching, which caused a great deal of bleeding, swelling, pain, and other unsavory results. Big oops! He spent weeks in bed, in pain, following his surgery, and many more months to fully recover.

Let's talk about pain specifically for a moment: "There are two major types of pain: nociceptive and neuropathic. Nociceptivepain is associated with tissue injury, and responds to anti-inflammatory drugs [like Ibuprofen] and opiates [narcotic pain medication]. Neuropathic pain, caused by injury to the nervous system itself...is much more difficult to treat" (Infinite Mind: Pain). Unfortunately, the major pain I was experiencing was in the later category. Just how difficult it would be to treat became one of life's hard lessons for me.

"When you have an injury the nervous system establishes a memory of the pain." Ever notice that the areas around a previous injury can often remain tender indefinitely? "If pain goes untreated, the pain can stay because the memory of the injury continues.... You must treat pain aggressively" (Infinite Mind, 2003). So what might "aggressive" pain treatment be like? The answer to that and many other fascinating questions, lies in the pages to come.

Chapter Four

I've Never Seen This Happen Before

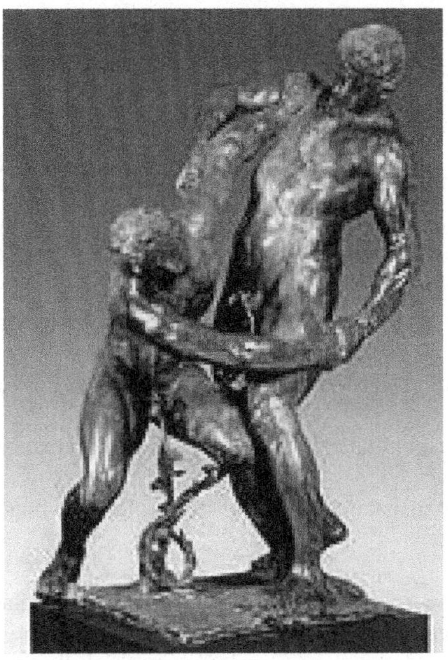

"Hold still so I can examine you!"
(Actually, The Wrestlers, by Adriaen de Vries, 1625)

By the time a month had passed, my moment-to-moment experience of pain was not improving, and my patience with the situation was wearing thin. My internist was equally mystified as to what was going on and helped me with blood tests and whatever else she could. The medications took the edge off the pain a little, but it was still ever-present and quite limiting.

I took my wife and family to dinner for her birthday about five weeks after the vasectomy. I awoke that night doubled over with terrific abdominal pain, and increased testicular pain and nausea, which led to vomiting and diarrhea. Something was drastically wrong. By morning the diarrhea had turned bloody.

My wife called our internist. Go to the emergency room she advised, and she'd see me there soon. "But I hate hospitals, and especially all those needles," I implored. I called my urologist too, and he advised me not to go to the hospital. I wondered whose interests he was looking out for.

"Get in the car" my wife insisted. I complied because I knew that as much as I was hurting at the time, she knew how to hurt me more.

The ER doctor couldn't figure out why I was having so much pain either, since I didn't have any apparent infection or food poisoning.

"I've never seen anything like this before. This is quite an unusual reaction to a vasectomy," he professed, "You must be one-in-a-million."

One-in-a-million? Why did I have to be so damned special? Just this once, couldn't I be just like all the other guys?

It felt like my intestines were exploding with the stress of the pain. Evidently that was what was happening. The emergency room staff started pumping me full of morphine, saline and several other substances that day. Pumping me full, that is, after trying to drain all of the blood and every other fluid out. I was quickly reminded of why hospitals are not restful places.

It seemed like every five minutes someone was coming into the room to check some aspect of my anatomy or to extract something.

The first nurse commented "My you have a great tan" as she lifted the gown.

"Thanks," I replied trying not to be too self conscious, "I swim a lot, and would much rather be doing that right now."

Another nurse five minutes later repeating the process: "My, you have a great tan."

"So I've heard, can we just get this over with and I'll get out of here so I can get some rest?"

My internist visited me in the hospital later in the day and was perplexed as to why this was all happening.

"What did you do to him?" she insistently asked of my urologist when they ran into each other in the hall. He shrugged in disbelief.

They sent me back to that very demure young lady for another testicular ultrasound. The head of the radiology department chaperoned this time and I later learned that he had experienced some long-term pain after his vasectomy. Less than three percent, huh? One-in-a-million, huh? I was beginning to think that the only guys who got counted in that less than three percent statistic were the ones who died on the operating table.

With a little morphine in me it wasn't quite as painful this time, and the images revealed epididymitis, an inflammation of the epididymis structures attached to the back of the testicles. Since this might have been due to infection, I was put on a course of antibiotics along with the painkillers. By the middle of the night I learned what a whopping headache morphine can give you, and by morning was begging to be released like a man trying to make bail.

Chapter Five

On Pins and Needles

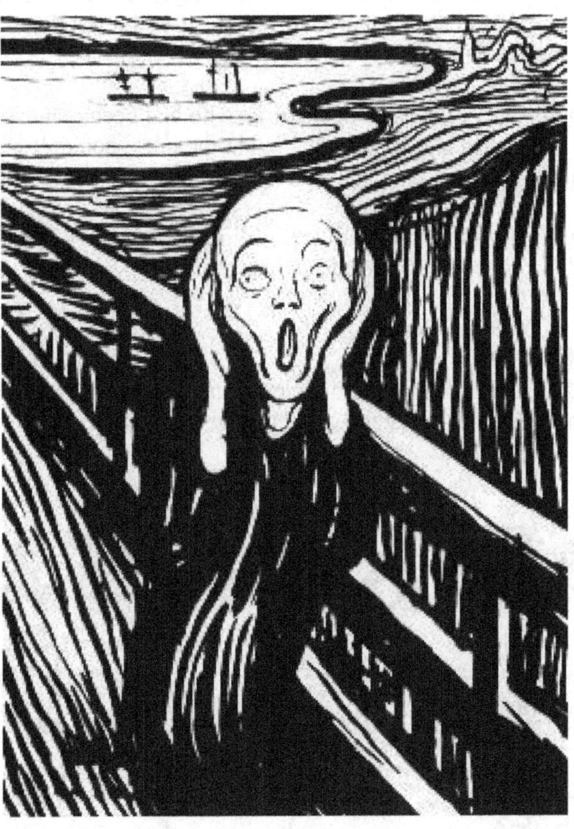

It took four different phlebotomists to draw blood from me that day in the hospital since I was so dehydrated combined with my vein's natural ability to hide in the presence of needles.

"Come try to draw this guy," one phlebotomist asked of another after her fourth or fifth try, "this guy is a hard stick."

"If you knew what was going on, you might phrase that differently," I responded.

I was reminded of the joke about the two young boys who were in the same hospital room. One boy asked the other, "Are you medical or surgical?"

"I don't understand," the other boy replied.

"The easiest way to tell is," the first boy said, "were you sick before you got here, or did they make you sick while you were here?"

The hospital staff wouldn't let me eat since everything was going through me like Grant going through Richmond. I learned what a "clear liquids only diet" was, and it wasn't much. The starvation diet ended late in the second day when I was finally allowed to eat. I think the sound of my stomach growling like an angry dog was keeping the other patients awake, so something had to be done. Once the pain lessened, I was allowed to make my escape. I did receive wonderful treatment from everyone involved. It was just the intensity of the hospital atmosphere that I needed to get away from.

Upon being sprung, I mean discharged from the hospital, I determined that treatment solely under the medical model was not benefiting me in the greatest way. I began to wonder what other forms of treatment might help. Several people had mentioned success with acupuncture for nerve pain in the past. I knew that acupuncture involved needles, and I had an inherent, long-standing distaste for needles and everything that goes along with them. My wife, in fact, reminds me to this day that I passed out during my blood test for our marriage license. I insist that the prospect of marriage at that time was at least as scary as the needle, but that's another story.

So, in desperation, I went to see a Chinese acupuncturist who had been recommended to me. After discussing the unusual aspects of my situation, she felt that she could help. What the heck, couldn't hurt worse than it already did, right? So she began to place needles from my ankles to my legs and knees and finally in numerous locations throughout my groin.

She then proceeded to pull out a small box with lots of lights and switches on it. The box had a number of wires hooked to it, which she proceeded to connect to the needles in my groin.

"What are you doing?" I inquired nervously.

"Just a little electricity" she stated as she turned the machine on and ran pulsating currents through my genitals. I felt like the X-rated version of Frankenstein's monster (would that be Frankensack?):

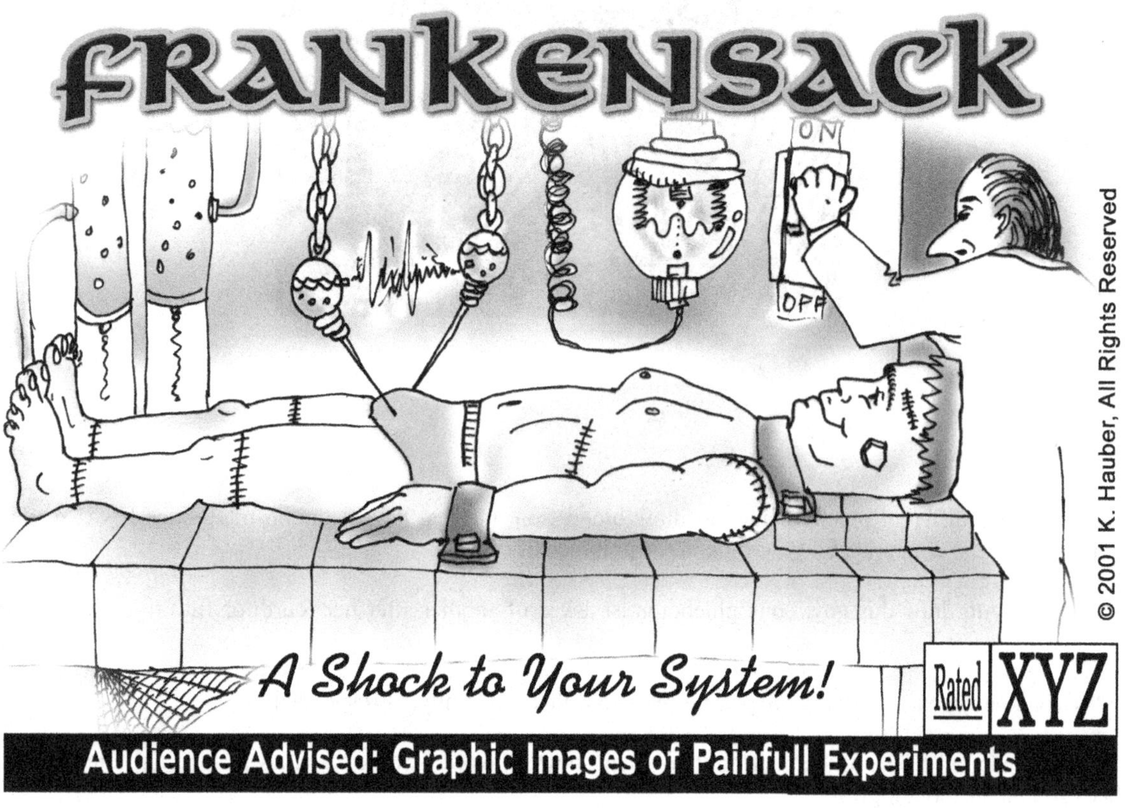

"Do you feel that?" she asked.

"Who wouldn't?" I wondered.

She left me alone and wired. Strangely enough, or perhaps not strangely enough, after several minutes of being a human genital electrical conduit, I felt a significant relaxation response begin. This continued over the twenty minutes or so of the treatment and led to substantial relief that lasted for several days. Maybe all those thousands of years of Chinese medical practice could teach us Westerners a little something after all. Upon completion of the treatment, the acupuncturist gave me several herbal medications to try and we agreed to do all this again the next week.

The pain and tension built up again during the following days, but was substantially relieved again by the next acupuncture treatment, furthering my conviction that this was a good avenue of therapy. Surprisingly, my urologist and internist agreed with this approach, acknowledging that the medications were not very effective, and if it provided relief and promoted healing, why not give the acupuncture a try? I continued to see this particular acupuncturist until an incident in which the assistant who was responsible for removing the needles overlooked taking one out of my lower quadrants, which I found as I hoisted my pants back up. Ouch! This object lesson taught me to never leave the final needle check to someone else. As Ronald Reagan used to say, "Trust and verify." I saw several acupuncturists as time went on, one of whom also helped me with diet counseling as a means of pain management and health promotion, which was of tremendous benefit.

Next came the inevitable question to my urologist, "So, Doc, when can I give this vasectomy a road test? If I can't sleep, walk or sit comfortably, I might as well be able to have sex. After all, my original intention in being cut on was to actually be able to do that again."

"Don't try to be a hero, and bring in that semen sample as scheduled," he admonished me.

Okay, at least he didn't say not to try. I'll interpret that as free license, and just refrain from the more energetic moves guys can be inclined toward. Like that would work now anyway.

However, in beginning my practice as the world's gentlest lover, I found that yes indeed, this too increased the pain sensations I was experiencing. Without being too graphic, let's just say that experiencing stabbing and tearing sensations in your testicles and groin while attempting lovemaking can have a deflating consequence. As a matter of fact, that kind of pain will make all of your equipment want to hide in abject terror.

Not to worry, there's plenty of chemical assistance out there these days for that kind of thing. A little of that and a guy can go all day and night. Only now, attempting sexual activity not only led to pain for longer periods of time, but no big finish, no orgasm, no semen sample, nothin'. That was a new frustration to add to the growing list.

When the urologist's office called to inquire as to why my semen sample was overdue, I roared that I'd get around to it when I damn well could. Obviously, there was a little tension surrounding this issue.

I finally mustered the courage to discuss this with my internist, and learned that the nerve medication that I was on while attempting to quiet the pain sensations from the nerves in my loins was also having the effect of blocking nerve impulses from other functions in my body, namely sexual response, digestion and probably more. That, plus chronic pain, overshadows other nerve sensations. I had wondered why I wasn't able to sense appetite, or bowel pressure, or bladder pressure. In fact, my indicator for those bodily functions had shifted to pain, instead of the normal sensations I had known all my life.

About this same time, my medical insurance company sent me a letter saying that the painkillers I had been taking were potentially addictive, contrary to what I had been told, and they refused to pay for continued prescriptions. Huh? Time for a change! I was quite ticked off by now and insisted on a different approach.

My doctors decided that I needed to be on bigger, stronger medication. This took the form of steroids in hefty doses to combat the apparent inflammation. My mind flashed quickly to stories from high school and college of guys who took steroids to bulk up, but resulted in their testicles shrinking, their breasts growing, and their talking like Michael Jackson. This was not exactly what I had signed up for. I was assured that this wouldn't happen, and I would taper off the Prednisone over several months. I moved past those old fears and agreed to try it.

Then my urologist suggested that if the steroids didn't work that we could try a cord block. Really, what's a cord block? I was told that they would go through the groin and disable the nerve that was carrying all the pain signals. Wait a minute! I start out with a simple vasectomy, and now you want to numb me from the groin down permanently? Not in this lifetime! I'll try the steroids, thank you.

I did as my doctors ordered for several weeks and learned that if you give steroids to someone who's already angry, depressed, and in chronic pain, the steroids can make those emotions BIG. In this role as Steroid Man, I wanted to kick locomotives off the tracks and knock over tall buildings.

It got so bad one night that I had to go outside into the backyard and sit in the cold away from my family, because I feared how the unfocussed rage I was feeling might erupt. This was the moment that my urologist chose to return my phone call. Bad timing! Fortunately, I chose not to take the call, knowing what might fly out of my mouth at that moment.

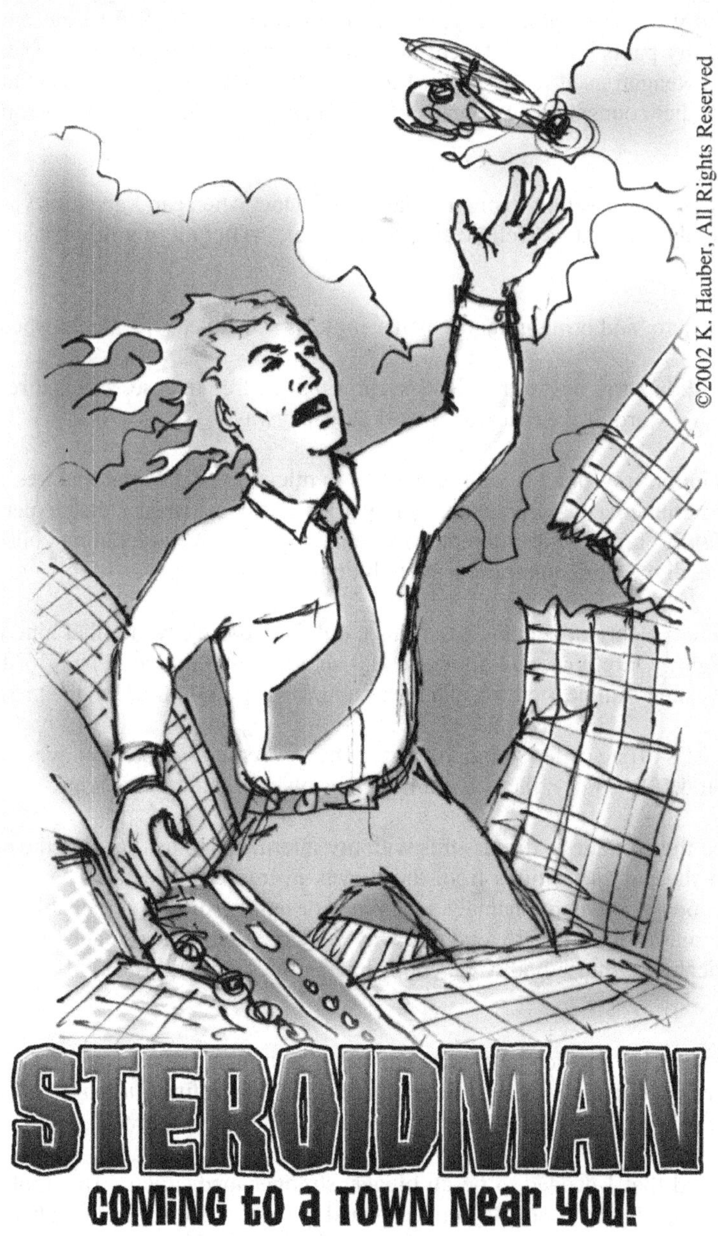

The next day at work, as I was slamming file drawers and swearing under my breath, my boss came to me and said, "Let's take a walk." Fine, a change of scenery would be good.

"You need to get off those steroids," he warned, "I was on them myself for quite a while, and they can really screw you up."

I went back to my internist and said, "I'm stopping the Prednisone."

"No you're not," she replied.

"Why the hell, I mean heck, not?" I insisted.

"Because if you stop taking steroids cold turkey, you can become suicidal," she warned me.

"I'm already there. How fast can I get off this stuff?"

"Taper off over two weeks," she advised.

That was hell time, not only for me, but also for my family and everyone around me. I was not a pleasant person to be around. I finally realized this when my wife invited me to take a few weeks retreat at the New Camaldori Monastery I had talked about visiting up in Big Sur.

Around this time a minister buddy of mine observed that these kinds of "creative center" issues in the body surely would get one's attention. I'll say! When the temporal part of you is in agony, you tend to seek help and guidance from the more eternal parts of your being.

Initially for me, this took the form of confident affirmative prayer: "God, I know that there is some good in this somewhere, and I am ready to move on with my life."

As the pain continued, this would digress to desperate, beseeching prayer: "PLEASE GOD, LET THIS END!"

Finally I resolved to look for the blessings in this situation, in whatever twisted form they might have taken. So how had I grown in this experience? Well, I had certainly gained a new and deeper empathy for anyone in chronic pain. I had been forced to deal with anger, depression, and other strong emotions and find a way to make peace with them. I had to reach out for help and advice with a degree of frankness and honesty that I had never experienced before. In the process, I had also learned to rely more than ever on my own internal guidance as to what was beneficial to my body and my health. My guidance at this point was saying, "Get off the drugs!".

Since every visit to the doctor's office felt like urology by Dr. Mengele, I decided that I'd had enough of that approach for a while. In retrospect, he was probably doing everything he thought was appropriate to help me. It just didn't feel helpful, and in fact usually hurt like crazy during the exams and more than usual for days.

I don't want to say I fired him, but I asked my urologist to focus his efforts instead on those patients he might actually be able to benefit, and we'd talk when needed. Besides, it was getting to the point that some of the medical providers I was seeing didn't recognize me with my clothes on. At one point my urologist commented that he hadn't realized that I was as tall as I am at 6'2''. I felt that this must have been because I always needed to lay down in his presence. Some distance from this brand of medical attention seemed appropriate.

I also talked to my internist about what alternatives were available other than what I was already doing beyond the medical model. She suggested I try another medication called Neurontin, which had been mentioned by several sources. I appreciated the suggestion, but having the experiences I had so far with drugs, I asked that we look up the potential side effects of Neurontin, this time before I started experiencing them. In checking out the PDR, it turned out that Neurontin is mainly used as an anti-seizure medication.

We read on. When the discussion in the text started quoting percentages of side effects including impotence and sudden and unexplainable death, I said stop, close the book, and let's go home. The way things were going, I didn't care how "rare" the chances of problems were since I felt exceedingly rare all of the time.

In a later discussion with another physician friend, he reminded me that medications are all "selective poisons", which is why you don't take too much of them or eat them like food. The Neurontin in particular didn't sound too good.

"How will I know that this is over and I'm in the clear?" I asked my internist.

"I think you'll be safe when you haven't experienced any pain for two weeks straight," she replied.

Two weeks, heck, I'd have been satisfied with two hours, heck with that, two minutes, without some kind of pain sensation at that point.

After making the decision that I wasn't going to be able to be on more and more drugs for the rest of time, I determined that I was going to need to do something to moderate the pain as best I could without medications. Since most medications did nothing for me or seemed to make matters worse, this made sense. As I discussed earlier, I began regular acupuncture treatments, which helped a great deal, especially with the more severe episodes of pain. My regular massage therapist worked with me to relieve a lot of the muscle-guarding and tension that accompanied the pain.

Since the nerves going to the testicles run up through the groin and into the lumbar portion of the spine, along with the testicular pain, groin pain, and digestive distress that I experienced, I would consistently have a low back ache as the other sensations increased. This motivated me to see a chiropractor specializing in nervous system work, rather than the skeletal adjustments. These were all quite helpful therapies, and were effective in giving at least partial relief from the increasing spiral of the pain. They allowed me to get around for several hours at a time before needing to be horizontal again to let the pain settle down.

A friend suggested that I do some journaling since the experience of pain was bringing up so many strong emotions for me. This writing process and the research that followed actually became the basis for this book.

During this time, my father-in-law, a retired veterinarian, offered to help me solve my problem surgically. I told him that, while I appreciated the offer, I just wasn't ready for the method he had used on all those dogs and cats in his many years of practice. It was nice to know that I could count on family for support when I needed it though.

I would meet friends in passing who would inquire how I was. "Nauseous, and my balls ache like hell, and how about you?" was the honest reply that I wanted to give. Somehow though, that just doesn't work in social settings.

But I still needed to deal with the aching and shooting pains every day, all day long, and the indications were that those symptoms might go on for a long time. Through a few fortuitous coincidences, the kind that seem to happen often in life just at the time that you need them, I was introduced to Dr. Mark Schecter who taught a pain and stress management course. Even though Dr. Schecter was in the middle of teaching an eight-week course at the time and didn't have another one scheduled for several months, he offered to start me off on the practices taught in the course and counsel me through until the next course began.

It must have had something to do with the visible distress I exhibited, along with a very helpful and open nature on his part. The course itself is based on the work of Dr. Jon Kabat-Zinn at the University of Massachusetts Medical Center Stress Reduction Clinic. Kabat-Zinn wrote a book entitled <u>Full Catastrophe Living</u>, which I heartily recommend, outlining the program and his experiences as well as those of patients at the Clinic. I was beginning to understand how being in pain all the time makes your life feel like a catastrophe, and I was getting glimpses of how to deal with it.

This program has been duplicated across the country at numerous medical facilities, and is based on mindfulness training that helps you learn to be more at peace with whatever is going on in your life, such as job stress, or relationship stress, or in my case, chronic pain. The concepts are quite helpful, if not easy to learn, and made a tremendous difference in being able to make it through the experiences that were ahead of me. It was a lot like learning to ride the waves of the pain sensations as they came along, instead of fighting them.

In <u>Full Catastrophe Living</u>, Kabat-Zinn discusses an appropriate approach to the treatment of chronic pain. "In the best of cases," he states, "which is probably still the exception rather than the rule, a person with chronic pain will receive the ongoing support of a highly trained multidisciplinary pain clinic staff. Psychological assessment and counseling will be integrated with the treatment plan, which might include everything from surgery to nerve blocks, trigger-point injections with steroids, intravenous lidocaine drips, muscle relaxants, analgesics, physical and occupational therapy, and, with luck, acupuncture and massage. The goal of counseling is to help the person work with his or her body and to organize his or her life to keep what pain there is under some degree of control, to maintain an optimistic, self-efficacious perspective, and to help the person engage in meaningful activities and work within his or her capacity (Kabat-Zinn, 1990)." He seemed to be speaking directly to me and to my situation. Now I was on the right track.

The heart of the pain and stress management program teaches several meditation and yoga practices that are used in the cultivation of mindful awareness. I had spent many years in various meditation practices prior to this, and had tried yoga several times. I can truly say that the approaches taught in the course were an entirely different experience from anything that I had up to that time.

Everyone in the course seemed to gravitate toward certain parts of the practices that worked best for them, and I found the yoga to be particularly helpful since I needed to restrict most of my other exercise routines because of the pain I was experiencing. I even developed an idea for a special post-vasectomy yoga position, as shown:

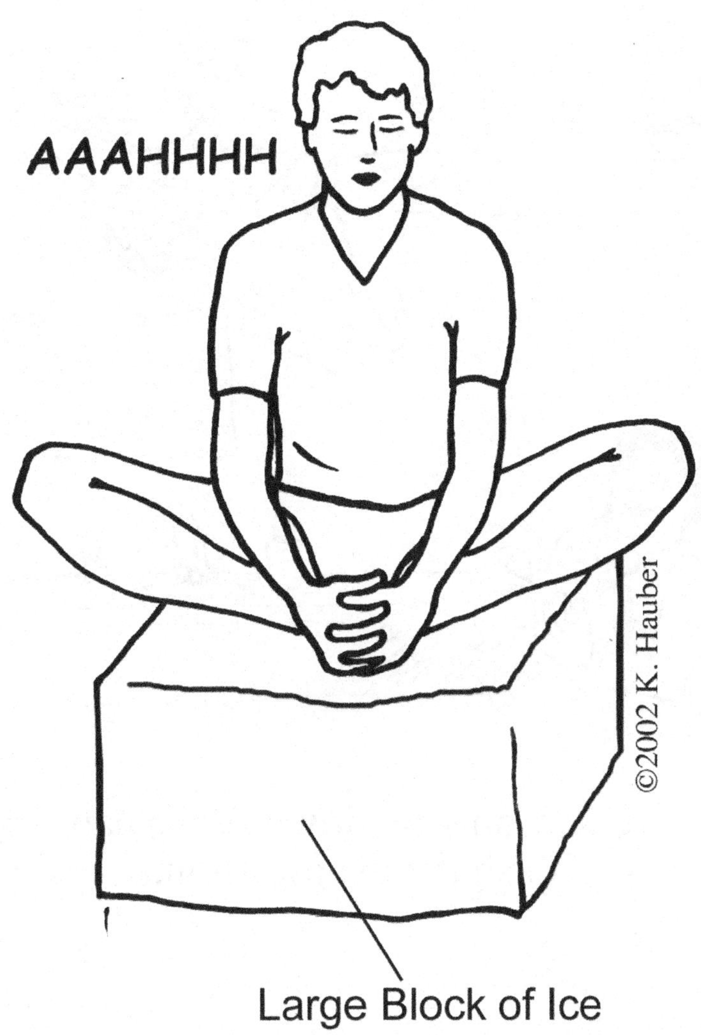

Even though I knew that I was going in the right direction as far as treatment was concerned, and my doctors agreed, getting my HMO and insurance to buy off on this was far more difficult. This battle is the beginning of the chapter titled "I'm Sorry; That's Not a Payable Benefit," the details of which I will share with you later. Ticked off, but undeterred, I forged on and continued my newly discovered treatment modalities.

My internist eventually got me a referral to see a pain specialist physician with the intent of finding something within the medical model to help manage the pain in addition to the pain management training I was learning. By this time I was four months into the chronic pain experience, so I cautiously agreed to give this a try.

When I had my appointment with the pain specialist, he did most of the usual exam stuff, and then told me to lie down on the exam table. He took a safety pin, opened it and sterilized the tip. Huh? He then proceeded to poke the pin in various parts of my thighs and groin.

"Can you feel that?" he asked repeatedly.

"You bet your…err, yes, I can," I insisted.

"OK then, I know this is going to feel like torture, but…" he said as he went straight for my scrotum with the safety pin.

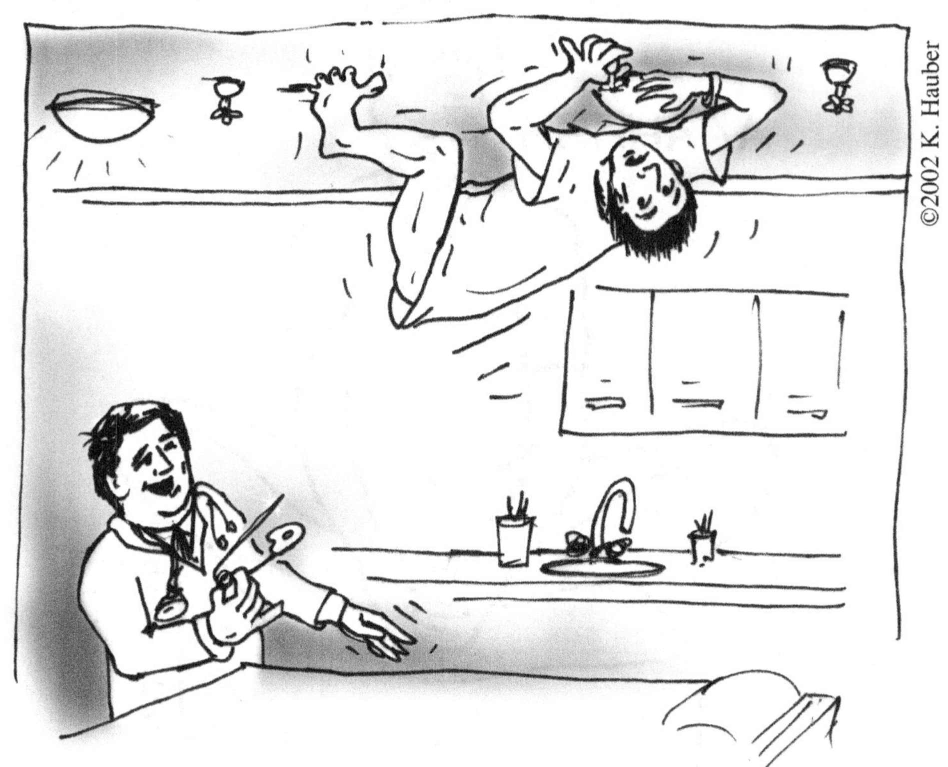

OK, Come on down so we can
finish the examination...

Until that moment, I thought that only Sufi mystics could levitate. I acquired that skill instantly. On my way back down to the table I wondered how long this guy had been an understudy for the Marquis de Sade. I had the mistaken impression that I was seeing a pain specialist to find a way to decrease the pain I was experiencing. Surprise again! Why couldn't anyone just believe me when I said I hurt a lot? I later learned in reading his report that this was termed the "pinprick" test. There was certainly a pin and a prick involved, and I'll leave it at that.

After all of this, when the pin was safely stowed away to await the next unsuspecting patient, we finally got down to what he might suggest to help with my chronic pain. He knew that drugs were out as far as I was concerned, given my experience thus far.

"I think you are a good candidate for a TENS unit," he stated.

So what's a TENS unit, and how could it help? Well, the idea is to run mild pulsating electric currents along the pathway of a nerve that is emitting pain signals, thereby effectively providing a white noise type blockage of those pain signals.

Okay, the electricity had worked pretty well for the acupuncturist, so how do I use the thing? He demonstrated how he wanted me to wear and adjust the unit.

"Wait a minute. You want me to tape electrodes to my groin and run current through my privates to try to quiet the cries of anguish from the twins?" I wondered out loud.

That was the idea. What the hell, might as well try.

I soon learned that you need to be quite careful about how you adjust the amount and frequency of the current when you are wired in this way. My wife then figured out a new form of discipline to keep me in line by simply threatening to turn up the TENS unit. In the long run, I found that using the TENS unit more directly on the groin like this was not as effective for me as trying to block and unwind the pain signals from the back. So I used the unit to provide some temporary relief before the stronger sensations would build and find another route for expression.

As you might have gathered by now, all of these pain management techniques were part of a delicate balancing act that I was learning. This allowed me to walk along at the edge of what I could tolerate without falling over into the abyss of pain and ending up in the hospital again, which I was quite motivated to stay away from. But there is a big difference between pain management and pain relief, and my search was on in earnest to relieve the problem, not just treat the symptoms. I had no idea what I was in for.

I knew I needed to continue with non-invasive modes of treatment, but finding the appropriate balance provided a new challenge every day. As an interesting note: my Chinese acupuncturist later told me of 10 or more men she had treated in China for chronic pain following their vasectomies. According to her, the Chinese medical journals contained numerous articles on the subject (unfortunately I don't read Chinese), and the problem was most prevalent in rural areas where rough surgery was more common. One-in-a-million, huh?

Chapter Six

I Think I Need a Creative Outlet

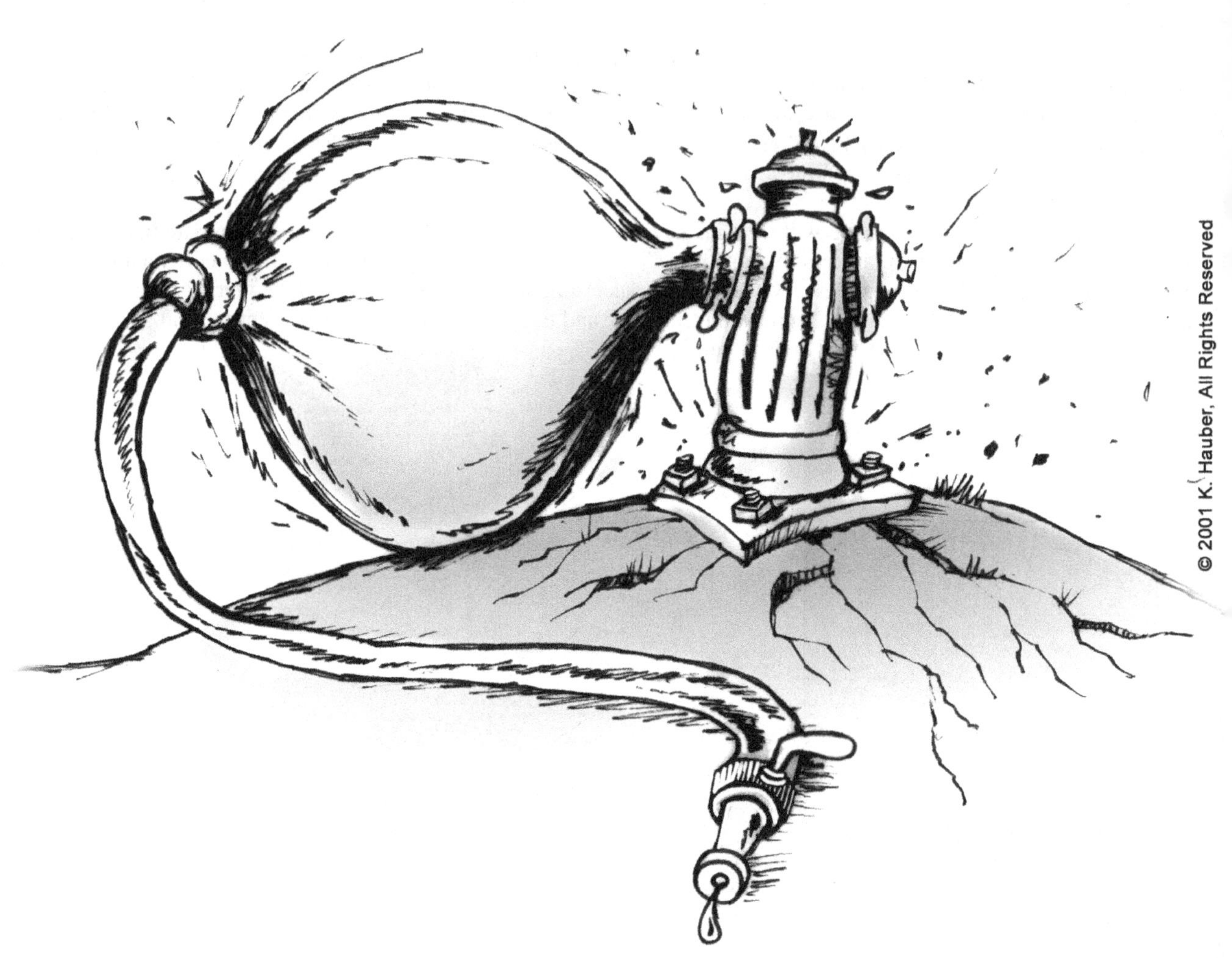

Let's try an analogy on for size: Take a 40-year-old fire hose and hook it up to a hydrant. Turn the water on. Let the hose represent the epididymis portion of the testicles and the vas deferens, which would measure some 20 feet in length if stretched out. Let the water flow represent the 50,000 sperm cells a minute that a man's body manufactures, even after a vasectomy.

Now, tie a knot in the fire hose. What's going to happen? Something is going to rupture, right? That's why fire departments don't use 40-year-old fire hoses, and why men develop ruptures in their testicles after the vas is tied off during a vasectomy procedure. How accurate is this analogy? Just keep reading.

45

When you are awake much of the night with pain for years on end, you find that there are several choices available to you as to how to spend the time. You can try tossing and turning and being angry. I did that for a while. Actually, it seemed like a v-e-r-y long while. Eventually, I found that if I ran a warm bath and used the meditation practice I was learning in the pain management course for an hour or two. That was a relatively effective way of dealing with the pain, and helped to sooth much of the strong emotion that accompanied it. So this became my nightly ritual between about 1am and 4am for many months. I became adept at doing this without waking the rest of my family.

The other thing I found out is when your body is experiencing pain, your adrenal glands start to kick in, giving you that old fight or flight type response. When you've got a lot of adrenaline coursing around in your body in the middle of the night, getting back to sleep is tough even after a long meditation. Finding myself in this circumstance with regularity, I tried to use these wee hours to better my situation. This became the time that I would correspond with my doctors, ask pointed questions, and question their answers. Most of this was by FAX, since I assumed that at 3A.M. they would prefer a FAX to a call or a page. Maybe I was being too courteous. I don't know.

I used the time in other ways as well. Not content to just sit around while receiving electrical charges, I determined that I couldn't be the only man among the 50 million or so who had vasectomies performed to have experienced what was happening to me. It took many months to find out how right I was.

I wasn't getting any terribly helpful information from my urologist at this point, so I started doing some research, and all I can say is thank God for the Internet. I was able to find a number of references on post-vasectomy pain that were real eye-openers.

The first article I found was put out by the U. S. Department of Health and Human Services titled "Facts About Vasectomy Safety." This article revealed that in a survey of 10,590 men who had undergone vasectomies, chronic pain in the testicles was more prevalent than in men who had not undergone the procedure (National Institute of Health, 1996). So I was one-in-a-million, huh? I was beginning to have my doubts. I continued the search.

The next item I ran across was a 1999 article by H. G. van der Poel and E. J. Meulman on the Internet titled "Post-Vasectomy Pain, An Underestimated Side-Effect." I read with interest. This report analyzed the data from several studies and found that post-vasectomy scrotal pain was present in up to 54% of patients in one study. Another study found *chronic testicular discomfort to be present in 33% of the patients four years after vasectomy, often during intercourse.* The veil was beginning to come off a very sore subject.

Another study showed chronic scrotal pain in 18.7% of patients after vasectomy. In yet another study, occasional discomfort was found in 70.6% of patients, and severe pain that affected quality of life was found in 11.8% of the patients. The onset of pain symptoms ranged from two months to twenty years (Van der Poel, et. al., 1999). So I was one in a million, huh? Two to three percent complications rate, huh? I don't think so!

The Van der Poel, et. al., (1999) article went on to describe the various causes of this pain syndrome. First, blocking the vas causes obstruction of the epididymis, which, in a healthy, sexually active man naturally gets cleared out on a regular basis. This results in "dilatation of the caput epididymis and interstitial fibrosis" (for all intents and purposes: swelling and scarring). So what's the big deal about scar tissue forming? How about this: "Interstistial fibrosis contributes to irreversible damage of vasectomized testes" (Shiraishi, et. al., 2002). Tell me, gentlemen, is this the area you want scar tissue to form in your body causing irreversible damage? This effect takes place mainly within the first year after vasectomy. Inflammation and ruptures were noted as a second cause of pain by Van der Poel.

A study characterized this phenomenon this way: "Vasal obstruction results in build up of epididymal back pressure and subsequent dilatation of the epididymal ducts. Ductal dilatation may be marked, even leading to the development of cysts. Pathologically, a combination of tubular dilatation, sperm packed tubules, sperm extravasation [outside the vas], with sperm granulomas and a relative lack of inflammatory cells characterize the post-vasectomy syndrome (Choe, et. al., 1996)." Let me translate for you: pressure builds up, parts of your testicles rupture, sperm ends up where it wasn't meant to be, and you hurt a lot. "Epididymitis is reported in up to 6% of vasectomized patients.... It is rarely due to infection but results from engorgement caused by continued entry of spermatozoa into the obstructed epididymal duct.... This 'congestive' epididymitis occurs mainly in the first few months after the operation" (McDonald, 1996).

Do you remember the diagrams of the testicle with that "friable" little crescent shaped epididymis? Here's another diagram specifically showing the epididymis and those delicate little tubules that start rupturing after a vasectomy due to this pressure build up. The testicle is on the right, and the now grossly enlarged epididymis is on the left:

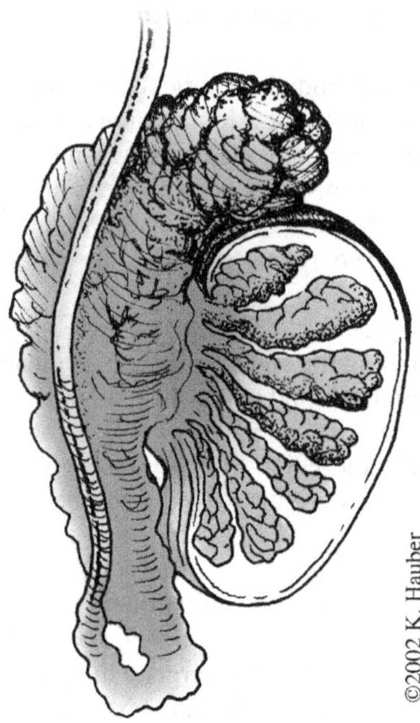

There's more. Choe, et. al., (1996) continues: "McMahon, et. al., (1992) found no correlation between early postoperative complications such as infection or hematoma and chronic pain complaints. [That means you can get by clean in the first few days or weeks and still wind up with long-term pain.] Sperm granulomas, however, a frequent finding after vasectomy, were associated with pain complaints in 54% of patients." I might add that aside from the pain associated with having these granulomas form in a man's scrotum, he will often get the pain associated with yet another surgical procedure needed to "excise" them. That means cut them out, otherwise live with the pain.

So what's the diagnosis, doctor? "A constant pain was reported in 9 of 10 patients in a study by Chen and Ball (1991). The majority of pain complaints were located to the epididymis. Pain is often exacerbated during intercourse and ejaculation (Van der Poel, et. al., 1999)." Not exactly the moment you want to feel the sensation of being stabbed in the testicles, is it? As if you would want that sensation anytime.

At the end of the Van der Poel article was a reference to yet another article by Kenneth D. Reda (1999) titled "Open-ended Vasectomy: Improved Reversibility with Less Chance of Chronic Pain." This piqued my interest. It turns out that while Mr. Reda was doing a little research in advance of his own vasectomy he found several different methods that can be employed. The method used by most surgeons is called a closed- ended vasectomy, in which both vas are cut and all four newly created ends are tied and cauterized.

There is an alternate method that was developed by Dr Edward Shapiro called an open-ended vasectomy in which the testicular ends of the vas are left open and the prostatic (upper) end is closed off in the normal manner. According to Reda, "If you read the relevant literature, you will find that the latter (open-ended) procedure leaves the testicles relatively unaffected with improved reversibility and less chance of long-term chronic pain." How much of a decrease in chronic pain, you might ask? How about a three-fold decrease in chronic post-vasectomy testicular pain with the open-ended procedure?

Now I was even more interested. " 'A nodule, i.e. a granuloma quickly forms at the cut end of the testicular end of the vas containing the sperm.' (Dr. Shapiro)… The idea of the open-ended vasectomy is to reduce pressure, allow a single granuloma to form at the testicular end, and thus prevent pressure-induced pain, ruptures and granulomas, which block the

47

epididymis. Painful complications clearly occur less frequently with the open-ended technique.... Studies confirm no increases in failure due to recanalization if the closed vas end is covered by the sheath [of tissue] after it is cauterized.... These combined studies evaluated over 10,000 vasectomies (Reda)."

Reda's article went on to recommend requesting the open-ended vasectomy technique in conjunction with the no-scalpel technique to further reduce the possibility of complications. Well, at least I knew half of what to ask for when I had my procedure done, since I had originally asked for the no-scalpel technique. Unfortunately, it was the half I didn't know that bit me.

Reda explained that by closing the testicular end of the vas, "blocking the normal exit of sperm in a [closed-ended] vasectomy can cause pain for a number of reasons: 1) elevated pressure within your testes; 2) swelling (i.e. dilation of seminiferous tubules); 3) thickening sperm debris; and 4) interstitial fibrosis [scarring]." He also noted that, "Reversal becomes less successful with time as conditions foster potentially painful complications."

I began to wonder about what in fact, had been done to me during my procedure, so I requested a copy of the surgical report from my urologist's office. I had received a closed-ended procedure, and the doctor had used a scalpel to make the incision, which he closed with a stitch. Why would a no-scalpel vasectomy that supposedly requires no stitches be done with a scalpel and a stitch you might ask? This seemed like a reasonable question. The report also indicated that I had received Valium as sedation, when I had specifically refused it. Hmmm. Discrepancies were beginning to surface.

A statement by a patient on the Prostatitis Web Site (Vasectomy Page) seems to summarize the situation I was experiencing quite well: "If any of you out there in cyberland have had a vasectomy and then developed acute and chronic prostatitis or epididymitis, your treatment needs to be handled a lot differently. Your doctor will probably not recognize the correlation between the two for medico-legal reasons. It can be an awful condition.... The truth is out there!" Okay, Kevin, full speed ahead, and damn the torpedoes!

I presented this data in writing to my urologist. Why hadn't we discussed the information about post-vasectomy pain syndrome and some of the possible treatments for it? Why was a scalpel used in what was supposed to be a no-scalpel procedure? A stitch was used when all of the information I had read indicated no stitches were required. What was the deal with the sedation note, anyway? And speaking of drugs, why did he tell me that the pain medication he was prescribing was not addictive, and my insurance was writing me back telling me that the medication was in fact potentially addictive? What gives? When he responded over a week later, he offered the best explanations he could.

He claimed that he went back and forth between using a scalpel and a hemostat to make the incision, but often preferred the scalpel and a single stitch to close because, aesthetically, it left a less noticeable scar. Up until that point, I had never considered much about scrotal aesthetics, but this again was one of those "beauty is in the eye of the beholder" issues. I guess if you have to look at scrotums all day long, you want them to be as aesthetically pleasing as possible.

I suppose it could best be termed that he had performed a modified version of the no-scalpel procedure. The sedation note was an error, and he didn't know how that crept in. As for the formerly non-addictive, now addictive pain medication, evidently the most recent Physicians Desk Reference showed the medication as having potentially addictive properties, whereas prior editions had not. I found these representations and errors disturbing, but decided to let them pass for the time being and focus on my healing.

I extracted a promise that he would research the issue of further treatment and the various studies and get back to me soon. By the time a month had passed, I was more than a little impatient with this definition of "soon".

According to Einstein time is relative anyway, but come on! I'm sure Einstein wasn't working on his Theory of Relativity while his nuts ached, or he would have called it the Theory of Urgency. I took a get-in-your-face approach and scheduled an appointment. At the appointment, the urologist shared some journal articles with me about post-vasectomy pain syndrome and potential treatments.

So we developed an action plan to deal with what he now was willing to acknowledge I was experiencing: *post-vasectomy pain syndrome*. Why I had to find all this out on my own, I still don't know, other than possibly a severe case of butt-covering on my urologist's part while mine was being continually bared. I wondered how many other men have had vasectomies and who have suffered similarly, but in silence? I wondered also how many have been told that they are one-in-a-million and believed it, feeling like some kind of freak in the process.

According to my doctor, first he would try a temporary spermatic cord nerve block to see if that would break the pain cycle. Sounds innocent enough, doesn't it?

If that didn't work, then an open-ended vasectomy or a reversal procedure were possibilities. Of course I could always consider having various pieces that were hurting taken out he noted calmly. Hold the phone, we're not going there! We agreed to take this one step at a time and do the cord block the next day.

By this time I had numerous friends and acquaintances, all perfectly reasonable and loving human beings, singing a chorus of "Sue, sue!" to which I responded, "But I don't want to be in a lawsuit, and have my genitals become a matter of public record. I just want to feel better. Besides, I live in a small town, have mutual friends with this guy and would just as soon get on with my life!"

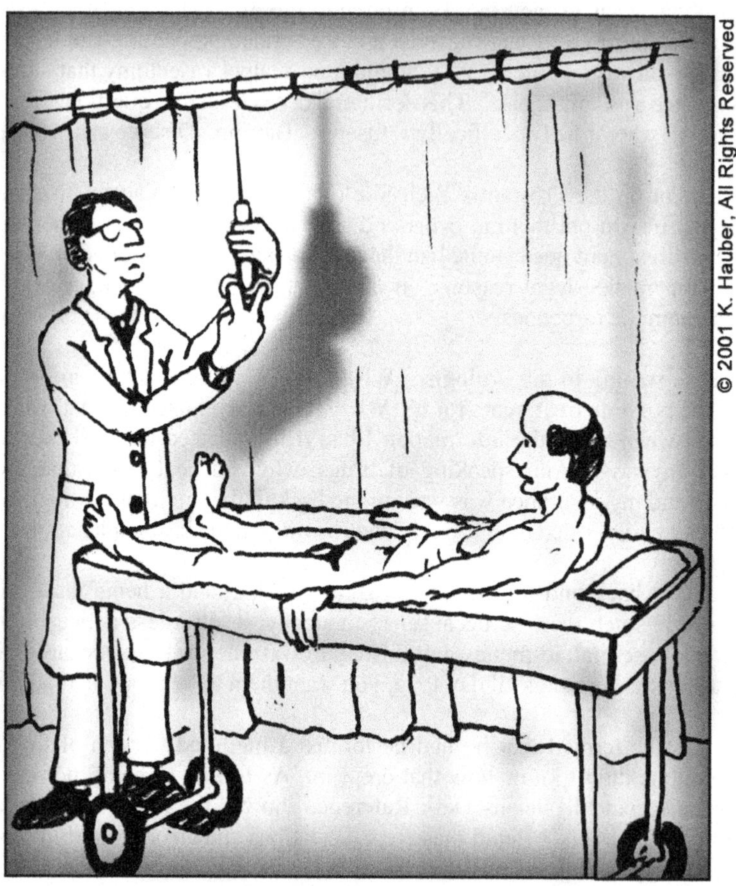

"Now hold still, this won't hurt a bit."

When I arrived for the cord block procedure, I was conducted to the now familiar procedure room, and given another of those large paper napkins with which to cover myself. Like it really made a difference? When the doctor entered he asked if I was ready to do this. Why did he always start off that way? Nothing like instilling doubt!

"Yeah, I think I am. Shouldn't I be?"

Since the end of the workday was approaching, the doctor sent the rest of the staff and patients home. Uh-oh. I think he didn't want anyone else to hear this. It was time to lie down. He pinched up the cord through the skin of my groin next to my penis.

"You're going right for the sorest parts, aren't you?" I asked.

Without comment, he tried inserting the needle. While procedure report states that "the patient had a moderate to severe amount of discomfort during the infiltration with local anesthetic," what he should have noted was it was agonizing and he barely kept me on the table.

"Was that a needle or a spike you were using?" I begged for clarification.

"Just a one and a half inch needle," he replied.

"Well you sure know where to put it to get the greatest effect!" I observed. I think I'm going to puke!"

"Don't do that!" he implored, knowing, I'm sure, that he was the most likely moving target.

Damn, this was supposed to help? He did likewise on the other side with similar writhing results. This put a total of 10cc of lidocaine into me, a little over three times what he had used for anesthesia in the original vasectomy. Seemed like he was loading for bear. He left me for a few minutes to allow the bleeding to stop and the anesthetic to take effect.

After 15 minutes or so, nothing was numbing up appreciably. "Strange, I've never seen this happen before," he commented. Not that line again!

He offered me the option of going home and cutting our losses, or getting another set of injections with 6cc of Marcaine this time, which was a little stronger, longer lasting stuff. I'm not sure why I took the "I'm here, I might as well try" attitude, but I did. This set was only mildly less agonizing than the first, and created bruises that would take weeks to go away. Why should I have expected anything less?

Breathe, Kevin, just breathe. This was no way to start a weekend.

Another 15 minutes passed and although I was full of medication, I was only about half way numbed out. I went home before he could come up with any other helpful ideas. The effect of the block increased somewhat as I drove home and lasted for a few hours, relieving enough of the aching to be temporarily helpful if not pleasant. But what a price to pay! This had been the most unsavory procedure yet.

I describe what went on with the cord block as a warning to you, sincerely hoping that you never find yourself in a similar situation. If you do end up with this recommendation, my advice is this: As the doctor walks toward you, quickly grab the syringe and stab him in the leg with it so he can't chase you, then run as fast as you can for the nearest exit. Don't worry about your clothes, they're not worth taking the time to collect: just get out. I think you can tell that I'm only half kidding.

I went to see the pain specialist again the following week, who thought that the results of the cord block warranted at least a little further experimentation and suggested doing a caudal epidural procedure. This time he would use a three-inch needle inserted up my tailbone to inject various pain medications and some dye. The idea once again was to try to break the nervous system's pain cycle and send some dye through me to see how things were circulating. Another innocent idea, right?

The epidural procedure was not too bad. Notwithstanding a couple of uncomfortable moments, everything seemingly went well. Until the procedure was over, that is. I stood up, my blood pressure went down and so did I. When I came to, one nurse was speaking impatiently to the other nurse she had relieved just before I passed out. Why did she deserve a crisis when she was trying to do her a favor? Later, I apologized to the doctor for causing the drama, observing that my body must have taken exception to yet another needle. Especially a large needle. Especially a large needle stuck up my…well, you get the idea.

The pain relief from the epidural was significant. Now I know why they are used so often during childbirth. The effect lasted about eight hours and I felt more normal during that time than I had in months. All of the pain sensations did return when the medication wore off (which was more than a little disappointing). Once again, this was a lot of drama and effort for little relief.

According to my urologist, this was a good indicator that performing the vasectomy over again using the open-ended method could relieve the pain. I suggested, since he was needing to get in there so darn often, he should install a zipper to make the process easier, just in case I needed to have a reversal done later on. I figured it was far easier to use a zipper than all these incisions, and better than the sound of Velcro ripping in that region. I offered to let him patent the idea:

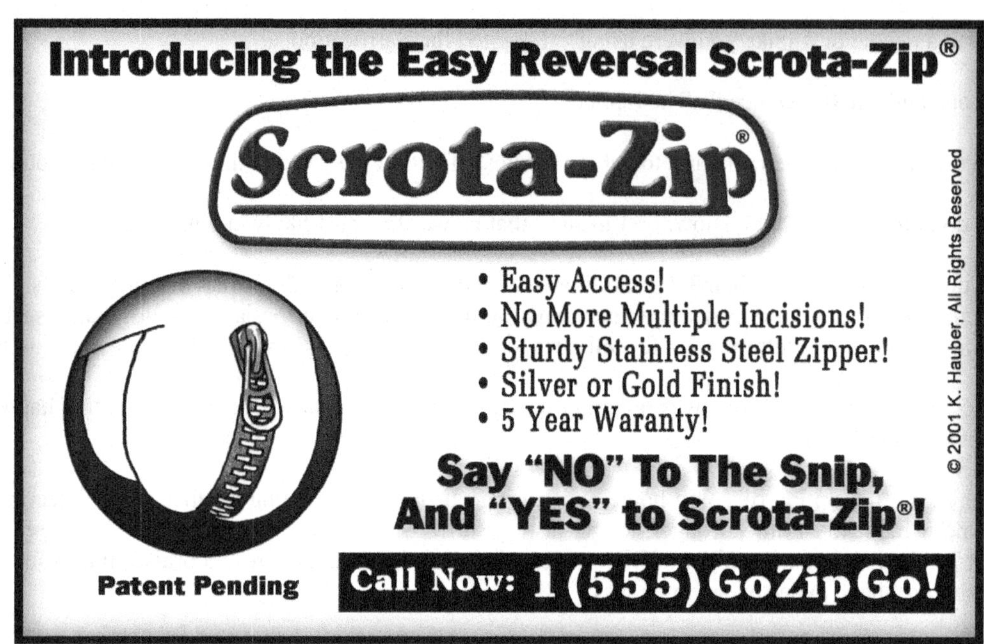

Chapter Seven

Once Is Not Enough

I continued to research my condition. Post-vasectomy pain has been studied for quite some time, even if it's not commonly publicized. An article published in the Journal of Urology in 1985 discussed epididymectomy (surgical removal of the epididymis portion of the testicle) as an often-successful solution when "conservative" treatments had failed.

Quoting from the abstract of this article: "A group of 20 surgical specimens in 18 patients with a previously unappreciated syndrome of unremitting epididymal pain and induration of 5 to 7 years [!] after vasectomy was collected during a 2-year interval.... Total unilateral or bilateral epididymectomy and partial vasectomy led to complete relief of symptoms, usually within 24 hours.... *Recognition of this late post-vasectomy syndrome, which represents a major complication of vasectomy*[emphasis added], might be expected to increase as cohorts of vasectomized individuals age" (Selikowitz, et. al., 1985).

Another idea offered along the invasive front (quite literally) by my urologist was to cut into my groin and surgically strip the nerves from my spermatic cords. This might alleviate the pain, but leave me permanently numb. Sounds fairly severe, doesn't it? A doctor at the University of Pittsburgh had success with this method in two cases, or so he claimed in one of the medical journals (Bruning, 1997). I had no interest in becoming the third case. While the prospect of pain resolution sounded attractive, the idea of permanently removing significant pieces of my various genital apparatus with unknown consequences had very little allure at that point. Put the scalpels away for the moment doctor, I'll just keep looking, thank you.

Eventually, my Internet searches yeilded a transcript of an Australian radio program titled "Long-Term Complications After a Vasectomy Operation," in which "late post-vasectomy syndrome" (another name for post-vasectomy pain syndrome) was discussed. The program aired in 1997, and featured a gentleman named Richard Barcham, who had (pardon the expression) the balls to talk about his vasectomy experience on national radio.

After his surgery, Barcham experienced pain that lasted for months. At first he thought he was going crazy, but the pain continued. "The kind of experience that I've had, any man will relate to the feeling that you get when you get a blow to your testicles, or when pressure is applied to your testicles, a feeling of nausea and that kind of sickly feeling that you get in your lower belly.... Three months later, I went back to my surgeon and said, 'Look, I'm still having a fair bit of discomfort with this. Is it all normal? Is everything OK?'

"He had a little quick check, and said 'Oh yes, it all seems fine. Forget about it' (Radio National, 1997)." This was sounding familiar. Not wanting to be a "whiner," Barcham went on as best he could, but continued to experience a lot of pain, especially when "getting it on" as he phrased it.

Barcham went on to say, "I had a terrible experience of pain over a period of a few days, just continuing to get worse and worse... until I reached the point where I was writhing on the floor in agony; it was dreadful.... I admitted myself to casualty at our local hospital, and began to explain to the doctor who was on duty at the time that I thought that this was a result of my vasectomy.... He dismissed that idea completely, that 'No, no, no, there are no complications of this type or this magnitude associated with vasectomy.'"

This was sounding more familiar all the time. Barcham was told that he probably had a kidney stone, which was never found, and he was treated for pain and released. Barcham's pain experience continued for two years. Despite his reluctance to undergo more surgery, at the time of the broadcast he was considering having an epididymectomy done. I can tell you from personal experience that you need to experience a lot to consider this.

So why don't more doctors alter the procedure method they use, or disclose or recognize the possibility of chronic pain after vasectomy to begin with? The same radio show that featured Richard Barcham also interviewed Dr. Geoff Brodie who provided some interesting answers to these questions. Dr Brodie was Managing Director of Australian Birth Control Services at the time, and had performed over 6,000 vasectomies. He was also a strong proponent of the open-ended vasectomy method.

Here is what Dr. Brodie had to say about post-vasectomy pain syndrome, "usually GPs think it's an infection, so they try them on a few courses of antibiotics. And sometimes this condition is intermittent, so it goes away for a while, and they think it might have been the antibiotics that made it go away…and then it comes back, and then it gets worse…. So after a while they [the patients] get sick of taking the antibiotics and get passed down the chain." This was sounding familiar, too.

Dr. Brodie continued, "by opening the [testicular] end [of the vas] up, we find surgeons who change their technique from closed-ended to open-ended vasectomy have noted a threefold drop in the incidence [of chronic pain from] this operation. Secondly, microsurgeons have shown to relieve the pain by rejoining the vas up. So that we would say I think from there you could assume that the primary mechanism is backpressure into the testicle. It's also suggested there's an interruption to the nerve and blood supply as the operation is performed initially. On top of that, it has also been noted that the higher up on the…vas deferens that you actually cut and tie, the lower the incidence of this problem. So there are ways of avoiding it."

But what do you do when you are already experiencing post-vasectomy pain syndrome? According to Dr. Brodie, "if it doesn't respond to anti inflammatories, then you've got surgery as the next step, whether you remove the epididymis, do an open-ended vasectomy and create a leak, or you go for a microsurgical reversal of the vasectomy. There are several options…all of them fraught with a level of uncertainty of whether it's going to work or not, and it could cost you an arm and a leg to have a reversal, just to relieve testicular pain, and you're fertile again if it's successful. So you rob Peter to pay Paul, so to speak."

So why don't more doctors use the open-ended technique? Dr Brodie offers, "Surgeons choose to tie both ends [of the vas] because a) that's how they were taught; and b) they may fear litigation or criticism for failure. If you remove a portion of the vas 2-centimeters or more approximately, you reduce the likelihood of failure, but you also reduce the likelihood of…successful reversal. And if you remove up to 7-centimeters of the vas, it won't fail and you can't reverse it. So I think some surgeons do the proverbial arse-covering maneuver…somebody's asked them to do a vasectomy, we know that's where litigation occurs is to do with failure, and failure to warn, so they basically take as much out as possible and no complaints." Surgeons who look out for their own best interest first? Well I suppose that is human enough, but shouldn't the rest of us be told?

This reminds me of the story of the guy who took a tour of the Mercedes-Benz factory in Germany. When he asked an engineer about why they designed one of the particularly quirky aspects of the car the way they did, the engineer responded, "Because vee haf alvays done it zat vay!" I guess if you have something that people continue to buy despite its quirks, you have very little incentive to change.

The advantage of the open-ended vasectomy was exemplified in the case of another man who experienced severe post-vasectomy pain for eleven days following his initial closed-ended procedure. His surgeon then opened the testicular end of the vas and the pain ceased. Reynolds (1997) states that the open-ended procedure "proved easy to perform and may be useful in resistant cases of post-vasectomy obstructive orchitis. This case may support the more widespread use of not occluding the testicular end of the vas."

Armed with the information I had gathered thus far, I scheduled an open-ended vasectomy with my urologist, which I assumed to be far less painful or complicated than a reversal or an epididymectomy. Given the extreme discomfort I had experienced during the cord block attempt, I told my urologist that I wanted to have my acupuncturist present to help with pain control in addition to the local anesthetic he might choose to use. I figured that as long as I was expanding his concept of what could go on with vasectomies anyway, why not continue to do so. At this point, I was firmly convinced of my need to make choices that were in my best interest, listening to my gut instincts in the process.

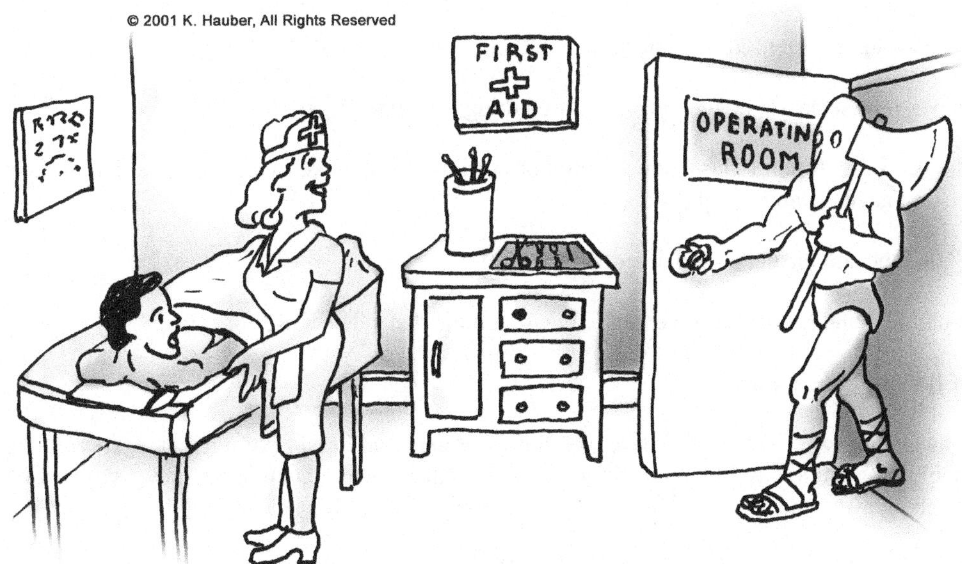

Oh goodie, Here comes your surgeon now.

This time the doctor opted for the "classic" no-scalpel vasectomy technique, and used a sharpened hemostat to make the puncture in my scrotum. This did eventually leave a more noticeable scar than when he used a scalpel the first time. Maybe there was something to his theory on scrotal aesthetics after all.

As he started to cut and snip again, he commented that the literature on performing the open-ended vasectomy that he had read recently made reference to judicious use of cauterization of the tissues in the process.

My mind raced, "What!? You're operating on me now after just reading the flippin' instruction manual!? I thought you said you had done this upon request for other guys in the past! I know it's probably only variations on a theme to you, but this is not confidence inspiring! OK, this is not the time or place to panic, but can we talk about those disclosure issues again?"

When I finally had the courage to question this some time later, he stated that he had only been asked about the open-ended procedure once or twice in the distant past, but was certainly reconsidering offering the option given his experience with my case. Much later, he admitted that to his recollection he had *never* performed an open-ended vasectomy prior to mine. Nice way to find out.

In doing the open-ended procedure, he started on the right side by cutting back the testicular end of the vas, and then squeezed my testicle firmly to try to get sperm to come out of the tube. I thought I was going to explode, acupuncture needles and local anesthetic or not.

"Oh my God!" I exclaimed as my body tightened in response to the pain.

"Hmm," he said in a dissatisfied tone.

"What, not an agonizing enough response for you?" I thought. "Just keep breathing, Kevin," I told myself.

He cut back the vas some more and did the squeeze thing again with a similar sensation resulting. Nothing emitted from the now twice shortened tube though. I didn't think I could take much more, and this was after asking him to use whatever local anesthesia was needed? This guy needed to review the chapter on pain control during surgery before looking at the open-ended vasectomy section!

"Hmm," he said again as I tried to regain my composure. So he started to probe the vas with a sharp instrument to try to open it up.

"Please do whatever you need to while you're in there to get this to work," I begged.

"That may not be so easy," he replied, and closed things up on the right.

On to the left side. I didn't know how much more of this I could take. OK, suppress that thought. He found the vas, made the cut, and gave the now familiar squeeze.

"Ohhh," both he and the nurse exclaimed.

"You sound like Old Faithful just went off. Please tell me that side is OK," I begged.

"Lots of flow here" he replied.

There was an almost instantaneous sense of relief of pressure and easing of tension, even with the discomforts of the cutting and snipping going on at the time. Maybe all these other doctors knew what they were writing about after all. Time to tuck everything away and close up.

Did I want a stitch this time since I had questioned that as part of the "modified" procedure he did the last time? Scrotal aesthetics aside, he recommended using a stitch to minimize bleeding. Evidently, one of the partners in his practice had recently done a vasectomy for one of the other partners. During the procedure they got into one of those "my method is better than your method" debates about whether to use a stitch or go the traditional no-scalpel method without. Of course the doctor performing the procedure won out, and no stitch was used. The receiving doctor bled quite a bit for the next few days. Enough said, use a stitch again this time around, doc.

As badly as I wanted out of there, I took a couple minutes to slow my breathing down while my acupuncturist took out the needles. I didn't want to pass out again as I got off the table like after the epidural. That would have been so unseemly. All told though, it was still easier to take than the cord block had been, even though this was much more invasive and lengthy. I credit this to the moderating effect of the acupuncture, and better mental preparation on my part. Since the 20-minute procedure had turned into the better part of an hour, my family was already there waiting for me. I dressed, thanked everyone involved, had a brief discussion with the doctor and my wife, and went home.

I was pleased to find that I was less uncomfortable than after the first vasectomy, even after only a few hours. My appetite started to return that night and the following day. I took it easy and was able to avoid taking many painkillers. By the next night, I felt much better and was elated with the return of my energy and appetite that had been absent for months.

I called family and friends and joyously proclaimed, "I'm cured!"

I puttered around the house the next day, and while I experienced what seemed like typical post-surgical discomfort, it was nothing like the aching and shooting pains from before.

By the third day, I was beginning to feel a little sore again. Hmm, no big deal, I'll just take it easy. By the next day, I was back to being quite achy again and was having doubts. Damn it, not again, please!

As the week progressed all the previous pain sensations came back. By the time I saw my urologist again at the end of the week, I was limping around as before. And as before, he made me writhe and turn with a simple examination.

So we discussed the options. He felt that it was time to see about a reversal, and by the way, I would need the deluxe version because of what had happened during the open-ended vasectomy with only one side being open. Had he mentioned that this was a four or five hour microsurgery?

He was quite up front this time, and said the deluxe version, called a vasoepididymostomy, was not a technique at which he was proficient, and that there were only a handful of sub-specialists in the country who were. At least I didn't find this out after I was already on the operating table. He happened to know one such super-duper specialist who was a friend of his from residency who had a "high profile" practice down in Beverly Hills.

"If I don't like and trust this guy, he's not cutting on me," I insisted.

Not to worry, my doctor insisted, this guy had the best hands in the business for the kind of work I was going to need. That wasn't completely reassuring, but my options seemed a little limited.

"Let's wait a few weeks and see…" my doctor started to say.

I stopped him in mid sentence. "Let's get this going now," I insisted, "At the rate this process has gone it'll be weeks before I get in to see him anyway."

He reluctantly agreed. By the way, the deluxe version ran about $12,000, according to my urologist.

"Any other good news that I need to know about, Doc?" I inquired.

Oh yes, I would need to wait at least six weeks before having the reversal to heal enough after the second vasectomy.

Shit! Pardon me, but there really isn't a better way to express it. So, ship me off to Beverly Hills to see the guy who works on the scrotums of the stars.

Before I made that trip, however, it seemed appropriate to get a second opinion about this surgery, which promised to be quite unpleasant and quite expensive if it was really needed. I arranged to see another urologist not affiliated with my original doctor, and he said the same thing. Yes, in fact, I did need to have a reversal done.

He gave me the name of an alternate sub-specialist to contact at UCLA and wished me luck. Why was I seeing all of these solemn, long-faced looks on every doctor I saw? What did they know that I didn't? These long-faced looks seemed to be saying "This guy's gonna lose his nuts!"

When I received the information about the first sub-specialist, I began reading the brochure about his practice. It turned out that he dealt with many types of infertility and other sexual issues than reversals, such as I was presumably in need of, to low sperm counts, penile curvature correction, impotence, premature ejaculation, and on and on. I hadn't realized that a practice could be built on such things, but if you have the need, you will go to great lengths. One curious service mentioned in the brochure was a state of the art technique called "electroejaculation." There's an item of interest for your next party!

This technique was apparently used in the artificial insemination process somehow. I had a picture in my mind of a missile shaped capsule like the "orgasmatron" in Woody Allen's movie "Sleeper," a virtual sex machine where you climbed in and set the dial settings to "Low," "Medium," or "Oh My Goodness."

In case you never happened to catch this forgettable little gem in the theaters, Woody Allen plays a guy who goes into the hospital for a routine surgery only to have complications set in and be put in cryogenic freeze for 200 years. When he is revived, he finds that everyone he knew is long dead and he's immersed in a strange new world. Perhaps this helps to explain my hesitancy to be put under general anesthesia.

At one point along the way, a doctor I saw for an appointment jokingly asked, "Gee, I wonder what you did to deserve this." Rather than commenting on this enlightened form of bedside manner, I responded that I was trying not to view this as some karmic payback, but rather some very twisted form of opportunity, that I didn't fully understand yet. Maybe I'd write a book.

Chapter Eight

I'm Off to See the Wizard

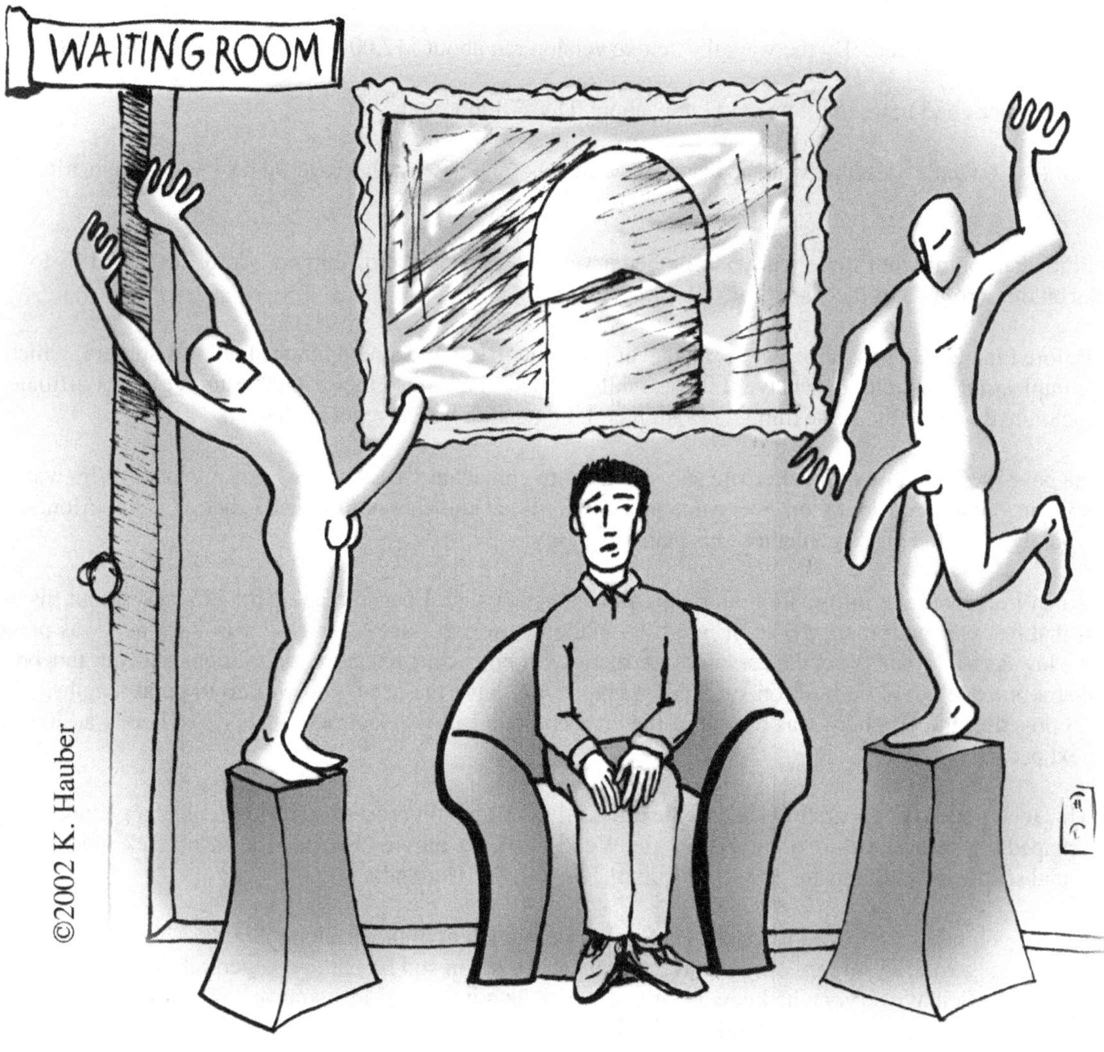

When I went to see the Leaps-Tall-Buildings-With-a-Single-Bound-Type Specialist, I found that his office was, in fact, in a tall building, adjacent to a very expensive looking hospital in Beverly Hills. The office had an assortment of stone fertility god statues with oversized genitalia. Hey, this was L.A., and in that line of work, you need all the help you can get. The doctor introduced himself as Phil. According to Phil who, incidentally, was a very nice guy with compassionate hands and a twisted sense of humor, yes, I probably was going to need the deluxe version of a reversal.

He pronounced this, of course, after testing my current standing high jump capabilities with a testicular exam. It appeared also that I had now developed a sperm granuloma on at least one side, and that would need to be removed during the operation. Was there one problem that I wouldn't develop in this process? I was beginning to have my doubts.

57

He stated that the pain I was experiencing may have been the result of pressure and congestion in the epididymis, or might be a immunological response to the presence of sperm antibodies, or the result of an infection, or a combination of these factors. There was no good non-surgical way to tell.

But I couldn't have the surgery for at least another month and a half. Why the heck not? Hangin' out wasn't much fun these days, ya know! Well in his words, I hadn't healed enough from the second vasectomy a month earlier, and if he were to operate now, it would be "like a grenade went off in there" lowering the chances of a successful surgery.

I thanked him for the colorful image, and begrudgingly accepted the need to wait, making a mental note, once again to talk to my original urologist about these kind of disclosure issues before he started to cut. I sure was glad to be enrolled in a pain management course, because it appeared I was going to need it more than ever.

After returning my pants to their upright position, we moved our discussion to his desk. In looking around the room, I noticed a brass and wood cylinder with a tube and bulb type pump sitting on a shelf.

"Phil," I asked, picking up the device, "what is this, an Austin Powers-style decorator penis pump?"

"It's a kaleidoscope," Phil said in matter of fact tones. Evidently nothing phased him.

I looked down through the top of the tube and pressed the bulb, and saw all the little crystals jumping around.

"Oh, so it is," I observed, "this is probably much nicer to look through, anyway." Rule number one: make no assumptions.

So, how many cases like mine had he seen?

Not too many actually, especially where the pain lasted this long, but notably he had encountered one man referred to him who had seen a doctor to have a mole removed from his scrotum. This guy must have been concerned about scrotal esthetics too. Evidently, the doctor picked up the wrong chart, because instead of removing the mole, he performed a vasectomy. And I wonder why I want to stay conscious during my procedures?

Realizing his error, the doctor quickly referred the patient to my super-specialist who said, yes, he could do a reversal, but the guy had to wait at least two and a half months to heal from the vasectomy before the reversal could be done successfully. In the meantime, guess what? He developed post-vasectomy pain syndrome. I never did find out if the poor guy got his mole removed. The man's pain continued even after his reversal. I might add that the he was just getting married wanting to start a family at the time. What a way to start.

In doing the reversal, aside from reconnecting the plumbing, Phil would try to clean up any scar tissue or other damage along the spermatic cords. Presumably, this would alleviate the effect of scarring causing nerve trauma. He assured me that I would only end up with a three or four inch scar on each side of my scrotum.

Huh? Only three or four inches on each side? So much for my chances of a centerfold modeling career with appropriate scrotal esthetics!

He also informed me that other surgical options, such as removing the epididymis, carry more risk. This is because the blood supply to the epididymis and the testicle are the same. When the epididymis is removed, the blood supply to the testicle is often restricted. This causes the testicle to shrink, eventually necessitating its removal.

So now I was only a few surgical steps away from having my testicles removed? This reversal idea had better work the first time. I later found out that, indeed, Phil was right. In a report I read on a particular series, nine out of ten patients who had their epididymis removed to relieve chronic testicular pain had to subsequently have their testicle(s) removed (Davis, et. al., 1990).

Was there anything else to do in the meantime? Prayer was a good option according to Phil, which was as good a prescription as I had heard yet. As long as we had to wait anyway, he wanted to augment God's work and try me out on a course of the new generation, more macho-type anti-inflammatory drugs and an antibiotic. Fine, why not? I waddled back to the car and drove the 200 miles home, picking up my 37th and 38th medications on the way, continuing my stint as the post-vasectomy pain poster boy.

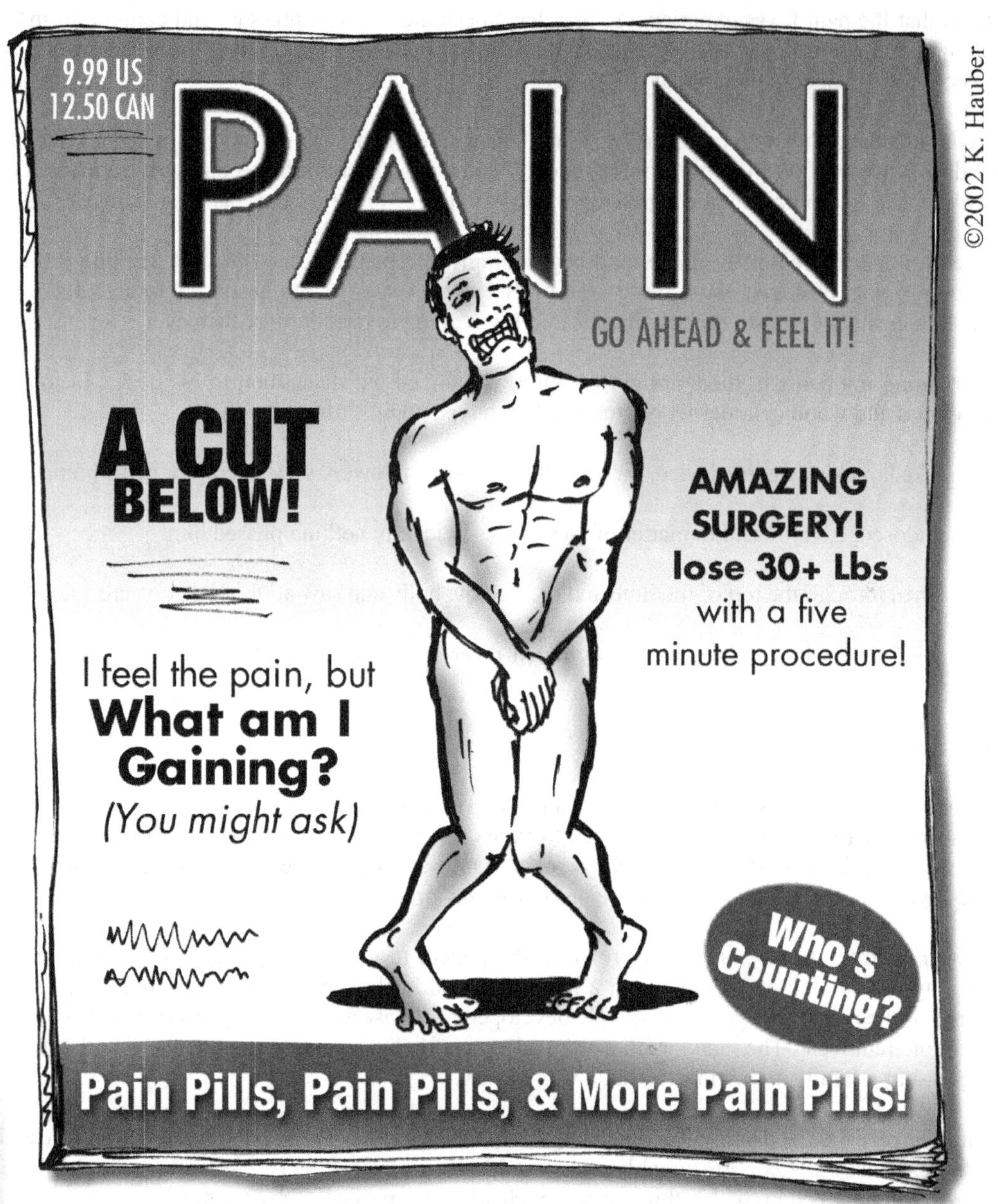

By this time I was at month seven of this little drama, and my wife Kristen was beginning to resort to bribery to keep my spirits up. Promising sex wasn't particularly effective at this point given the nature of what was going on, so one day she offered, "When you're done with all this, we're going to get you a new Porsche Boxster."

"I'm really feeling a lot better now, honey," I replied.

"Really? Let me check."

"No, no, that won't be necessary, we can just go to the Porsche dealer another time," I insisted.

Valentine's Day was fast approaching and Kristen wanted to have our annual party to blow off a little steam. I found the perfect tacky musical tie for the occasion with hearts all over it. It played "Love Me Tender", which had become my theme song by that time.

I have never been overweight. I was 6'2" and 198 pounds at the time of my physical two months before my vasectomy. Now, months later, I stepped on the scale at the doctor's office again. 168; well, I think losing 30 pounds is enough. It was time to do something about this. Kristen started buying and making all kinds of goodies for me including pumpkin pies and peppermint ice cream, my all-time weaknesses, which unfortunately, were not very enticing since I was nauseous much of the time.

As time went on, it seemed as if several people each day would ask, "Kevin, have you been losing weight?"

Now when people ask that question, my interpretation is that they're really saying either "Gee, you look great," or "Holy shit, what's wrong with you?"

Their intonations indicated the latter. "Yes, I have lost weight," I would state factually.

"Really, how much are you trying to lose?"

"I'm not really trying to lose weight, I just don't feel like eating much these days," I would reply.

"Why not?" inevitably followed.

"It's called Post-Vasectomy Pain Syndrome. Would you like any other details?"

Usually an awkward silence signaled the end of the conversation if another subject couldn't be determined quickly. Answering questions isn't always easy.

I met with the pain specialist again in advance of the reversal surgery, keeping my pants firmly on this time and watching closely for any safety pins. I wanted to get his advice on the best way to manage the pain that would be part of the reversal surgery and subsequent recovery.

I was surprised when he recommended that I take a weeklong course of narcotics like Codeine or Vicodin, beginning three days before surgery and continuing four days after. He said that opiates used in this manner would often help to break a chronic pain cycle in a person with a sensitized nervous system enough to lessen the pain response from an invasive procedure.

What about the fact that narcotics make me stupid beyond my normal levels? To this inquiry he replied that I would just need to allow for that since my system was "opiate naïve." If I have to be naïve about anything in life, I can't think of a better thing to be naïve about than narcotics. But what exactly does that "opiate naive" term mean?

He responded that for those who don't take narcotics often, their systems tend to react more strongly than those who take narcotics frequently, like an addict. So in this case, naïve is good. For me, maintaining consciousness during this narcotic test run might be an issue, but, what the heck? I was already losing so much time at work; what could another week out hurt?

Chapter Nine

Here, Eat This Root

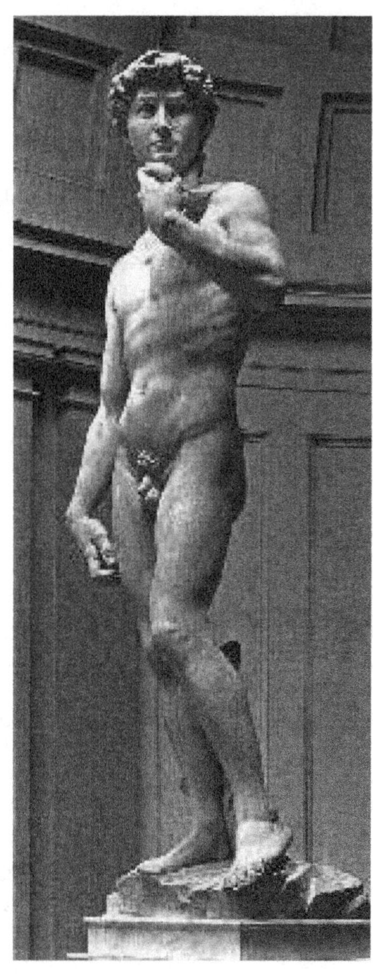

While doing my research for the various treatments I was receiving, I happened to run across a cute little item that seems to summarize the gist of the evolution of medical knowledge. Here it is:

"Doctor, I have an earache."

2000 B. C. "Here, eat this root."

1000 A. D. "That root is heathen. Say this prayer."

1850 A. D. "That prayer is superstition. Drink this potion."

1900 A. D. "That potion is snake oil. Take this pill."

1950 A. D. "That pill is ineffective. Take this antibiotic."

2000 A. D. "That antibiotic doesn't work anymore. Here, eat this root."

And the article went on to discuss soybeans and their use in treatment for various disorders (Prostate Forum, 1997). I took this all as interesting and entertaining at the time, and didn't think much more of it.

While I was healing from the second vasectomy and waiting to be able to be opened up again to do a reversal, my phone rang at home one Sunday afternoon. It was the UCLA urologist and researcher to whom I had been referred. I had briefly spoken with him weeks before when trying to determine if I should proceed with the reversal.

"I can't believe you are calling me at home on a Sunday afternoon," I said, wondering what was up.

After a lengthy discussion of my situation and symptoms, he asked me to come to UCLA the next week and begin a trial of a new medication, at no expense to me. Not to be suspicious or anything, but what gives, and why all of the sudden interest in me?

The medication was called Quercetin, which is a soy-based "bioflavenoid" herb that he thought might be helpful.

"Just try it for thirty days," he said, "and let me know if your pain goes away."

Let me think, thirty days of eating an herb, versus five hours of microsurgery on my testicles. OK, what do I have to lose? I agreed to meet with one of the doctor's associates the next week.

Here, eat this root.

But the curious and, by now, slightly distrusting part of me had a few questions still unanswered. So I called a pharmacist friend of mine. Tell me about Quercetin, and what the heck is a bioflaveniod anyway? Sounds like something out of a biological warfare lab.

He didn't know right off the top, but offered to help me with the research. He did comment however that he had seen many cases come through the pharmacy over the years with prescriptions for medication to combat chronic epididymitis in men who had undergone vasectomies. Sounds curiously familiar, doesn't it?

Bioflavenoids are plant-based substances, many of which have antioxidant characteristics. A class of bioflavenoids, called Isoflavonoids, had been used with some success as hormone balancing therapy in women who experienced loss of their sex drive and other symptoms during menopause, but couldn't take estrogen for a variety of reasons, or preferred not to. Other uses included treatment of skin irritation, coronary heart disease, and anti-carcinogenic applications (Holman, et. al., 1999).

Quercetin in particular was noted for its anti-inflammatory properties. Sounds like pretty good stuff. Then, things became a little clearer. My pharmacist friend found an abstract of a study co-authored by the UCLA doctor and his associate in which Quercetin had recently been used to treat men with chronic pelvic pain, termed category III prostatitis. This category evidently included a number of symptoms, but use of the Quercetin therapy was quite effective in improving symptoms in many cases (Shoskes, et. al., 1999). OK, now I get to be a lab rat. But if it would stop the pain, then "Squeak, squeak, squeak!"

As it turned out, I happened across some information indicating that contracting chronic prostatitis is quite common after vasectomy. The prostatitis encountered following vasectomy can evidently be either infectious or non-infectious but inflammation of the prostate gland is a common element (Prostatitis Web Site). By all accounts, this is a particularly unpleasant and painful situation for a man to encounter. Add chronic prostatitis to the growing list of potential negative results of that simple snip, snip.

I went to UCLA Medical Center at the appointed time and found it to be what you might have expected: large, cold, with lots of long corridors leading nowhere, and orange lines on the floor to lead you where you needed to go. Now I did feel like a rat in a Habitrail.

The Urology Department was in the bowels of the building, as you might expect, and had a distinctly clinical feel to it. When I met the doctor, he had that distinctly clinical feel about him too. We reviewed my case and the records I had brought.

"Go ahead and put on this gown," he said, and left for a moment.

I should have known that I wouldn't just be picking up the pills and leaving. Not to worry, this guy is trying to help me out, right?

This is where the material gets more personal and explicit for a while, so be forewarned. The doctor then proceeded with the now familiar groin and testicular exam in a particularly rigorous manner that left me writhing on the examination table. Couldn't anyone just take my word for it that this stuff hurt like crazy and just let me point to the spots? No, they all had to feel for themselves!

"Please put your leg down," he requested at one point.

You're lucky I haven't kicked you with it, asshole, I thought. Let's switch positions and see if your leg doesn't do a little involuntary movement.

This was just the warm up. He went on to check me for a hernia in this rigorous manner too, stopping only when I finally became light-headed. I was beginning to understand how lab rats feel.

"I want to get a specimen," he said, disappearing again.

Good, I thought, I needed to urinate by then anyway after all that mashing. He returned with assorted cups and vials.

"Turn around and put your forehead on the corner of the exam table," he said.

Uh-oh, I think I'd heard about this once before. I was suddenly reminded of David Letterman's admonition to be suspicious of any doctor who tries to take your temperature with his finger. I later learned that this little venture into my depths was termed a digital rectal exam. "Digit" you might expect to mean "finger" or at most fingers. Actually it felt like he went in up to his elbow.

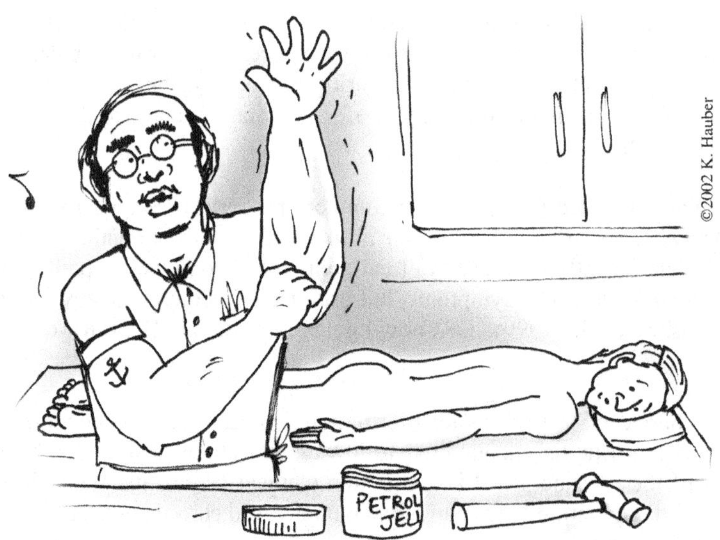

He then endeavored to find out just how much pain I could experience from the inside. I'll spare you all the details, but after what seemed like an eternity of asking "Does that hurt?" as I tried to respond intelligibly, he mashed on various glands from the inside and out. When he finally relented, he stated in a somewhat surprised way, "Gee, I'm usually pretty good at that massage."

"You call that a massage?" I asked incredulously.

Man, I needed to take this guy for lessons by my regular masseuse if he thought what he had just done was a massage. My body eventually stopped spasming, and since he had extracted everything he wanted from me, it was my turn to extract some information from him.

So how many cases of post-vasectomy pain syndrome had he seen?

"A lot," he replied. Evidently, he was a man of few words and many fingers.

Would he care to expand on that?

According to this doctor, many men who had undergone vasectomies would come in for regular exams and he would note inflammation and painful reactions to pressure in their epididymis during the exam. Often, they had previously been treated for epididymitis repeatedly with antibiotics. This was sounding like what my pharmacist friend had told me.

He felt this was often a misdiagnosis, and that the pain and inflammation experienced by many men was not due to infection, but instead to the pressure and rupturing associated with post-vasectomy pain syndrome. This is why the condition was not responsive to antibiotics for permanent resolution in many cases.

The severity of symptoms varied from patient to patient, of course, but the doctor had observed that pattern. He couldn't offer me any further guidance as to whether I would benefit from a reversal at this point (he gave me 50/50 odds) but agreed to get me his lab's results in a few days and discuss them.

Anything else? Yes, he wanted me to ejaculate every three days and track the volume.

"You realize that is a painful proposition at this point, don't you?" I inquired.

"Yes," he responded tersely.

I found it hard to believe that I was expressing resistance to doctor's orders to have an orgasm on a regular basis (Wait 'til I tell my wife about this one)! I hobbled off with my little bottle of free herbs that I had certainly paid for, even if no money changed hands.

In what had been an extremely unpleasant experience since its inception, I had been through several highly memorable and unsavory procedures and events. The abdominal pain and bleeding that put me in the hospital certainly qualified for the list. The pain specialist going after my scrotum with a safety pin was right up there too. The spermatic cord block left an impression, quite literally so, as did the second vasectomy surgery. I now could add this exam to that list of "peak" experiences.

Subsequent discussion with the doctor from UCLA after the lab results came in confirmed that I didn't have gonorrhea or any other infection (thank God for small favors). He also revealed that he had seen one other patient who experienced post-vasectomy pain syndrome to the extent that I did. Finally, someone who isn't saying they've never seen this before.

So how did things work out for that guy? He had to have his epididymis removed. Couldn't anyone give me some good news in this process?

Part II

Fixing "the Fix" (or Trying To)

Chapter Ten

Tied to the Cross

"Isn't it a bit unnerving that doctors call what they do practice?" - George Carlin

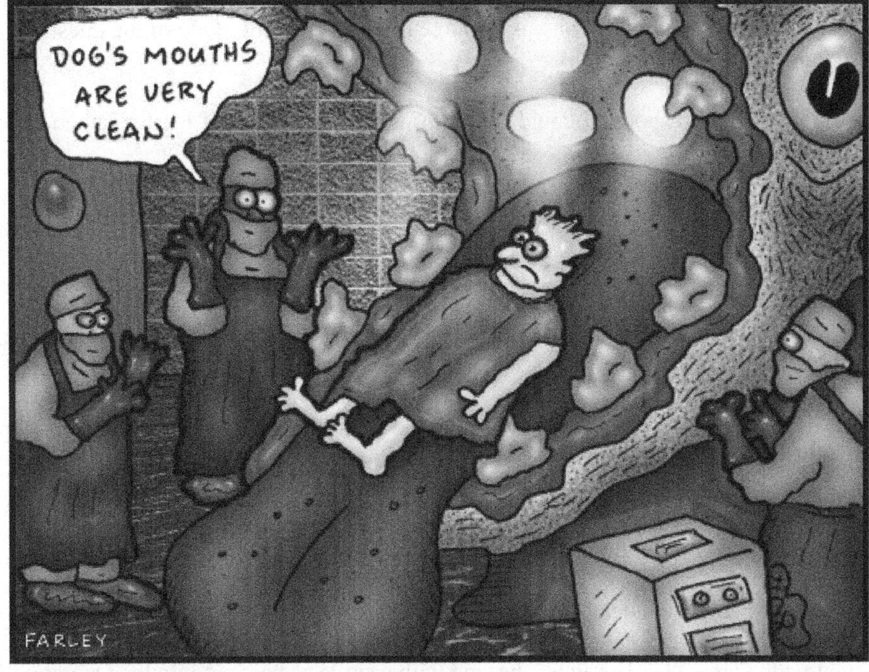

Innovative new equipment designed to make operating rooms more reassuring.

Time was growing short before the appointed date for my next dicing, I mean, surgery. I wanted to talk to another man who had a similar circumstance and experienced a successful resolution. Since all of the stories I had heard were more grim than I cared to focus on, trying to find a positive result seemed like a valid way to bolster my hopes for success. Even my proposed surgeon was unable to give me the odds considering the complications involved.

I heard through the rumor mill about the relative of a neighbor who had a similar experience and a successful reversal. When I mustered the courage to make the "this may sound like an odd question" phone call, I found that yes, this neighbor's brother-in-law had a reversal done, but it was because of a remarriage and a desire to start a new family. In fact, the story went that the brother-in-law didn't have any pain before the reversal, but experienced significant pain for a long time afterwards. This was about as reassuring as the story of the guy with the mole, therefore I decided not to make any more calls. I proceeded on faith alone.

My surgeon's office advised that I pre-register with the hospital, give them my insurance information, pledge my first born as payment if my check were to bounce, and so on. The processing clerk pulled up my file, took all the information imaginable, and then told me to bring my insurance card and a photo ID on the day of surgery.

"Photo ID, what for?" I had to ask, "Do you know what I'm having done? This is not the kind of procedure where you have a friend stand in for you."

It turns out that some inventive people with substance abuse problems had begun stealing other people's insurance information and would go to hospitals to get drugs. To me, this was yet another demonstration of the twisted power of addiction. My interest, however, was in accomplishing this venture with the minimum amount of drugs possible. Was this an unrealistic expectation? Time would tell.

My wife and I made the 200-mile trek to Los Angeles early on the morning of the surgery with the intent of spending as little time away from home as possible. Phil had advised that we stay at a nearby hotel the night after surgery just in case something was to go wrong. This, besides the prospect of a four-or five-hour car ride after spending four or five hours on the operating table, probably wouldn't have been much fun anyway. I had no idea how right he was.

The paperwork I had to complete upon arrival was a source of entertainment. One of the questions was, "Who do you rely on for emotional support?"

"God" was the most appropriate response I could come up with. I hoped for at least a cameo appearance during surgery.

"Is there anything about being in the hospital that makes you anxious?" was the next question.

Well, let's see....

Honesty overcame me again, and I wrote "Yes, having my testicles cut on for four or five hours today makes me a wee bit anxious."

We finished the rest of the paperwork, making our way to the room that was to be my launching and landing pad for this flight. From there I was wheeled to the elevator and given a moment to express my love to my wife one last time before being taken upstairs to the operating room.

I waited outside as several guys busied themselves cleaning the operating room in advance of my surgery. As this was going on I heard an ominous thump, thump, thump, emanating from the stereo in the OR. Rap music! Anything but rap music! This could be a very long surgery indeed.

The surgical assistant walked by. "Hi, I'm Pete," he said with a smile as he went into the Operating Room.

A charming redheaded nurse came on the scene, introducing herself as Dorene.

Next entered the anesthesiologist who said he preferred to be called Norm. Great! Everybody's on a first name basis. I always like a nice, intimate setting for this kind of exposure!

Norm set up my I.V. and asked what I wanted in the way of anesthesia. An epidural would be fine, but he should know that the last one I had took a while to set in. Fine, and for sedation?

"No sedation, thank you," I replied.

"Do you realize what you are saying?" Norm inquired.

I assured him that I preferred to be a conscious participant in the process. After all, I had tried to be as conscious as I could all the way along and my trust level was not that high. Besides, general anesthesia had always made me feel awful afterwards. Dorene walked by again inquiring of Norm as to what type of sedation to pull and have ready.

"None, this guy just wants a bullet to bite," he responded. Believe me, I'm not that brave.

Phil came to see me and go over the surgical consent form. We confirmed our understsnding that this little venture had no guarantees and was as much exploratory in nature as it was repair-oriented. I might feel better, or the same, or it could make my pain worse.

"Just do your best, Phil. You know what you're doing," I told him, appreciating his honesty.

It was one of those "speak now or forever hold your pieces" moments.

They wheeled me to what looked like a very narrow operating table, and I was instructed to roll up on to my side as Norm began the epidural. This one was much less pleasant than the last, and in fact caused my left leg and hip to cramp. Norm placed the catheter in my spine so he could keep me in medicated bliss as long as necessary.

I was then rolled onto my back. This table was a little narrow, as it had looked. Not to worry, the OR crew added two wings to the table making it into the form of a cross. My arms and legs were tied to this crucifix form. With Easter being just a few days away, I hadn't anticipated celebrating it in this manner.

Was this how it was going to end?

Time for a prayer: "Please God, don't let my life end this way; tied to a cross, and forced to listen to rap music!"

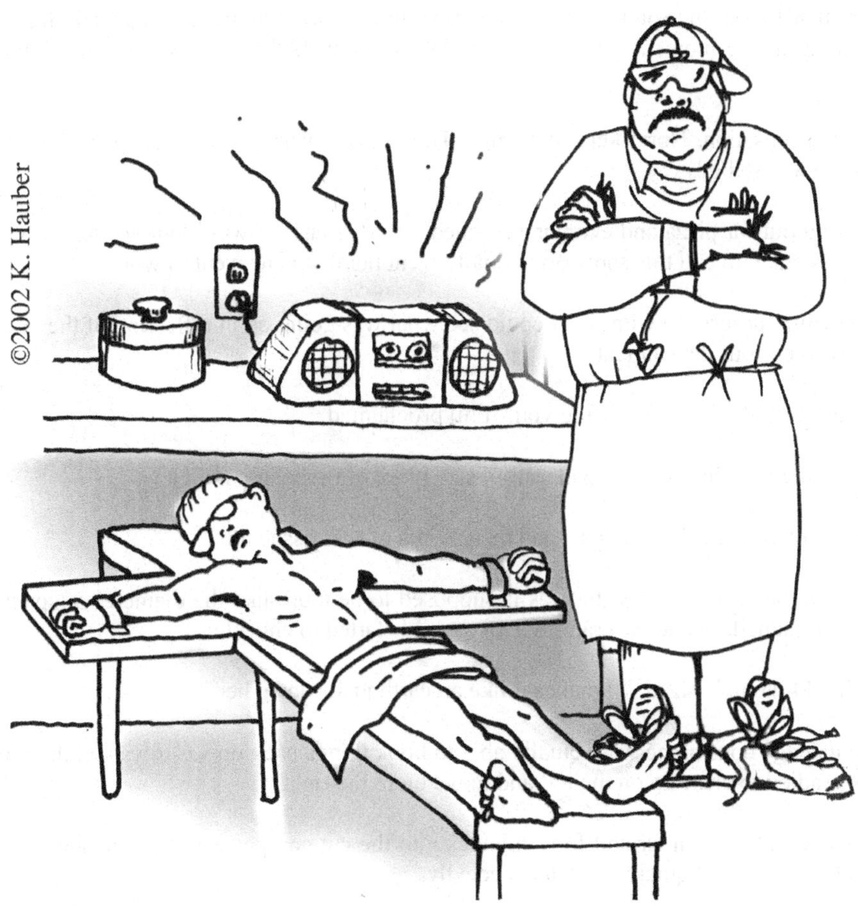

Norm and I had a chance to talk a little to compare musical preferences. We decided to make a preemptive strike with some cool jazz while the rap fans weren't looking. Thank goodness! Somehow music made being strapped down more tolerable, even without sedation.

This of course was the time that my cheek began to itch. I instinctively tried to raise a hand to scratch the itch. Oops, tied down. I tried every meditative technique I knew, but after several minutes, I succumbed.

"Norm, need a little help here!" I begged. It was a good thing that Norm and I were buds by now, because he grabbed a piece of gauze and started scratching furiously.

"A little to the left," I guided "...yeah, right there! Great, thanks Norm." This was all part of the process of waiting for my honorary saddle block to kick in. After a few minutes, Phil came into the OR.

"Can you feel that?" he asked as he poked around various parts of my lower anatomy.

"Sure can," I replied, "Thank you for not cutting yet."

Phil went back to the doctor's lounge to return calls, buy stocks, or perhaps order a Mercedes with the money this was going to cost me, or whatever doctors do in those lounges. All the while, Norm filled me with more Lidocaine. On the next trip Phil removed the stitch from the last vasectomy that hadn't fallen out yet after two and a half months.

"Looks like you tend to throw stitches," he commented.

I wasn't sure that I liked the sound of that but wasn't in a position to argue or question this opinion. Plus, I was unable to throw anything at the moment given my position. I could think of many other more pleasant reasons to be strapped down.

Since I still had sensation, Norm kept injecting. This process was repeated for over an hour, as more and more lidocaine found its way into my body.

I offered to send out for pizza and everyone laughed. They thought I was kidding. Actually, I was starving. Just at the point that Phil was ready to call this show off, I finally went numb and he went to work.

It was a fascinating process to witness. I could see what was going on in reflection of the operating light. I found myself able to watch with curious detachment.

"Here's at least part of what was hurting you," Phil proclaimed.

"Show me," I asked, as Phil brought a macaroni size piece of tissue into my view.

"This is a piece of your vas," he stated, "and there's lots of scar tissue too."

Continuing with the pasta analogy, the vas is supposed to be more like the diameter of spaghetti. This piece was obviously significantly inflamed. Someone cracked a joke, and I started to chuckle.

"Don't laugh!" Phil emphasized, "It makes it like an earthquake down here!"

After all the damage control, he was actually able to hook things back up vas to vas on the left, which I knew was a good sign. He then readied to close up on the left and move on to the right.

We were approximately an hour and forty minutes into the cut and paste part of the show. This turned out to be the time that the anesthesia wore off quickly and unexpectedly.

"Phil, I'm starting to feel some cord pain on the left," I stated while breathing calmly into the pain. The pain rapidly intensified.

"Uh, Phil, now I'm feeling a lot of pain on the left," I updated a few moments later.

I could see in the light's reflection that he was attempting to put the pieces of my testicle back in the scrotum where they belonged. This was getting really uncomfortable, and I mean *really* uncomfortable. I might need that bullet after all, if only to put me out of my misery.

Phil turned to Norm. "This is no place to stop! Can we do something about this?"

"I've already got three times the normal amount in him," Norm exclaimed, "I've never seen this happen before."

Not that old refrain again!

Later, I was to find out that I had received three bottles of lidocaine in the process, which is far more than is normally needed, along with other medication that was intended to lengthen the effect. For whatever reason, all this medication was not having the intended result and I was burning through it in a hurry.

We all agreed that I needed a little sedation in the IV, which turned into a lot of sedation quickly. This put me to sleep for the rest of what would be a four-and-a-half hour surgery.

The last memory I have of the surgery was Dorene looking me in the eyes and saying in a comforting way, "It's all right, we're going to take good care of you."

For whatever reason, I believed her. At that moment, I let go of my desire for conscious participation and just took the ride that all those substances were taking me on. I trusted that I was in good hands.

As I awoke, the recovery room attendant watched me nervously. I tried to focus on him and the room just spun.

When my wife walked in. He gave her a look like, "What kind of horse are you married to?"

Evidently. one that hurt a lot.

He explained to her that he had to administer six times the normal amount of pain medication during recovery to keep me comfortable. Actually, I'm not sure I would characterize it as comfortable. Probably more like stupefied so that I didn't feel like I'd just been horse-kicked in the groin. I started to throw up but there was not much left in me by then.

Man, that was lousy. If I had known it was going to hurt this much beforehand I would have asked for some kind of enhancements. After all, shouldn't you end up better off than when you started?

My wife's friend, who also happened to have been the maid of honor at our wedding, spent the day with Kristen while I was in surgery, and saw me in recovery. I must have been speaking in tongues.

The next day she teased me, "You're funny when you're stoned."

I still believe I'd make the world's worst junkie, given the fact I can't stand needles and don't tolerate medications well, but I'm glad to have been of some entertainment value.

Phil came into recovery and had a concerned look on his face. The "just-been-kicked" sensation took a long time to go away, as did the nausea from all the drugs. Phil convinced me to stay the night in the hospital to be near all that "good pain medication" since the surgery had been more extensive than expected. The surgery had turned out to be more of a reconstruction than a reversal. He told us that he'd never seen so much scar tissue from a simple vasectomy before and was sending the removed tissues to get a pathology report. He had been able to hook up both sides vas to vas, which improved the odds of the reversal working.

Now all I needed to do was take it easy and not have any scar tissue reform. He and the whole operating room crew had really done a great job under what must have been rather unusual circumstances, and I thanked him profusely. He said he would come by and see me first thing in the morning.

When I got up the courage, I took a look at what had been done. Wow, I was going to have some award winning scars from this one. I should have had that zipper installed while I had the chance. This wasn't even something I could show off at parties; most parties that is. I wondered what Phil's signature was on his work, kind of like the Mark of Zoro. You just know all surgeons must pride themselves on that kind of stuff.

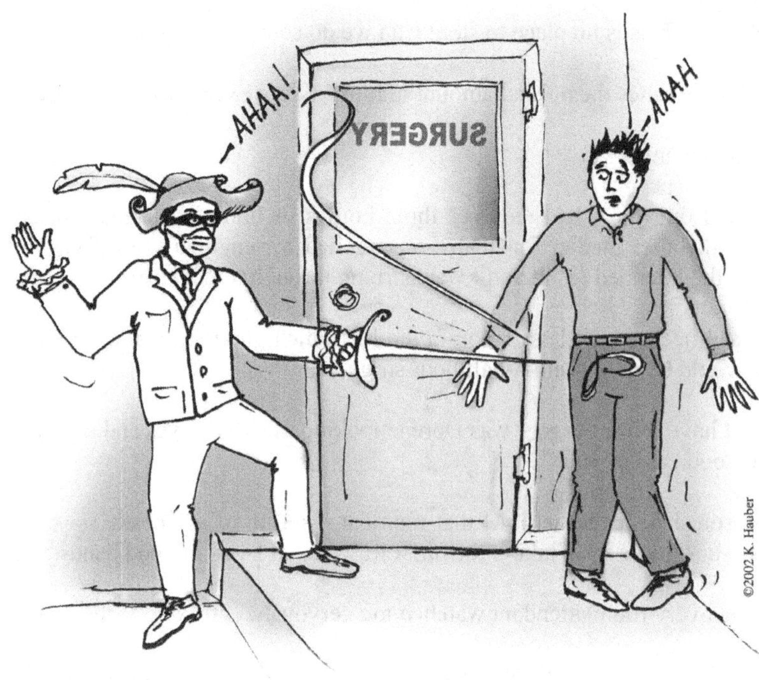

I was moved to a double room with a roommate who was a very congenial 75-year-old gentleman named Rocky. He gave me the "So what are you in for?" line of questioning, and I told him, not being in a mood to mince words. Later, when I moved to get out of bed and go to the bathroom, he got a glimpse of what had been done and visibly cringed. Here's what Rocky saw (looks like I was ready to go out and play basketball, doesn't it?):

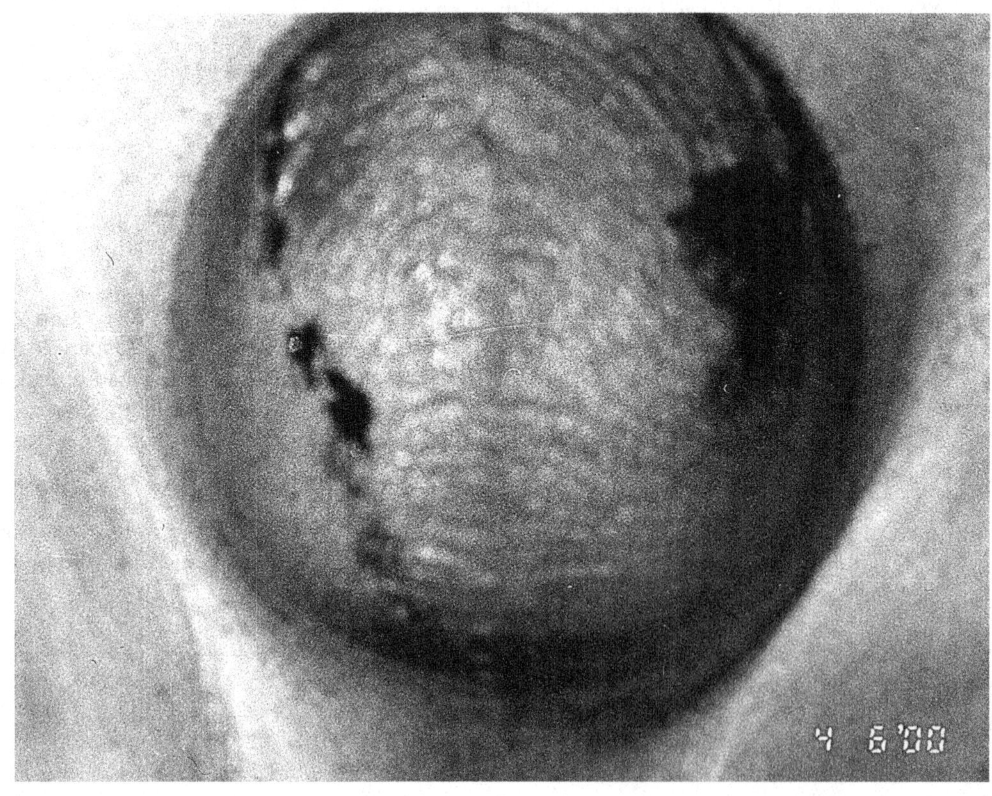

In Rocky's opinion, what I had just gone through made the polyp he was having removed from his colon the next day seem like a walk in the park. I'm not sure that I would want to choose one over the other, but I can attest to the testicular surgery being far less than fun.

Later in the evening, it turned out that Rocky's doctor had kinda-sorta overlooked telling him that the polyp he was having removed was cancerous. Rocky found that out from a nurse in the course of going over paperwork. This was quite upsetting to him, understandably, and I listened off and on most of the night while several doctors tried to backpedal and reassure him that it was no big deal.

This seemed like a lot to throw on a guy to process less than 24 hours before his surgery. Rocky didn't have any family in the area, and this whole scene was very distressing for him. My heart went out to him, even with what I was dealing with at the time, and I tried to be the best comfort I could and listen.

"Good pain medication" turned out to be morphine, which once again gave me a roaring headache. After a night of minimal rest, I was more than ready to go home. Phil came by to check on me and write my release papers at ten minutes after six in the morning.

"How do you feel?" he asked.

"Other than feeling like a truck has run over my genitals? Okay, I guess."

Thankfully, that was good enough to get my release papers signed.

"Please make bail and spring me, honey," I begged of Kristen a moment later over the phone.

Wisely expecting this kind of response, she had awakened an hour earlier and was ready to come get me.

"Have I mentioned that you're wonderful and I love you?" I asked her.

"Not lately, but you can keep reminding me," she said.

I practically made a wheelchair race of getting out the door. I believe Keith was the name of the guy who guided me to the exit.

"Being in the hospital will sure give you a spiritual experience," he commented.

"And gets you in touch with your mortality, too," I observed, knowing I'd had enough of the experience to last a lifetime.

By 7 a.m., we were on the road. I may have been heavily medicated, but at least I was on my way home. After reaching home four hours later and resting for a while, I decided that getting showered up would probably be a welcome sensation. As I was getting out of the shower, Kristen excitedly brought me the phone.

"Phil's on the phone," she said, and thrust the receiver into my dripping wet hand.

According to Phil, the pathology report had come back, and showed that not only were there large granulomas that he had removed, but within the scar tissue on each side were neuromas that had been extracted. Normally, I don't like hearing that there was something in my body that ends in "oma."

"This was a good thing that you found these things and now they are out, right Phil?" I confirmed.

Absolutely, this was probably the source of quite a bit of the pain according to him. That explained a lot, because even though I was still in a lot of pain, I wasn't having as much shooting pain as before. Phil and I wished each other well, and agreed to talk the next week.

Now how does a healthy guy who goes in for a routine vasectomy end up with neuromas on each side? This question kept running through my mind as I resolved to get a copy of the surgery and pathology reports. I was able to do so the following Monday. Meanwhile, I found out what a bliss-filled, drifting lifestyle one can lead on Vicodin. When I did venture out on my short leash while being chauffeured by my bride, friends and acquaintances would typically see me dressed in very loose shorts and a Hawaiian shirt.

"Gee Kevin, looks like you're on vacation," they would say.

"That's Vicodin, not vacation," I would reply, receiving somewhat puzzled looks.

My appetite was returning, and even if I couldn't get up and walk around very well, at least I could eat. This was good, because a number of family friends banded together to make dinners for us over the following week. All of a sudden it seemed like I had eight to ten Jewish mothers. It was one of those experiences that makes you feel loved, and gives a sense of connection to others that you might have thought died out several generations ago.

During the next week, when I wasn't horizontal, which was not very often, I began examining the surgery and pathology reports, asking some pointed questions of my doctors. How did I wind up with "traumatic neuromas" on both sides at the vasectomy sites if there was nothing exceptionally injurious that had occurred during the original vasectomy? After all, trauma relates to injury, doesn't it, and neuromas form around injured nerves, right?

No one seemed to have a good answer for me. And why did the epidural become ineffective so quickly? Was the pain level just too intense? No good answers here, either. Hmm, it seemed as though I needed to widen the search.

Phil was excellent at calling to check on how I was doing. Since I was still hurting quite a bit and having to use painkillers at regular intervals now, I asked how long this might go on.

"People are beginning to think I've lost brain cells because of this surgery since I'm so drifty from the drugs, Phil," I said. "I know all the old wisdom about where a man's brain really is, but I hate to be proving that right."

He tried to reassure me, "The inflammation should start going down when we can get you ejaculating again."

I strained to remember what sex without pain might be like. "Didn't your post surgical instructions say no ejaculating for at least a month, so as not to blow up all your good work?" I inquired.

Yes, that was right. It was feeling like a long recovery already. I guess the "Free the Imprisoned Sperm" movement would have to wait. At least he was being honest with me. But as good as he was, I doubt he could have prepared me for what was ahead.

Chapter Eleven

I've Got a Lovely Pair of Coconuts

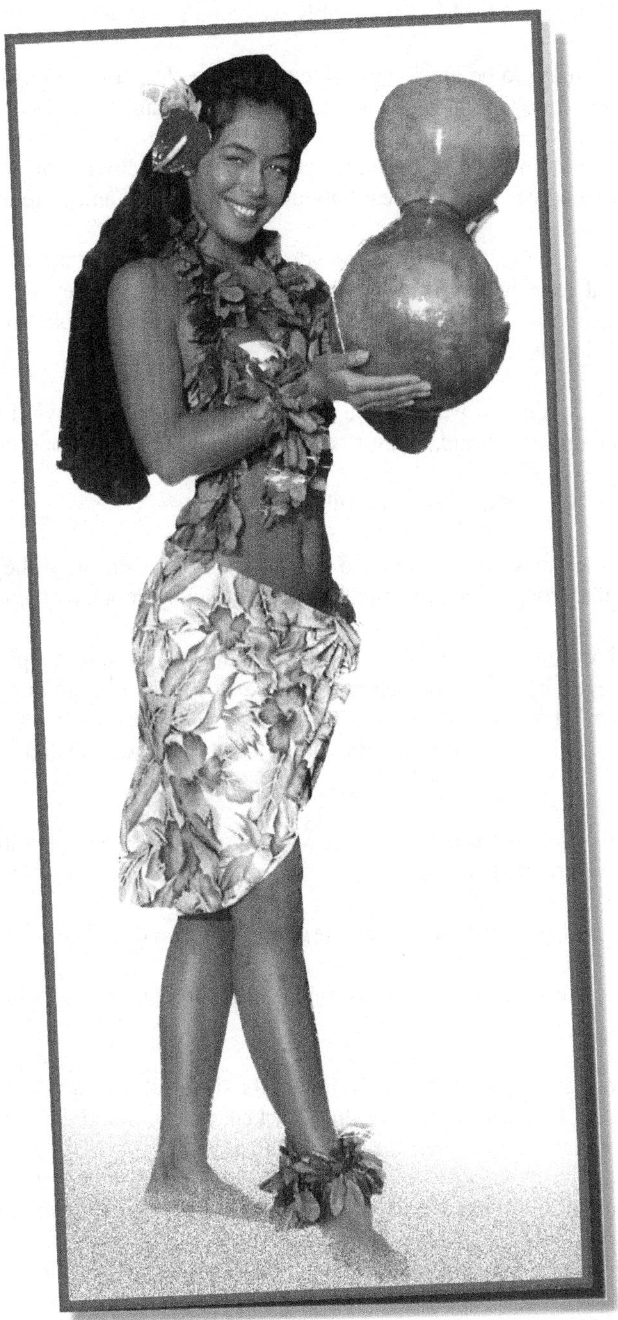

Here's one of the nurses from my reconstructive surgery (I wish)!

Actually, this was a get-well card sent to me by a friend who also had complications after his vasectomy.

Insightful friend, huh?

Have you ever noticed that when you *have* to lie around and relax for any reason, you find it extremely difficult to do so? This was surely the case for me, and it went on for weeks. Generally, I don't sit still for long. There seems to have always been a fair amount of inertia in my life. I'm sure this is not an experience unique to me.

Soon Kristen began to hide the catalogues, the phone, the computer, and whatever else I might use to get into mischief. And I found that I could get into mischief remarkably well, and used the medication as an excuse.

"Is this what retirement is going to be like?" my bride asked one day, "Because if it is, I don't know if I can stand it." It appeared as though retirement for us might be accompanied by significant amounts of counseling.

During this time another friend of mine was going in to have his vasectomy done at the same urology group I had originally gone to. He and his wife had watched and heard about my experience, and were quite concerned.

Not feeling fully justified in saying, "For God's sake don't do it!" I tried to take the middle path and suggest that if they wanted to proceed, that he at least have an open-ended procedure done. They went ahead with the consultation, primarily because they had just gotten through another pregnancy and now had enough kids to fill a Chevy Suburban. I sensed there was a certain urgency in this for them.

When they brought up the subject of wanting the open-ended procedure to avoid the possibility of chronic pain, the doctor (a partner of my original urologist) said, "Don't you worry about it; that's a one-in-a-million problem."

The wife responded, "But I know that one-in-a-million person."

"Oh", the doctor said, and reluctantly agreed to do the procedure the way they asked. It seemed as if the disclosure practices in that particular group of doctors might not have changed much by then.

By the time four weeks had passed since my reconstructive surgery, some of the post-surgery pain finally began to subside. This was replaced, however, by a stinging sensation that took the lead in the discomfort hit parade accompanied by a new variety of swelling. I called my new local urologist with whom I had previously consulted and he saw me that day. I inquired as to why I was swollen up like I was growing a third and fourth testicle, and why I was extra tender to boot.

He did some tests and observed that I had developed what turned out to be Staph infections at the surgery sites on both sides. "Scrotal Abscesses," he termed them.

Special. I told him that I was scheduled to see my surgeon again two days later.

"Stay on some antibiotics in the meantime," he advised, "your surgeon will probably need to lance these infections and let them drain."

My radiologist friend was good enough to redo my MRIs since all this was going on, and he noted swelling, cellulitis (infection), and multiple hydroceles, which are fluid pockets that can, and did, cause lots of discomfort. Here I was again, experiencing other potential maladies first hand. Special, again.

I FAXed all this information to Phil in advance of my appointment. He called me that night unexpectedly.

"Please tell me that the infections are superficial and not deep inside," he implored.

"Why, Phil?" I questioned.

"Because if the infections are deep I'm going to have you checked back into the hospital, put on intravenous antibiotics, and then fillet you open to get the infection out," he replied.

Surgeons, always wanting to cut! This guy certainly had a way with words that made an impression.

"Let's go with superficial for now and you can see the films for yourself the day after tomorrow," I responded hopefully, not wanting to be treated like prime rib once again, or maybe more accurately like Rocky Mountain Oysters.

I tried to reassure Phil that, other than this medical situation, I generally led a charmed life, and I didn't hope to have all this medical attention on a permanent basis. I'm not sure he believed me. So I began mentally preparing myself to have my scrotum cut on again for the fourth time, to go along with the other associated invasions in the region. Just call me lucky I guess.

Most swelling after scrotal surgery occurs due to infection such as I experienced, or due to bleeding under the skin (hematoma) which has nowhere to escape, and gives that eggplant-like appearance. Other problems associated with vasectomy can result in infections or infection-like symptoms. Randall, et. al., (1983) found an overall post-vasectomy infection rate of 32.9% in their study. That seems a lot higher than 2-3% doesn't it?

Infectious epididymitis after vasectomy is a common problem and can be quite persistent and painful, as I'm sure you have gathered by now. Also, "many patients report that their chronic prostatitis problems began after they had a vasectomy (Prostatitis Web Site/Vasectomy Page)." One patient noted "I've been suffering with pain and a 'non-bacterial' prostatitis diagnosis for five years now, following a painful vasectomy." It is interesting to note that recent theories about chronic prostatitis include autoimmune causes of this consistent and painful malady. You will learn a great deal more about vasectomy and autoimmune reactions shortly, but you can find an interesting article on the subject in the references section by Gowers from the LATimes.com web site.

Doctors at the Mayo Clinic reported on several serious infections in vasectomy patients. In particular, the report detailed the case of a man who developed a Staph infection after his vasectomy. Unlike me, though, his Staph infection settled in his heart, requiring a seven-week series of antibiotics, and a subsequent mitral valve reconstruction surgery performed for "severe mitral regurgitation. The present case further supports an association between vasectomy and S. lugdunensis endocarditis" (Fervenza, et. al., 1999). Yuk! I'm not even sure what all those words mean, but still, yuk! Other research has examined the relationship between vasectomy and other cardiovascular diseases, namely myocardial infarction, a.k.a. heart attack (Chi, et. al., 1990).

The heart is not the only area where serious infections can set in. A friend of the family had a recurrent infection develop in one of his testicles following his vasectomy. It became so bad that the testicle had to be removed. This had major hormonal repercussions for him, which led to lots of physical and mental stress. It has taken years for him to begin to unwind these effects.

Of an even more serious nature is the occurrence of gangrene following vasectomy, which has been reported several times in medical literature. This is typically termed Fourier's gangrene, and is particularly difficult to treat, often requiring that "filleting open" approach as Phil mentioned, and can be deadly. Infections of this nature are treated "aggressively" according to the literature available on the subject.

Here's an example: "A 35-year-old male with no remarkable previous history, who underwent vasectomy…developed a clinical picture compatible with Fournier's gangrene 7-8 days later. The patient required wide, aggressive surgical debridement on several occasions with broad-spectrum antibiotic coverage. After a long stay at the hospital, the patient was finally discharged and referred to another hospital for plastic surgery (de Diego Rodriguez, et. al., 2000)." Bigger yuk!

Without getting too gory, what kind of "aggressive surgical debridement" do you think would necessitate a lengthy hospital stay followed by plastic surgery? Do you think he left the hospital with the same number of parts he went in with? I was beginning to feel lucky that I only ended up with Staph infections that could be treated with antibiotics and drained, despite how uncomfortable they were.

There's more. Most sources will claim that no one has ever died from a vasectomy. Those who make this claim must have missed this article published in the Journal of Urology: "A case is presented of a healthy young man who had Fournier's gangrene after standard bilateral vasectomy. Despite maximal treatment, including extensive necrectomy [i.e. removal of dead tissues: I wonder what tissues were dying with scrotal gangrene?] and broad-spectrum antibiotics, this complication was lethal (Viddeleer, et. al., 1992)." No wonder surgeons are so anxious to find ways to minimize chances of infection, even in "simple" procedures like a vasectomy.

Seven other men died from vasectomy over a 15-month period in a population sampling reported by Grimes, et. al., (1982). Three of those deaths were attributable to the same surgeon on the same day. In the surgical world that is what is known as a bad day.

While most sources claim no deaths, or exceedingly low death rates due to the procedure, "a report from the 1971 Family Welfare Festival [another vasectomy party!] in India indicated a death-to-case rate of 8.1 deaths/100,000 vasectomies...." Another report from Bangladesh "found a death-to-case rate of 31.1[/100,000]" (Grimes, et. al., 1982).

Fortunately, most infections are not so severe, but many are still preventable. Do you remember that I mentioned that my urologist didn't do any exams or tests before my first vasectomy? This lack of testing is actually quite common. Of course, there are ways to avoid these types of problematic infections if a few basic checks are performed.

Research has shown that most infections which become evident after vasectomy procedures were actually present beforehand, and were somehow exacerbated by the procedure and its inherent trauma on the body. Doctors who perform simple checks beforehand like urinalysis and semen analysis have been able to substantially lower the incidence of post-vasectomy infections with antibiotic treatment before surgery (Sharma, et. al., 1983). But doctors would have to be willing to take the time and effort for these simple checks, wouldn't they? Insurance companies would have to be wiling to foot the bill. This seems to be as much of a challenge as fighting the actual infections.

Chapter Twelve

**All the Kings Horses and All the Kings Men,
Couldn't Put Humpty-Dumpty Back Together Again**

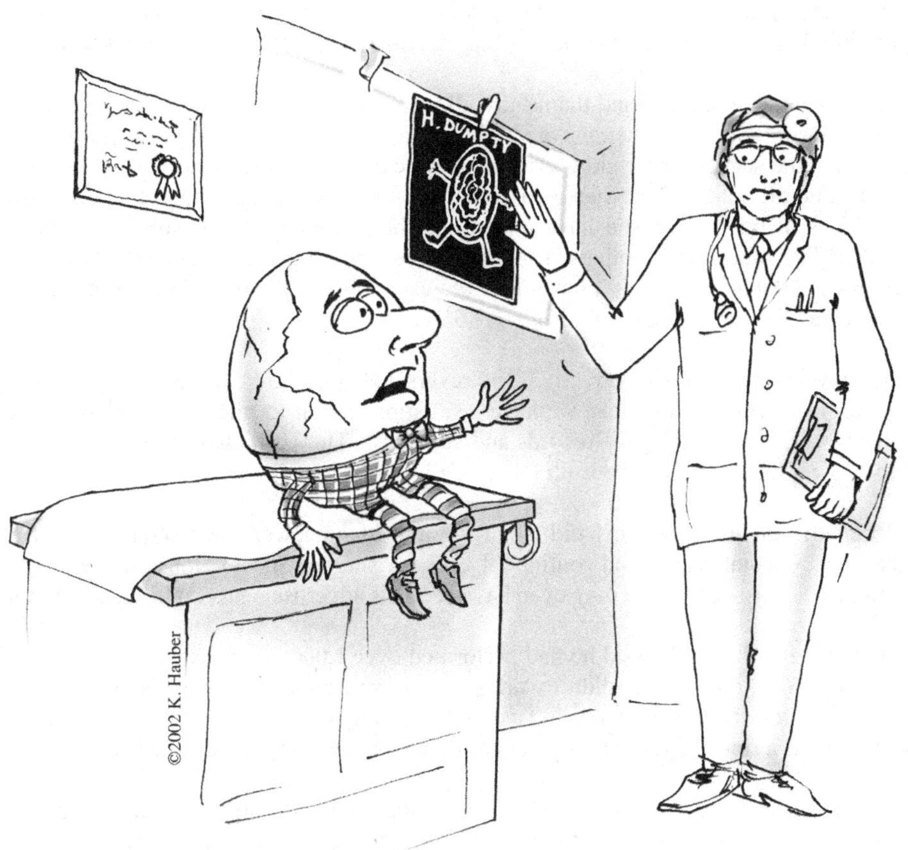

Ever since that fall, Doc, I just feel all scrambled inside.

"As surgeons we are always on shaky ground when we advocate additional surgery that is obviously of direct monetary benefit to us without first demonstrating that it benefits the patient" (Kevin R. Loughlin, M.D., 1999).

There is a very popular concept among men who have had vasectomies and their partners that if they ever want to have children again, they can just have a surgical reversal performed. It's kind of like taking a trip to the body shop to get the old car shined up like new. In fact, the demand for vasectomy reversals is increasing dramatically (Witt, et. al., 1994). However, studies report between 30% and 80% of men who seek vasectomy reversal to restore fertility are still unable to father children afterward (Simon, et. al., 1998). Sounds like another area that might deserve looking into, doesn't it?

This proposition of vasectomy reversal can be more complicated (and more expensive) than one might think. Let's look at the complicated part first, and talk about expense later. "There is confusion about the reversibility of the procedure" (Sandlow, et. al., 2001). These researchers determined that the confusion was probably due to the way pre-vasectomy counseling about the permanence of the procedure was done. I recall this as being the biggest emphasis in the pre-vasectomy counseling I received, and the news of the commonplace occurrence of reversals came as a surprise to me.

There are numerous reasons that men seek vasectomy reversals. Chronic pain after vasectomy such as I experienced is just one of them. "The most common motive that leads patients to request vasovasostomy is a remarriage. Less common reasons include loss of children, change of heart in a patient with no proven fertility, and rarely[?], chronic testicular pain or concern about the adverse effects of vasectomy, most commonly atherosclerosis" (Kessler, 1982).

"Caveat Emptor" (Let the buyer beware) applies in this area of vasectomy reversals. It is important who you choose to have do a reversal, the technique they use, and the experience they have. Even being informed in this area, there can still be unanticipated difficulties. This is well demonstrated by the story of Dr. David G. Williams who offered this account in his October, 2002, issue of *Alternatives*: "I make a very concerted effort to steer clear of conventional medical practices, if at all possible [I like this doctor's attitude already!]. Guinea pigs in that field don't seem to fare too well....

"I've had four surgeries in my life and thankfully all were elective. My first surgery was a vasectomy about five years ago. The other three surgeries were attempts at vasectomy reversals. I say attempts because they were all failures.... When I had the vasectomy, the standard procedure was to simply cut the vas deferens (the 'tube' leading from the testicles to the prostate gland) and tie off both ends. When a vasectomy is performed, little, if any, thought is given to reconnecting the vas. Just like millions of other men who have undergone the procedure, I was sure at the time that I didn't want additional children. And like thousands of others, I later changed my mind. If the surgeon had known that there was a chance I would want more children, he wouldn't have done the vasectomy in the first place, or at least maybe it would have been done with greater care. But, as they say, 'hindsight is 20/20.'

"My vasectomy was actually done correctly. The reversal attempts are another story. As in many other areas of medicine, when it comes to vasectomy reversals, we have a situation similar to 'the fox guarding the hen house.' Doctors who do reversal procedures generate their own records and statistics. They can claim to have whatever success rate they want, and it's hard to know if they're telling the truth [!].

"When I decided to do the reversal, I did a fair amount of homework, but obviously not enough. I honestly thought the procedure was uncomplicated and routine. I chose a surgeon in the Houston area that specializes only in reversals, and even guarantees his work. You may even have seen his advertisements on billboards around the country.

"In my first meeting with him, he said he had performed over 1,000 reversals, and was so confident that he could guarantee his success rate. Well, it obviously didn't work the first go-around. Not only was it a huge disappointment (and pain in the groin), I can tell you that a vasectomy is far less expensive than trying to reverse the procedure. The money-back guarantee, by the way, is a rip-off structured so that hardly anyone gets his money back.

"Contrary to what I read and was told, reversing vasectomies isn't routine. It requires a great deal of skill and 'microsurgery' because the vas is such a small tube. Unfortunately, and since there's no one to regulate the doctor's advertising, everyone performing this procedure claims to perform true microsurgery and have extraordinary skill in this area. It was a year later before I found out just how untrue these claims were and just how botched my surgery was....

"Many surgeons doing vasectomy reversals 'cherry pick' the individuals they'll operate on, and then deem the procedure a success if sperm passes through the reattached vas. Tricks like these allow them to claim higher 'success rates.' It's not uncommon, however, for blockages to occur shortly thereafter from swelling, adhesions, scar tissue, poor surgical procedures resulting in inadequate circulation to the area, and a dozen other reasons. All of that's irrelevant to the doctor. Even if such a blockage occurs, the doctor can still consider the operation a 'success.' That's how surgeons can make money-back guarantees and never have to refund money, even though the surgery is a total failure from the patient's point of view."

Dr. Williams eventually found a surgeon in Australia who pioneered the vasectomy reversal technique and was willing to perform the reversal for a third time. "As he does with all his surgeries, he [Professor Owen, the operating surgeon] videotaped the procedure. Two days after the surgery, we reviewed the tape. That's when I saw just how crude my prior 'microsurgical' procedures were. One re-attachment was no longer even together. Under magnification from Professor Owen's microscope, the stitching from the other surgeon looked like it was sewn with rope and very poorly done.... The prior reversal surgeries had damaged the small tubules so badly the damaged portions had to be removed prior to an attempt at reattachment. There wasn't much hope from the start, and, unfortunately, the operation wasn't successful."

Even those in the medical field are not immune to this kind of pain and heartbreak. Unfortunately, like Dr. Williams, many men will find a reversal more difficult as time goes on after their vasectomy.

Dr. Edward Shapiro, who pioneered the open-ended vasectomy technique, is quoted as stating, "The success rate of reversal after standard vasectomy decreases with time because the rise in pressure produces leaks of sperm in the epididymis resulting in granulomas that obstruct it so that no sperm reaches the vas" (Reda, undated). Other early observations confirm similar suspicions regarding vasectomy reversal: "A 40% to 50% vasovasostomy failure rate in formerly fertile males implies that normal physiologic characteristics of one or more components of the male reproductive tract have been altered" (Brickel, et. al., 1982).

That makes sense. But how and why does this occur? "Silber (1979), Lee (1986), and Belker (1991) are agreed that the rate of successful reversal decreases with time after vasectomy, particularly more than 9-10 years, presumably due to increased epididymal granuloma formation and obstruction of the epididymal duct in the longer term" (McDonald, 1996).

According to some sources, if an electric needle was used to perform the original vasectomy procedure, like the cauterizing done during my procedure, a reversal also tends to be more difficult. Perhaps this is one reason why my original urologist felt that I needed "the best hands in the business" for my reversal. Another factor from the original vasectomy surgery that will have a bearing on the outcome of reversal is how much of the vas remnant is intact. Witt, et. al., (1994) found that if the vas remnant was shorter than 2.7 cm., the chances of the sperm being present in the vas at the time of reversal fell from 94% to 15%. That's a big drop. These researchers recommended trying to measure the vassal remnant *before* reversal surgery to inform the patients of the likelihood of success. I have to wonder how often this recommendation is followed by surgeons.

Remember the regular and deluxe versions of a reversal that were previously mentioned? Most doctors use sutures finer than hair to tie the tubes back together. Some doctors are experimenting with special glues for this purpose. Here's a diagram of the "regular" version that will be attempted first by a surgeon in trying to hook the plumbing back up:

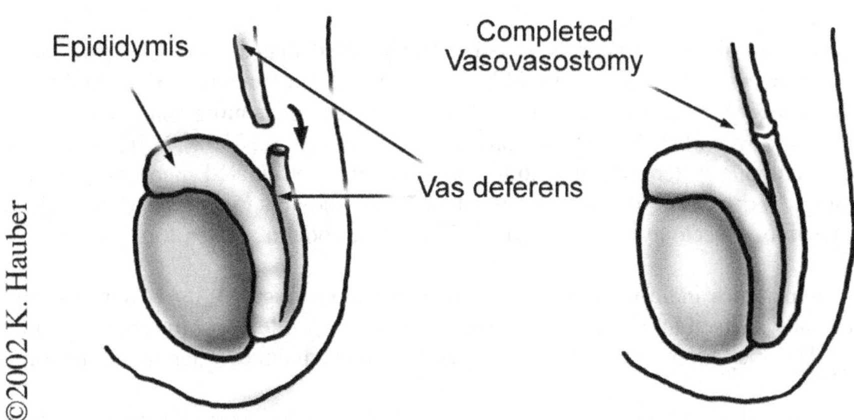

Sometimes this works, sometimes it doesn't. Do you remember the previous discussion about the congestion and rupturing that often occurs in the epididymis after vasectomy? This is quite common and may or may not cause pain, but will often have an effect on the success of vasectomy reversal. Pardanani, et. al., (1976) characterized the effects in this way: "It was shown in a large majority of cases the epididymides showed gross changes which could not be considered normal. It is believed that the process of sperm maturation may not proceed normally in these diseased epididymides.... This may explain the reported disparity between the surgical success rates (reappearance of spermatozoa in the ejaculates) and the physiologic success rates (occurrence of pregnancy) following vas anastomosis operations."

According to Harvey Simon, M.D., et. al., (1998), "If the sperm count does not recover within a reasonable period after vasovasostomy, epididymal damage may be responsible, requiring microsurgical bypass (vasoepididymostomy) of the obstruction. In the past, vasectomy reversal failed about three-quarters of the time because secondary blockages in the epididymis (which is 1/300th of an inch wide with a wall thickness of 1/1000th of an inch) could not be repaired using standard surgical procedures. This technique requires such precision and expertise that a surgeon who specializes in microsurgery should be sought if a first reversal procedure fails because of epididymal damage. Success rates are higher for repairing obstructions closer to the testicles because the epididymis is wider in this area."

If the surgeon cannot get enough sperm out of the vas after opening the testicular end because of scarring or congestion in the epididymis or the vas, the upper end of the vas will have to be connected directly to the epididymis. This procedure is much more involved (more expensive, too) and has a lower success rate. This can be due to a more difficult connection by the nature of the procedure, or to less mature sperm from the upper portion of the epididymis being rerouted into the vas before they are fully developed and motile. Here is a diagram of the deluxe version (vasoepididymostomy):

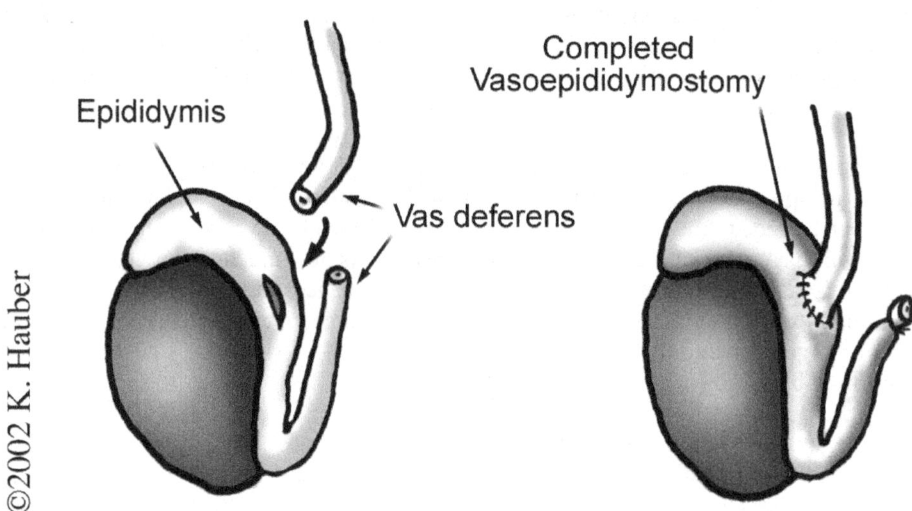

In examining the data about reversals, it is consistently noted that the longer it has been since a man had a vasectomy, the lower the chances that the reversal will be successful, at least in terms of his ability to impregnate. "After ten years the chances for recovery of fertility drop to 35%, and the procedure is more complicated, although some evidence exists that reversal may work even after 20 years in some men (Simon, et. al., 1998)." There are other factors involved, like the extent of a man's immune system response to the presence of un-ejaculated sperm, a subject that will be discussed at some length later. Surgical damage to the nerves that cause the epididymis to contract during ejaculation has also been found to be a common result of vasectomy (Pabst, et. al., 1979). More about that later, too.

Some doctors' experience indicates the problem with reestablishing fertility is that continued obstruction often exists in the epididymis and vas itself after reversal. These situations will often lead to repeating of the reversal procedure (Carbone, et. al., 1998). This may be combined with other fertilization techniques when impregnation is still desired.

If all of this cutting and sewing fails to make a man fertile enough to father children again there are a few involved techniques that can be used such as in-vitro fertilization, epididymal sperm aspiration (MESA) and intracytoplasmic sperm injection (ICSI). Big technical names like those sound expensive, don't they? They are, not to mention the fun of having needles stuck into your epididymis to retrieve the sperm in the process, usually after having been opened up one or more times previously for a reversal.

If you have any money left over from the second mortgage you had to take out for all this, there's an experimental procedure called round spermatic nuclear injection (RONSI). The term sounds like something done in a nuclear warfare lab, doesn't it? In fact, it costs about as much. This might bring into question your ability to afford to raise the child you are so desperately trying to create.

During the RONSI procedure, immature sperm are "aspirated" directly from the testes and injected into an egg using the aforementioned ICSI technique. Why all these methods have to involve scalpels and/or those damned big needles I don't know, but such is the case. Sounds pretty rigorous, doesn't it? The other problem is that the longer the time interval since your vasectomy, the less likely sperm obtained through ICSI are able to impregnate (Abelmassih, et. al., 2002).

These issues are summarized well by Turek (1999): "Assisted reproductive technology with ICSI offers impressive success in couples with immunological infertility; however, there are equally impressive burdens associated with the use of IVF and ICSI for this problem, including tremendous financial and emotional costs and unknown or incompletely described risks of developmental delay and sex chromosome abnormalities in offspring. All of these factors must be appropriately weighed and discussed with couples before such therapy is recommended."

My case was a little different in that I desired to remain sterile, if possible, to solve our contraception issue. I had sought a reversal as a solution to the constant pain I was experiencing. I was hoping that, somehow, I could end up without infections, still sterile, and out of pain with all my original parts in tact. Was this too tall of an order?

Nagler, et. al., (1999) speaks to this very issue: "Reversals were also performed because of changes in religious beliefs, scrotal pain, psychologic reasons, the loss of a child, or the desire to restore fertility for the future. In general, because there are no ethical, moral, medical, or surgical contraindications to this procedure, surgeons should be nonjudgmental regarding an individual's motivation for vasectomy reversal; however, reconstruction for the relief of a 'post-vasectomy syndrome' should be approached cautiously.

"Less commonly, vasovasostomy has been performed for post-vasectomy pain. Restoration of fertility may be an undesired side effect. McMahon and associates reported chronic testicular pain in 33% of 172 patients 4 years after vasectomy; 15% of the patients considered the pain to be troublesome. Testicular discomfort related to sexual intercourse occurred in nine cases (5%). Although the pathogenesis [cause] remains poorly understood, Myers and associates reported the relief of pain in 27 of 32 men who underwent vasectomy reversal for post-vasectomy pain syndrome. Despite this report, the surgical management of post-vasectomy pain remains controversial. A surgical procedure should be contemplated only as a last resort and should be performed only if the patient has a clear comprehension of an unpredictable outcome." I was becoming more familiar with these reports, and with the "unpredictable outcome" of the procedure.

By the time I went to see Phil again, it seemed like the infections were starting to get a little better. He looked at my most recent MRI films, pronouncing, "Yes, you still have two testicles." This was a fact that I was actually quite thankful for at that point, given everything that had transpired.

Okay, here comes another one of those explicit parts, so respond appropriately.

After examining me and once again skillfully finding all the tender spots, he said, "Looks like we should lance the largest of those infections, but before I do, can you give me a semen sample? I don't think you'll feel like it afterwards."

At least he asked instead of trying to mash what he wanted out of me as had been done by others.

"Uh, I don't know, Phil," I responded hesitantly.

My genitals still felt like a no-fly zone. He assured me that this was the best way to be sure that the reversal had worked. I expected him to open a secret door revealing that missile shaped orgasmatron, but instead motioned toward the bathroom.

Ah, the old-fashioned way. This was not exactly the kind of spontaneous and joyous sexual expression I was looking forward to. But, with the promise that in some strange way this was supposed to help, and having no pride left at all, I agreed.

I suppose I should inject a bit of humor here (I know, I need professional help). There is a story about a guy who goes back to get his "all clear" check by the doctor after his vasectomy.

The doctor handed the man a jar and said, "Here, take this jar home and bring back a sample tomorrow."

The next day the man came back to the doctor's office with a clean empty jar in hand.

"What happened?" asked the doctor.

The man explained, "First I tried with my right hand, but nothing. Then I tried with my left hand, but still nothing. Then I asked my wife for help. She tried her left hand first, and then her right hand, but still nothing. She then tried her mouth, first with teeth in, then with her teeth out, but still nothing. Then we called up the lady next door and she tried both her hands, and her mouth too, but nothing."

The doctor was astounded. "You asked you neighbor to help?"

The man replied, "Yep, but no matter what we tried, we couldn't get the lid off that darn jar!"

OK, enough for the story within the story.

After returning from bathroom, prize in hand, Phil asked, "Did that hurt?"

"Yes, but not as much as attempts at any kind of sexual activity before the last surgery," I replied.

He prepared a slide and put it under the microscope, switching on the video monitor, revealing lots of little swimming, struggling cells.

"Mondo sperm!" he exclaimed, "Well, I'm encouraged.

I assumed this was like hitting lotto for a fertility specialist since he seemed so happy about it. Let's see, first I'm fertile and not experiencing any pain, and in great shape. Then I'm sterile and in pain all the time. Then I'm fertile again, but still in pain and limping around on disability. I wished that I could have shared in his enthusiasm, but this was not the progression I was hoping for.

After he cut open one side of my scrotum to attempt to drain it, we talked for a while longer and agreed to give my healing more time. He tried to reassure me in the process. Numerous sperm cells were still wriggling about on the video monitor as we concluded our conversation.

"All those little guys desperately looking for a home. Seems like kind of a waste, doesn't it?" I observed.

Phil chuckled. It became apparent to me that this was nature's shotgun approach to the creation of life, and it was no wonder that each of us comes out as unique as we do.

I called my wife after I left his office. "Dust off your diaphragm, honey, I'm fertile again!" I pronounced as she answered the phone, trying to put the best spin on the situation that I could.

"Why? You're still too sore to do anything about it." she answered in matter-of-fact tones.

"Hey, a guy can dream, can't he? Let's keep a little optimism here." I implored.

As my hobbling and hurting continued unabated, I wondered once again if all this medical attention was in fact a good thing. According to my pain specialist, in fact, it wasn't, and the series of surgeries I had undergone were only worsening the pain response that I was experiencing. I decided it was time to take a break.

By now, it seemed as though most of the western world knew that something was drastically wrong with me. I had friends that I would see on the street or at the pool who expressed tremendous sympathy and openly offered prayer support, which I appreciated tremendously. The immediate reaction of most people was "I'll bet that really messes up your love life," and then typically "How do you stand it?" I would respond that this kind of situation messes up a lot more than your love life; it changes your whole life.

As for standing it, we all have to tolerate what life hands us and find the best coping tools we can, even in the face of the most unpleasant of situations. On the days when I was not handling the pain very well or found myself extremely irritable, I would usually deny myself contact with others, so as not to inflict my bad attitude on those around me.

Several friends knew that I was writing a book about my experience by this time. Some inquired as to when the movie would be coming out. The only problem was that I couldn't figure out who would be willing to play the male lead. Maybe Mel Gibson; he's always good for a few gratuitous butt shots. Then there was also the issue of who the lead would use as a stunt double. Decisions, decisions.

Chapter Thirteen

Life Finds a Way

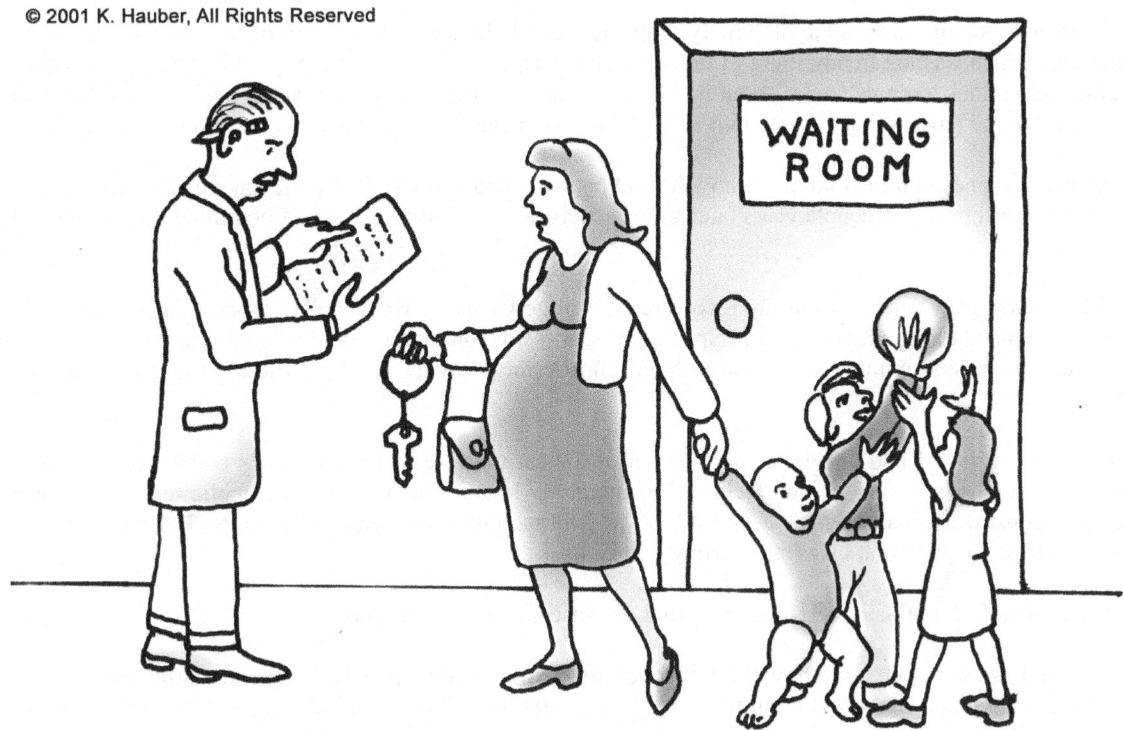

So, uh Doc... About when is that vasectomy supposed to kick in?

"Data on failure rates is limited as authors do not wish to publicize their failures" (Frances, et. al., 1983).

Remember the movie Jurassic Park? In the movie, Jeff Goldbloom plays Dr. Malcolm, a physicist working on a "chaos theory." While being shown the island, the dinosaurs, and the laboratory where the dinosaurs were genetically engineered, Malcolm and the other visitors are told that the dinosaurs can't reproduce because they have all been genetically engineered as females. Their technology was so advanced as to not allow for any unwanted births. Dr. Malcolm scoffed at this notion and replied, "Life finds a way."

I love that quote; life finds a way, because it is true about so many life processes that we can't control and just don't fully understand. Of course, in the movie, Malcolm turns out to be right, which leads to a substantial human buffet for the dinosaurs.

"Life finds a way" is a good thing to remember when it comes to vasectomies also. Todd is a friend my wife and I came to know as he would help cater parties at our house. He was a little older than most of the guys who worked for the caterer, and in talking one day, we found out that this was his second job, while his daytime job was as a school teacher.

When I asked why he was working two jobs he explained that he was supporting a wife and four kids at home. Hadn't he figured out what was causing this yet? As a matter of fact, he had, and that was why he had a vasectomy performed after his second child. He received clearance from the doctor, being told that he was now sperm free. Then he and his wife conceived again, twins this time. He and his wife are now very busy loving and tending to four kids instead of the two originally intended, and Todd works a lot of nights to help support it all. They love their kids dearly, even the "oops" babies. It's a lot more than they originally anticipated after a vasectomy.

Another friend of mine had a vasectomy after his second child was born. The doctor used staples at the time to seal off the vas, which was the trendy thing to do at the time. He says that he felt a pop while having intercourse on one occasion, but didn't think too much more about it. Not too long after, their third child was conceived. Evidently the pop he had felt was part of the process that allowed him to be "Pop" again, and he got to have his vasectomy done again to boot.

An acquaintance of mine told me of how he and his wife thought they were done having children after three, so he had a vasectomy performed. A couple years later they conceived their fourth. It was a good thing they loved and enjoyed all their kids too.

While I was convalescing from my reconstructive surgery, Spring Break rolled around for my kids. My in-laws had just bought a nice little condo in the Palm Springs area, so I was told that I would be continuing my recovery around a pool while the kids were swimming in the warm desert climate for a few days. Hey, who am I to argue with this type of therapy?

Upon our arrival, I had no sooner stepped out of the car than we met my in-law's realtor who had helped them with their condo purchase. "How are you feeling?" he inquired. I hadn't realized that the public service announcement of my testicular reconstruction had been broadcast all the way through the Coachella Valley some 300 miles from my home, but evidently it had. I replied that I was still hurting quite a bit.

"Yeah, I had a lot of pain for a long time after my vasectomy, too," he confessed.

Choosing not to inquire as to how the subject of my post-vasectomy pain had come up during the course of my in-law's real estate transaction, and deciding instead to gain a greater understanding of what a resolution might be like, I asked what happened with him. It turned out that he had experienced a lot of pain for months after his vasectomy.

Finally, the surgeon who had done his procedure numbed him up again and started trying to move and massage things around, I presume to try to alleviate granulomas that may have formed, but the man was unsure as to exactly what was done. The doctor evidently didn't say much about what was going on and the man didn't want to look. After this, he still experienced pain for many months. Then his wife became pregnant. Sounds to me like things were moved around a little too much the second time around. Years later, his pain finally subsided. Double whammy, wouldn't you say?

"Vasectomy techniques and failure rates vary among surgeons, and the criteria for failure are often not clearly defined" (Alderman, 1988). One doctor claimed that he had never had a failure in over 23 years of performing more than 4600 vasectomies (Schmidt, 1987). You might view this as a cocky claim, but it seemed to be quite a point of pride and was stated as if he was throwing down the gauntlet for his colleagues. It appears that admitting you've had vasectomy failures as a urologist is akin to taking the walk of shame.

At an appointment with my original urologist one day I asked him why he didn't offer the open-ended vasectomy to patients as an option.

"Because I don't have vasectomy failures," he stated emphatically. There was obviously a point of pride in this for him, too.

I told him to knock on wood, because even what I knew by then told me that vasectomy failures were only partially due to the surgeon's expertise and technique. The most significant reason that has become apparent to me is the pervasive reproductive process that goes on inside of us. When it comes right down to it, this is a really hard process to block, as a great deal of research has shown.

Some sources claim that vasectomies fail only 1/10th of 1% of the time (Bower, 1995). The technical term is recanalization, which normally means that, like a lizard growing back its tail, the vas spontaneously reconnects and the man is fertile again. Doctors take great pains to avoid this, and you'd think they were sailors with all the knots they tie to try to prevent a failed vasectomy. Since vasectomy failure is also the leading cause of litigation for urologists, they tend to be as thorough as possible and spend lots of time in knot and cauterizing class as medical students.

It is additionally proposed that vasectomy failures are due to not providing an adequate layering of tissues between the cut ends of the vas. This layering is an attempt to hide the upper end of the vas from all those persistent little sperm cells. You can imagine millions of suitors all around the base of a castle crying, "Rapunzel, Rapunzel, let down your hair." There goes my imagination again. But I digress.

I began to question the statistics on failures when I realized that by the numbers quoted, I would have to personally know four thousand men who had undergone vasectomies and who were willing to talk about it with me, for me to know four who had experienced failures. This didn't seem very likely. I like to think of myself as a social person, but I know I'm not that social.

My suspicions were born out (there's another one of those puns) when I obtained a copy of a report analyzing complications and failures at several facilities located in Canada. Now there are those who might try to convince you that Canadians are just different from everyone else, but I have a feeling that anatomically, we're probably all about the same. Canadian physicians do seem to be a little less optimistic in the statistics they quote, though.

Complications and failures were tracked for 1223 patients at a private clinic and a family planning clinic in Canada. Incidents recorded included such post-operative occurrences as painful granulomas, noninfectious inflammation, hematoma, infection, and undiagnosed pain. Failure rates were also tracked. All procedures were done by the no-scalpel vasectomy method, which you will remember is supposed to have the lowest complication rate.

For the patients of the private clinic, 2.8% experienced failures of the procedure, while at the family planning clinic the rate was 1.2%. This sounds like a lot higher than one in a thousand to me. It is also worth noting that the overall complication rate at the family planning clinic was 12.3%, while 5% of the patients at the private clinic experienced the aforementioned problems (Labreque, et. al., 1998). What happened to the 2% to 3% complication rates?

Dr. Choe and Dr. Kirkemo at Henry Ford Hospital in Detroit state, "It is well known that persistent fertility after vasectomy occurs in 0 to 6% of the cases." That is a pretty wide range and certainly quite different from the one in one thousand claims made elsewhere. Other research articles confirmed this "up to 6%" failure rate (Kenogbon, 2000). This made me wonder how effective vasectomy really is compared to other forms of birth control. Condoms are quoted as having a 1% failure rate under ideal conditions, and up to 6% in "real world" usage. Not much difference is there?

"In one British study, 5% of vasectomies had to be repeated- mostly because of persistent residual live motile sperm…. One study indicated that about 10% of men were still producing functional sperm at six months (Simon, et. al., 1998)." I don't think the Brits are that much more fertile than the rest of us.

Other research has shown that men can have occasional sperm in their ejaculate (O'Brien, et. al., 1995). This may be true even if the vas does not recanalize, i.e. join back up spontaneously. It just happens sometimes for no apparent reason other than the pervasive target-seeking nature of sperm, and the body's amazing ability to throw off an occasional live round. Sperm granuloma or vasitis nodosa that can grow and recede are often credited with this phenomenon.

Smith, et. al., (1994) studied six cases of DNA proven fatherhood after vasectomy. All of the subjects had consistent negative semen exams. The study concluded, "All vasectomy patients and their partners should be counseled about the small possibility of late failure, and warning of failure should be recorded."

Yet another example of the persistent seed was found when 5% of the vasectomies done during the study period had to be repeated within 6-36 months. "Of these [repeated procedures], 87% were performed because of persistent sperm in post-vasectomy semen samples (Benger, et. al., 1995)."

In a study published in 1997, 33% of patients still had nonmotile sperm in their ejaculate 12 weeks after vasectomy. The conclusion: "Reappearance of nonmotile sperm was found in an unexpectedly high percentage (De Knijff, et. al., 1997)." This type of phenomenon led Khan, et. al., (1997) to conclude: "The doctor must not automatically blame the 'milkman' if there are no sperm in the husband's semen after vasectomy and the wife becomes pregnant, unless DNA testing has confirmed that the patient is not the father." Can you see how this might lead to a little relationship stress?

A thorough discussion of the issue of vasectomy failures is found in the Journal of the American Medical Association by Philip M. Alderman (1988) in his article titled "The Lurking Sperm." Almost sounds like a movie of the week, doesn't it? He states "It is evident that a controversy exists as to which technique of male sterilization is the most effective in reducing failures as well as which is best overall." Dr. Alderman goes on to classify failures as early (persistent sperm within the first 12 months after vasectomy), and late (reappearance of sperm after proof of success of the procedure). This seems like a reasonable approach. Dr. Alderman's study group included 5331 men. Of this study population, there were a total of 97 failures including both early and late. That's 1.82% and is about average, that is, average among doctors who will admit to such things.

While this information is by no means universally agreed upon, it told me that the low complication and failure rate spin given for vasectomies is often quite misleading and downright inaccurate. I have learned to rely more and more on my own personal experience and that of those I have come in contact with as a better indicator. "Life finds a way" has taken on a new and deeper meaning.

Part III

Good Reasons for Not Getting a Fix in the First Place

Chapter Fourteen

How Do You Make a Hormone?

So, how would you make a hormone anyway? Well, you could find a deep-pocketed investor like a pharmaceutical company, set up a lab, spend millions of dollars and many years to get approval and bring the product to market. Or you can just perform vasectomies on millions of men and let their bodies start to change their hormone levels all on their own. What am I talking about? Hold onto your seats folks, we're going for a ride.

The National Institute of Health (1996) claims that, "Vasectomy does not affect the production or release of testosterone, the male hormone responsible for a man's sex drive, beard, deep voice, and other masculine traits." Interestingly, a great deal of research would indicate otherwise.

In fact, even if a man has no noticeable complications from a vasectomy, his body starts to change. The body, of course, is constantly producing many natural hormones in an attempt to balance its many internal functions. Vasectomies change that natural hormone balance. Purvis, et. al., (1976) found vasectomy to be "associated with significant changes in circulating and in seminal plasma levels of several steroids" including pregnenolone, dehydroepiandrosterone, androstenedione, dihydrotestosterone, and oestrone (Is that a bunch of 50-cent words, or what?). These changes persist for decades and can be indicators of elevated risk for many diseases. Do you want an example? "We believe that vasectomy may influence serum androgen levels by reducing the conversion from testosterone to dihydrotestosterone in the long term. The influence on this conversion would be different in the early and late long term (many years later) after vasectomy. If increased testosterone levels in men who underwent vasectomy 20 or more years previously is confirmed, it could indirectly support the hypothesis that the elevated risk of prostate cancer after vasectomy was notable among men who underwent vasectomy 20 or more years ago" (Mo, et. al., 1995). We'll continue the vasectomy/prostate cancer discussion later.

As we discussed before, the pituitary gland produces follicle-stimulating hormone and luteinizing hormone, which causes the testicles to produce sperm and testosterone. There are other hormones involved also, but let's keep things as simple as possible. All of you know good old testosterone, I'm sure, since it gets blamed for many of the world's maladies, but let's look at the reaction in the body for a moment.

According to Dr. Erik K. Seaman, M.D., "Vasectomy has been reported to increase serum [in the bloodstream] testosterone." The doctor adds the caveat that "such increases are small if they occur at all and serum levels stay within the normal range." Why the concern? After all, who couldn't use a little extra testosterone in making his way through the world?

By now I had learned to take a "thou protesteth too much" attitude and dig a little further when anyone claimed they could make surgical changes to the body with no effect at all. The concern is that elevated levels of testosterone alter a number of body functions, including causing enlargement of the prostate. Artificially elevated testosterone levels are also known to be a possible cause of increased risk of prostate cancer (Chan, et. al., 1998).

<u>Gray's Anatomy</u> takes another, more attention-grabbing approach to the issue: "The operation of castration has also been, during the last few years, performed for enlargement of the prostate; for it has been found that removal of the testicles is followed by very rapid and often considerable diminution in the size of the prostate. The operation is, however, one of severity, and is frequently followed by death in these cases, performed, as it necessarily is, in old men (Gray, 1995)."

Let me assume for a moment that the reader has an interest in avoiding castration followed by death and pursue this a little further. You have to ask the question, if the body's testosterone balance is so critical to health, and elevated levels of testosterone have been shown to have potentially dire results, why would anyone do anything that would potentially raise their testosterone levels? The human body constantly attempts to balance hormone levels to maintain homeostasis. That balance tends to change gradually as a person ages.

Medical science has established a normal range of testosterone in healthy men between 260 and 1000 nanograms per deciliter of blood plasma. Those figures will vary depending on who you talk to, but that's a good starting place. And no, it's not as if all of the guys at the high end of the range look like Arnold Schwartzenagger, with the guys at the low end all playing with the Easy-Bake ovens. It's more just a matter of where your body naturally settles out, and how well you process the substance.

Testosterone levels change throughout life. In fact testosterone is what makes boys become boys in the womb. Later, "Testosterone in the bloodstream of teenage boys can jump to as high as 2,000 nanograms, which helps explain teenage boys" (Lacayo, 2000). If everything is functioning normally, testosterone levels naturally decrease as life goes on. Testosterone levels even vary throughout the day, typically peaking around 8 A.M., which might help to explain why Mr. Happy greets you so often in the morning.

Overweight adult men tend to have lower testosterone levels than their more svelte contemporaries. However, "Once you get past the proven links between testosterone, libido and muscle mass, the benefits of having higher levels of testosterone become harder to prove, though no less interesting to hear about (Lacayo, 2000)." The normal increase and then decline in testosterone level throughout a man's life is linked to so many factors and processes that "fixing" the amount of testosterone in one's body becomes risky business, unless there is some proven deficiency.

Younger men are often enticed by the idea of testosterone therapy because of the muscular bulking up that occurs. Author Richard Lacayo (2000) states, "For teens in particular the dangers of testosterone overload are not just acne and breast development but a shutting down of bone growth-though they may be at an age that makes them almost deaf to the risks.... Married men tend to have lower testosterone. It's evolution's way of encouraging the wandering mate to stay home.... For older men, studies indicate that high levels of T [testosterone] do not necessarily cause prostate cancer but do fuel the growth of tumors once they occur, which is why chemical castration is one means of treating the disease in the advanced stages."

Do you get the same feeling I do that this is sensitive stuff? This is not too different from what Dr. Gray was talking about, is it?

Speaking to the issue of testosterone-replacement therapy, Lacayo goes on to ask the inevitable question, "Gee. Even putting aside for a moment the much-increased danger of prostate cancer, do we really want men to turn latter life into a hormonal keg party? The thought could be mildly exasperating to women, who might be forgiven for greeting the news with the same feelings china shop-keepers have for bulls."

Aside from the entertainment and behavioral aspects of the issue, what does all this have to do with vasectomies? Well, it seems that, like many other controversial aspects of the procedure, there are studies that have shown increases in serum testosterone levels after vasectomy, which tends to bring howls of protest and denial from those who's livelihood is built upon doing the procedures.

Research has shown that male reproductive tract hormone levels change following vasectomy (Oversen, 1995). Let's backtrack a second: luteinizing hormone produced in the pituitary gland stimulates the production of testosterone in the testes, which is part of a complex feedback loop. Follicle-stimulating hormone also from the pituitary gland is critical in sperm production.

Around the turn of the 20th century when vasectomies were first being done, doctors believed that the procedure did, in fact, raise testosterone levels, and stated such (Carruthers, 2000). This led to vasectomies often being done not so much for sterilization, but as a fountain of youth mechanism. It was only after the negative aspects of increased testosterone and other hormonal changes became better known that the tune changed. Did the biological basics change in the meantime?

Speaking of biological basic, take a look at the following diagram showing the oversimplified version of the hormonal feedback loop in men and women:

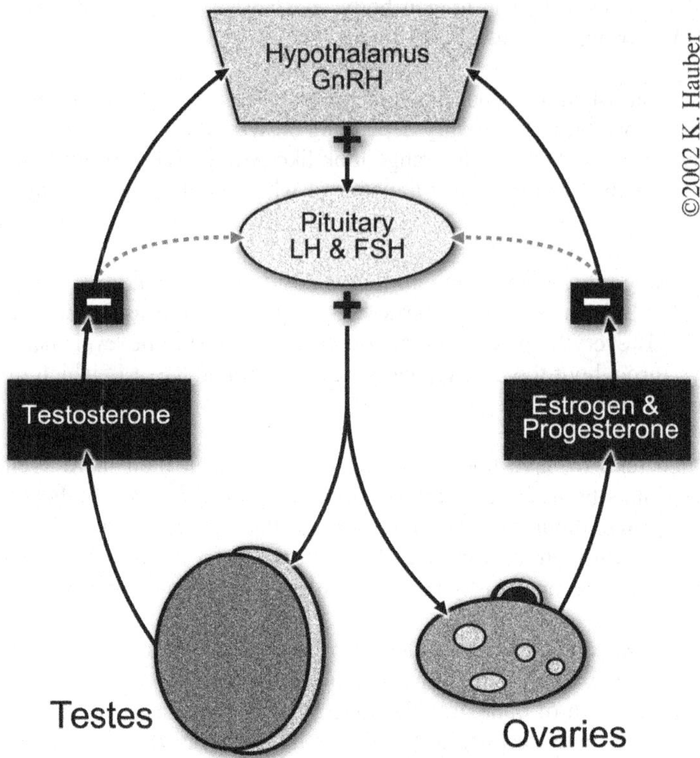

Gets a little complex, doesn't it? "The endocrine [hormonal] system is referred to as the hypothalamic-pituitary-testicular axis" (Sokol, 1999), as indicated by the diagram above. The diagram shows only a portion of what is actually going on, the major players as it were, and there are many other processes and sub-processes taking place at the same time. It is important to realize that the endocrine system is integral with the body's immune system, the importance of which will become more apparent as you read on.

What happens when you start to mess with this balance? Well, if it's any indicator, follicle-stimulating hormone therapy is one of the primary methods of treating infertile men. A study published in the Journal of Urology in 1989 showed that men who had undergone vasectomy had significantly altered follicle-stimulating hormone and luteinizing hormone responses compared to the non-vasectomized control group (Fisch, 1989).

Diminished or elevated secretion of luteinizing hormone or follicle-stimulating hormone can relate to low sperm production, gonadal failure, or pituitary tumors. Changes in these hormone levels also affect testosterone production, with the aforementioned potential results. How much change is there after vasectomy? That is one of the debated subjects, however "Any disruption of the delicately coordinated interaction between the components of the hypothalamic-pituitary-testicular axis may lead to hypogonadism [sub-normal hormone production by the testis]" (Sokol,1999).

Looking back at some of the research on the subject again, Smith, et. al., (1976) noted, "…beginning at 6 months after vasectomy, mean plasma testosterone levels demonstrated a statistically significant elevation… [and] mean plasma LH [luteinizing hormone] levels were elevated…. By 2 years after vasectomy…plasma testosterone and LH levels remained elevated." Do these changes in hormone levels have an effect on the body? What do you think?

A discussion of the long-term hormonal changes after vasectomy will ensue in several chapters. Before doing so, it is necessary to examine the immune system response to vasectomy.

Chapter Fifteen

Vasectomies and the Immune System

"The complex relationship between the immune system and the male reproductive tract is not well understood"
Turek (1999).

"The immune system provides us with a multi-layer defense against invading microbes and foreign intruders. It can recognize the difference between normal (self) and alien (non-self) cells, trigger a local or widespread inflammatory response, and retain the memory of the offending organism to repel it again if it should ever return. Like any finely tuned machine, however, the system can break down and leave us open to the threat of infection, or conversely, turn against our own healthy tissues, as occurs in such diseases as rheumatoid arthritis or lupus" (Gehlbach, et. al., undated). "In addition to specificity and destructive ability, the immune system has exquisite memory and mobility" (Turek,1999).

Let's look once again to the government for information. I realize that may be a scary proposition for many of us, but let's see what they have to say anyway. The U. S. Department of Health and Human Services and the National Institute of Health (1996) state, "Many vasectomized men develop immune reactions to sperm, although current evidence indicates that these reactions do not cause any harm."

Really? How many men can expect to have these "harmless" reactions? And what might those reactions be, anyway? Why is this important? Verajankorva, et. al., (1999) answers this third question quite nicely: "*The presence of sperm antibodies correlates with nearly every pathological condition of the male reproductive tract*" (emphasis added).

Quoting once again from the NIH report, "Ordinarily, sperm do not come in contact with immune cells, so they do not elicit an immune response. This is a good thing because sperm cells have very strong antigenic qualities. But vasectomy breaches the barriers that separate immune cells from sperm, and many men develop anti-sperm antibodies after undergoing the procedure." Research has indicated and several doctors relayed to me personally that, in fact, if a man doesn't develop these antibodies after vasectomy, they assume something is wrong with his immune system.

Sperm cells are haploid in their genetic composition, having half of a DNA strand, which is intended to join with the other half in an egg, making a new, genetically unique individual. Sperm cells also have very strong enzymes at their head since they need to eat through the outer layer of an egg to accomplish their mission. These are some of the reasons why a man's body will take exception to the presence of sperm cells in the blood stream.

The human body develops antibodies to fight off disease. When the body starts fighting cells and tissues of its own creation, it is known as "autoimmune." That word doesn't get bantered around the general public in the context of vasectomies very often, but in fact that is what happens, a man's body is likely to become autoimmune in response to the production and retention of his own sperm cells.

Autoimmune reactions in general are on the rise in Western countries (Guernsey, 2000), and it appears that this marked increase is lifestyle and environmentally related. To further clarify, most people are familiar with the opposite of autoimmune, which is immune deficiency, AIDS being the notable example. In that situation, the body is not making enough immune cells to protect itself. Autoimmune is just the opposite, where the immune system perceives a threat and overreacts like an army of recent converts. Autoimmunity affects 20% of the population in America (that's 50 million people or more), and there are more than 80 known autoimmune diseases. "Autoimmune diseases are not contagious or infectious, but they can causes major organ damage and be life-threatening." In fact, "Autoimmunity is the underlying

92

cause of most chronic illnesses," and "countless thousands of Americans die each year of these diseases" (American Autoimmune Related Disease Association).

Common allergic reactions are another example of immune responses and can vary quite a bit from person to person. Allergic reactions are traditionally considered to come in reaction to substances from outside the body, though often the terms "allergy" and "autoimmunity" get used interchangeably, despite the origins of the cause of one outside the body and the other inside the body, respectively. One person might be just fine eating nuts for example (the kind from the shell), but the oil from those same nuts might send another person to the emergency room. I've seen this happen with several friends, and it's not pretty. The body can react quite severely to a perceived attack.

Given the likelihood that vasectomy will cause a substantial autoimmune response would be enough to make most doctors not recommend the procedure, right? Wrong! Most sources claim that the autoimmune response to vasectomy is "harmless" and of no real consequence to a man's health. This is where you need to start thinking for yourself, and get beyond the sales information and agendas that would push you toward the operating table.

How likely is this autoimmune reaction after vasectomy, you might ask? In a study by Jarow, et. al., (1994) published results of a study in *Urology*, and found, "serum [in the bloodstream] antisperm activity was present in 74% of the vasectomized men but none in the control subjects." According to a 1983 study by Linet published in *Urology* magazine, 50 to 70 percent of vasectomized men have elevated serum levels of antisperm antibodies. Just to clarify, the terms sperm antibody, sperm autoantibody, antisperm antibody, and anti-sperm antibody are used interchangeably, often by the same individuals even in the same text.

Earlier studies in the 1970's showed the antibody incidence in vasectomy victims, I mean patients, at 55% to 75% two years after the procedure (Tung, 1975). Another study released in 1982 showed an incidence of antisperm antibodies in vasectomized men of 76.2% (Hattikudur, 1982). This is one of the primary factors assumed to contribute to low sperm motility (activity) in many men after an otherwise successful reversal procedure. Low motility, in turn, leads to lower than normal pregnancy rates because the little guys just can't swim as hard and do their job as well with all those antibodies hanging all over them. <u>Campbell's Urology</u> (1992) puts the percentage of patients with antibodies present following vasectomy at 60-80%. Most studies indicate increased incidence of sperm antibodies as time goes on after the procedure.

How does this relate to the population in general? The incidence of sperm antibodies in fertile men who have not had surgery or injury to their testicles runs less than 1%. Sperm antibodies have been reported in approximately 10% of infertile men (Gehlbach, et. al., undated). Compare this to a presence of antibodies that jumps dramatically in men having undergone vasectomy, with most current estimates in the 75% range of men having undergone the procedure. It is worthwhile to note that the means for detecting these antisperm antibodies is under constant development and has improved substantially in recent years. "Antisperm antibodies are found in three locations: serum [blood], seminal plasma, and sperm-bound" (Turek, 1999). The three types of antisperm antibodies tested for are IgG, IgA, and IgM.

Shearer, et. al., (1982) authored an article published by the National Cancer Institute titled "Is sperm immunosuppressive in male homosexuals and vasectomized men?" Most vasectomized men would probably be surprised to find that the reactions their bodies were having have been compared to the repeated exposure to sperm that homosexuals experience, but that in fact is the case. "Vasectomized males represent another population [besides homosexuals] whose immune potential may be compromised by leakage of sperm into the vascular system" (Shearer, et. al., 1982). So, the next time you tell a vasectomized man to go screw himself, you may be speaking more literally than you think.

So why doesn't significant autoimmunity to sperm occur for many men besides those who have vasectomies? Turek (1999) addresses that question as follows: "Leaks of sperm antigens are considered tolerogenic; immunity is reduced in a manner similar to desensitization treatment for common allergens. On the contrary, large doses of sperm antigens, such as following vasectomy or testis trauma, would incite a pathologic immune response." So vasectomy overwhelms the body's ability to reabsorb its own sperm products.

This immune system response to vasectomy normally starts in the epididymis, which, coincidentally is where most men with post-vasectomy pain experience their greatest symptoms. According to Turek (1999), "The epididymis is likely to be a major site of immune regulation within the reproductive tract. Clinically, this idea is corroborated by the finding that vasectomized men show significantly fewer (75%) white blood cells in the ejaculate than do normal men. The epididymis is considered to be the most likely source of antibody secretion and cellular immunity and autoimmunity in the male reproductive tract."

But the autoimmune responses that vasectomy causes don't stop at the epididymis unfortunately. The realization of the extent to which autoimmune responses occur after vasectomy "has given rise to concern on the part of doctors and researchers, because immune reactions against parts of one's own body often cause disease. Rheumatoid arthritis, juvenile diabetes, and multiple sclerosis are just some of the illnesses suspected or known to be caused by immune reactions of this type. Immune reactions can also contribute to the development of atherosclerosis, the clogging of the arteries that leads to heart attacks (National Institute of Health, 1996)."

What? The potential for increased incidence of arthritis, diabetes, multiple sclerosis, and heart attack all as a result of vasectomy?

Quoting from yet another source: "Experts are concerned that changes in the immune system might cause damage in other parts of the body, including hardening of the arteries, blood clotting, kidney disease, and arthritis" (Simon, et. al., 1998). Other accounts by medical professionals included patients experiencing "a prolonged and debilitating flu-like illness within the first few months after vasectomy, which is when the immune reactions would be expected, and granulomas appear.... Some patients show active generalized immune process as shown by raised levels in the blood of a protein called 'immune compliment' which has been linked to the possibility of increased heart and circulatory disease after vasectomy.... The majority show anti-sperm antibodies. In fact it has been widely recognized and accepted for many years that anti-sperm antibodies are found in up to three-quarters of vasectomized men. One medical researcher on the subject cheerfully says, 'Vasectomy can be considered a particular form of experimental autoimmunization' (Carruthers, 1997)."

I happened across a quote by Dr. H. J. Roberts (1993): "Antibodies also have the potential for causing much harm and serious autoimmune disease in some individuals...no other operation performed on humans even approaches the degree and duration of the multiple immunologic responses that occur in the post-vasectomy state." There's another attention-getter!

How did Dr. Roberts arrive at this determination?   While he was practicing as an internist a number of years ago, Dr. Roberts noticed that a number of relatively young men coming to him had developed serious and otherwise unexplained diseases within months or years following their vasectomies, after previously being in good health.

Dr. Roberts' examples of patients included:

- "A 43-year-old man suffered multiple chronic major illnesses, especially severe joint pain, for 12 years after his vasectomy."

- "A 32-year-old man developed severe allergies for the first time within one month after undergoing vasectomy."

- A practicing internist wrote Dr. Roberts and offered "I had a vasectomy at age 27 and did not have phlebitits. But now I recall that about six to twelve months later I noted one morning I could not touch my right heel to the floor without sharp pain in the calf of my leg. Being a physician, I recognized this as a positive Homan's sign" (phlebitis, or inflammation of the vein).

- "A 27-year-old salesman who experienced recurrent attacks of thrombophlebitis [blood clotting in the extremities] in his lower extremities during the 11 years after a vasectomy, despite many measures, including medications."

- "Arthritis symptoms were experienced by a 42-year-old man only one week after his vas had been cut accidentally during a hernia repair. Symptoms recurred at least once a month over the next year."

In all, Dr. Roberts treated or studied the histories of 74 such patients. Among the maladies noted, "Serious infections occurred in 20 patients from six weeks to five years after vasectomy...Multiple and recurrent infections were common in these patients. Other physicians have been impressed by the increased frequency of post-vasectomy infections involving the prostate, epididymis, seminal vesicles [storage glands for sperm near the prostate], and kidneys. Such susceptibility to infection probably reflects a weakening in the body's immune system caused or aggravated by vasectomy. Also, there may be a cross-reaction between antibodies to bacteria (or other germs) and antibodies to sperm."

What does that "cross-reaction" part mean? Anderson, et. al., (1982) tested antibody reactions in vasectomized men and compared them to both cancer patients and non-vasectomized men as control subjects. The results were fascinating, but alarming. "These tests revealed that vasectomized men had significantly higher antibody titers [levels] than did the controls in most antibody assays, and that significantly more vasectomized men responded to melanoma I, squamous cell carcinoma, and breast carcinoma extracts... the degree of reactivity to melanoma extract was positively correlated with antisperm antibody level."

The authors went on to state that "Sperm antigens can also be found on malignant tissues.... Our preliminary observation that many cancer patients have high titers of antisperm antibodies is interesting in the context of this report because it further reports the hypothesis that sperm and malignant cells express immunologically cross-reactive antigens that readily stimulate a host autoimmune response."

In a subsequent article published in the *American Journal of Pathology* (1983) by Anderson, et. al., the authors continued their investigation into the effect of vasectomy on tumor growth: "Both the initial stages of tumorigenesis and subsequent tumor growth may be affected by conditions associated with the vasectomized state. It is possible that sperm degradation products directly affect tumor initiation and development or have an indirect effect, such as interference with immunosurveillance mechanisms."

Let's look at a couple of the studies that have shown the types of disease links mentioned thus far in a rough chronological order:

A study published in 1978 concluded that, "the immunologic response to sperm antigen that often accompanies vasectomy can exacerbate atherosclerosis" [hardening of the arteries that causes most coronary heart disease] (Alexander, et. al., 1978). These researchers didn't stop, but "followed up this early work with longer term studies which showed even more marked changes. This was largely confirmed in studies on primates by several other groups of researchers, particularly where the monkeys were overfed and underexercised, like the average Western male" (Carruthers, 1997). "The major clinical problem associated with vasectomy is that monkeys and rabbits that have been vasectomized have been found to have enhanced incidence of atherosclerosis. The causative mechanism for this phenomenon is purported to be the presence of sperm autoantibody in association with circulating soluble antigens forming immune complexes, which result in immune injury to the artery. For immune complexes to form, the presence of sperm antibody is required" (Curtis, et. al., 1982).

Then, a study was published showing a 370% increase in the incidence of arthritis, rheumatism, and connective tissue diseases requiring hospitalization. This occurred nine years or more after vasectomy (Walker, et. al., 1981).

The risk of kidney stones forming in vasectomized men ages 30-35 and requiring hospitalization was found to be 2.6 times higher than normal in one study (Kronmal, et. al., 1988). A later study found a twofold increase in the risk of kidney stones for men under the age of 46 who had a vasectomy. "This increased risk may persist for up to 14 years post-vasectomy. Given the large number of men who undergo vasectomy worldwide each year, the increased risk for urolithiasis [kidney stones] among vasectomized men may result in substantial excess morbidity" (Kronmal, et. al., 1997).

Various other studies have examined the association between vasectomy and an increased risk of myocardial infarction (heart attack) (Chi, et. al., 1990). These factors can relate to hardening of the arteries as mentioned previously, or other factors related to hormonal and blood fat level changes.

As if that weren't enough, three separate hospital-based studies published in 1990 reported positive correlations between vasectomy and prostate cancer. Speaking of cancer, "Additional concern had been raised about the possible association between vasectomy and testicular cancer (National Institute of Health, 1996)." There are reports of "an increased number of cases of testicular cancer within the first four years after vasectomy, reaching a maximum after two [years] (Carruthers, 1997)." This is theorized to relate to the surge in hormone levels following vasectomy, as was discussed in the last chapter. All this wasn't sounding any better to me.

A study published in the *New England Journal of Medicine* in 1992 noted increased risks of lung cancer, non-Hodgkin's lymphoma and multiple myeloma in vasectomized men 20 years after vasectomy (Giovannucci, et. al., 1992)."

There's a lot more, but I'm sure you have the idea by now. Other reports included numerous incidents of thrombophlebitis, pulmonary embolism, narcolepsy, multiple sclerosis, migraine and related headaches, hypoglycemia, and numerous allergic reactions all occurring within a relatively short interval after vasectomy (Roberts, 1993).

We have already touched on the subject of vasectomy and an increased incidence of prostatitis (Prostatitis Web Site/Vasectomy Page), but what is interesting about this is that the most common form of prostatitis, by a factor of eight to one, is nonbacterial prostatitis. Research has determined that the chronic inflammatory and scar tissue responses that occur in this condition have an autoimmune basis (Keetch, et. al., 1994). Researchers have not yet determined the precise mechanism that causes this autoimmune response, but the potential link to autoimmunity to sperm antigens is an obvious one to consider. This is one of those situations where doctors will try to convince you not to be concerned even though they plainly don't know, but again, whose body is it that's on the line here?

Here's another item to consider while we're on the subject of prostates: "...30% of all American men over 50 show some evidence of prostate cancer cells. Long-term high-normal levels of testosterone are associated with an increased risk for prostate cancer. Because testosterone levels remain higher for a longer period in men who had vasectomy, experts have been concerned that such men have a greater chance for developing the cancer" (Simon, et. al., 1998.) It is also known that "several investigators have shown that the human prostate gland participates in antigen-antibody reactions" (Meares, 1977). You have obviously noted by now that vasectomy typically leads to a significant antigen-antibody reaction.

Let's look at this a bit further as long as we're on the subject of prostate cancer: "In 1993, a noted team of Harvard epidemiologists published findings from two large studies in the *Journal of the American Medical Association (JAMA)*. One of these studies was retrospective [backward looking], while the other was prospective and followed new patients. Both found vasectomy to be associated with a moderately elevated relative risk of prostate cancer that increased with time after the procedure" (National Institute of Health, 1996).

How elevated? And how "moderate" you might ask, as I did? "After more than 20 years, a vasectomized man appeared to be twice as likely to develop prostate cancer as a non-vasectomized man of the same age" (National Institute of Health, 1996). Another study had found the risk to be increased between 350% and 530% (Rosenberg, et. al., 1990). The typical observation has been an increase in relative prostate cancer risk as time elapses after the procedure.

The World Health Organization published this statement in 1993 as this debate was heating up: "Renewed concerns have been raised about a possible effect between vasectomy and cancer of the prostate many years after the procedure has been performed. These concerns are based on research conducted in the U. S. A., where there is a high and rising incidence of prostate cancer" (Farley, et. al., 1993).

Stop for a moment and ask yourself what really causes cancer anyway? Dr. Jon Kabat-Zinn gave the best summary I have found: "Cancer is a condition in which cells within the body lose the biochemical mechanisms that keep their growth in check. Consequently, they multiply wildly, in many cases forming large masses called tumors. Many scientists believe that the production of cancerous cells in the body is happening at a low level all the time as a 'normal' process and that the immune system, when healthy, recognizes them and destroys them before they can do any damage. According to this model it is when the immune system is weakened, either through direct physical damage or through the psychological effects of stress, and it can no longer effectively identify and destroy these small numbers of cancerous cells that the cancer cells multiply out of control" (Kabat-Zinn, 1990).

In the case of prostate cancer, this multiplying out of control claims 30,000 live per year (Simon, et. al., 1998). I might add that this is only a partial list of the many studies that raise significant questions about the safety of vasectomies. Doesn't this warrant at least some form of disclosure and discussion with the average man contemplating the procedure who has no idea about the possibility of such risks?

How does the medical community respond to this type of information in regard to vasectomy? Aside from those who don't respond at all and just keep on cutting and snipping, take a look at the response of Dr. Erik K. Seaman in his Internet article on vasectomy and prostate cancer: "In the past 10 years, there have been 14 major studies [published] investigating a possible relationship between vasectomy and prostate cancer...These studies were reviewed in the August, 1998 issue of *Fertility and Sterility* (Bernal-Delgado, et. al., 1998). Only 6 studies were found to have statistically significant association; however, all of the studies were found to have significant methodologic problems...."

Actually, that's not exactly what the article that Dr. Seaman is referring to says. If you were willing to take the time to read the research instead of relying on secondhand accounts, you would find the actual quote to be "Eleven of the 14 studies retrieved found an excess risk of prostate cancer in patients who had undergone vasectomy; this association was statistically significant in 6 of them" (Bernal-Delgado, et. al., 1998).

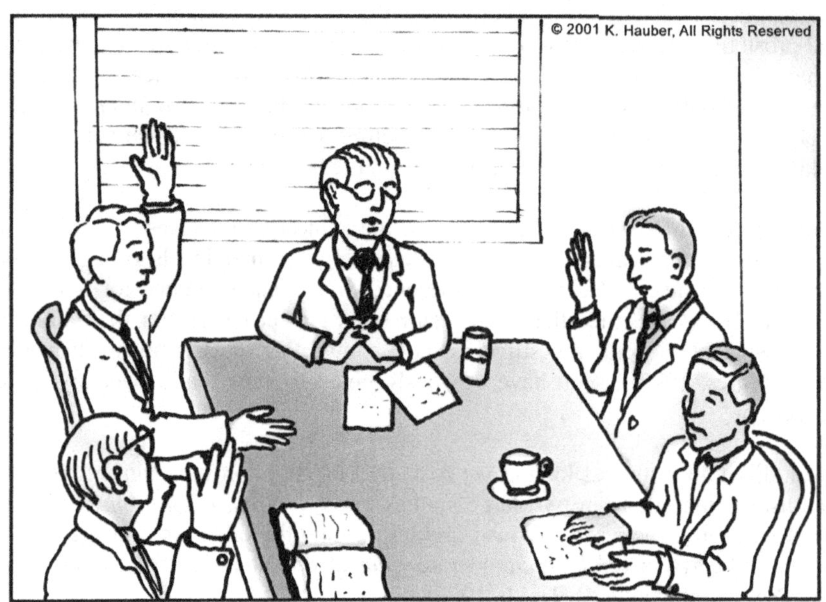

Now, I'm no statistical wizard but I can do the math and tell you that six out of fourteen is 42.9% of the studies that say there is a significant link between vasectomy and prostate cancer. Eleven out of 14 is 78.6% of the studies showing a positive association between vasectomy and prostate cancer. That's a lot of evidence that something is going on, wouldn't you say? And if the studies saying there is a link have "methodologic problems", then evidently the studies saying there is no link are also flawed. The bottom line is that most doctors either don't know or won't say for sure, but want to keep doing vasectomies anyway. "Pay no attention to that man behind the curtain; I am the great and powerful Oz!" Oops, there goes my imagination again.

As the heat from this issue was building, the National Institute of Child Health and Human Development (NICHHD) convened a meeting in 1993. An "expert panel" was formed to study the available data on the subject. It would be fascinating to examine the composition of the panel and find out how many members had a vested interest in continuing to do vasectomies. The panel concluded that associations between vasectomy and prostate cancer in particular may or may not be valid, and that further study was needed.

According to this expert panel, medical providers should continue to offer the procedure without any change in current clinical or public health practices while this issue is being studied. A statement was issued that "On the basis of much evidence, experts believe that vasectomy can safely continue to be used as it has been in the past, while further research is carried out (National Institute of Health, 1996)." Who is that "further research" being carried out on? That, my friends, would be you and me, or anyone else who has undergone a vasectomy, unwittingly becoming the participants in a mass study on human sterilization and immunology.

I've had a little experience with local government in the past, and I've noticed that the fastest way to kill off a hot issue is to "study" it. Public concern will undoubtedly shift to something else while the "study" process is continuing ad nauseum and the pressure to come up with definitive data and solutions will fade.

Since many of the reassurances offered regarding the safety of vasectomies rely so heavily on the aforementioned expert panel statement, I obtained a copy of the expert panel's report, entitled "Final Statement-March 2, 1993 Vasectomy and Prostate Cancer Conference". I found it fascinating reading, and noted that this had been published only two weeks after the two Harvard studies indicating a linkage were released in the *AMA Journal*. Do you think there was a sense of urgency on the part of the expert panel?

Evidently, the Harvard guys are like the E. F. Hutton of the research field; when they speak, everyone listens. Let's look at how that expert panel statement is composed: "Recent epidemiologic studies have raised important questions about a possible relationship between vasectomy and prostate cancer. Any relationship between vasectomy and prostate cancer, if proven, would be of great significance to individual and public health [no kiddin']. An estimated 20% [the highest number I'd seen yet] of men over 35 years of age in the United States have had a vasectomy... Prostate cancer is the most commonly diagnosed cancer in U. S. men and is second only to lung cancer in mortality among men. An estimated one in eleven U. S. men will develop clinical prostate cancer in their lifetimes. Little is known about the etiology [cause] and pathogenesis [progression] of prostate cancer.

"Findings from past epidemiologic studies investigating a relationship between vasectomy and prostate cancer have been conflicting.... Positive associations that have been found may be valid, or they may be due to detection bias, to other sources of bias, or to chance.... The credibility of a possible causal relationship between any disease and a particular factor is stronger if a biological mechanism is known to exist. In this case there is no biological evidence [yet] for an association between vasectomy and prostate cancer...." (National Institute of Child Health and Human Development, et. al., 1993).

Language is a curious thing, isn't it? Notice that what is said is that since no biological mechanism has been determined, it can be assumed that nothing is happening. That's like saying that because we don't know why the airliner crashed, killing all aboard, we can assume it didn't happen. This all means that they are not sure why or how prostate cancer forms, and they are not able to disprove the link between vasectomy and prostate cancer, but we should all continue to do things just as we have, fat, dumb and sterile. I'm not very reassured by this, are you? One has to wonder how long it took to prove the "biological mechanism" that linked smoking to lung cancer, and how many people died to help prove it.

Along those lines, if you look back at the Harvard studies, several conclusions are reached about causation: "The results support evidence from other epidemiologic studies that vasectomy increases risk of prostate cancer. A biological mechanism whereby vasectomy influences the rate of prostate cancer may be related to a diminished secretory rate of prostatic fluid following vasectomy, or, alternatively, to the post-vasectomy immune response to sperm antigens, which may cross-react with tumor-associated antigens and suppress tumor immunosurveillance mechanisms" (Giovannucci, et. al., 1993). It is also worthy to note that "Circulating antibodies diffuse from serum [blood] to seminal plasma via the prostate" (Upadhyaya, et. al., 1984), providing a pathway for these types of responses. That's definitive enough for me to have pulled in the reins, if only I had known in time.

The NICHHD expert panel report concluded, "Because of potential individual and public health implications, it is important that the question of any relationship between vasectomy and prostate cancer be fully and expeditiously resolved. Both epidemiologic and basic biologic research are needed to resolve existing questions.... Epidemiologic studies should be able to evaluate men at 20 years or more after vasectomy."

That is the "Final Statement"? Not very conclusive, is it? How about becoming a lifetime guinea pig? Do you want to participate in this research along with me? I thought not.

An interesting item to note: the Harvard epidemiologists wanted to test the objection that there was "detection bias" in their findings. The conjecture was that men who go to urologists for vasectomies are more likely to have prostate cancer detected since they see doctors more regularly.

So the researchers went to a place not well known for Western style preventative health care, India in this case, and did another study. Published in 1997, the study concluded, "The results of this hospital-based case-control study are consistent with the hypothesis of a positive association between vasectomy and prostate cancer. Because routine prostate cancer screening is not common in this population, detection bias was unlikely to account for this association" (Platz, et. al., 1997).

Have these warnings and the resulting call for further research taken hold? Not across the board, they haven't. For example, the World Health Organization (WHO), one of the proponents expected to lead the charge for further research, has a mixed record in this regard. WHO literature contained the following statement in 1994, the year after the aforementioned expert conference: "Even if there is a weak association between vasectomy and subsequent prostate cancer, we believe that large scale studies on this question should be of low priority in developing countries where vasectomy is widely practiced and where the incidence of prostate cancer is low" (Wildschut, et. al., 1994).

This relegation of further studies to a low priority was proposed despite other evidence of increased risk of prostate cancer in men having undergone vasectomy in places such as China (Hsing, et. al., 1994). A similar statement was contained in WHO literature in regard to vasectomies being performed in India: "Vasectomy acceptance has been declining in India during the past 20 years. Even if the risk of prostate cancer is marginally higher in vasectomized men, this risk has to be assessed against the immediate safety and other possible long-term benefits of this procedure…specific efforts to promote its acceptance must continue in India" (Tripathy, et. al., 1994). Is this an indication of a health concern, or of a social/political/economic agenda? Why don't the doctors here try asking the recipients of vasectomies how they feel about this information?

I was under the impression that one of the goals of the World Health Organization was to help people around the world live longer, healthier lives. Since the incidence of prostate cancer tends to increase as men age, and men in developing countries tend to live shorter lives than men in developed countries, why would you continue to promote a practice that could shorten life, and be hard to track given the lack of infrastructure in many developing countries? There are obvious political and economic agendas at work here that go beyond concern for individual health.

Not all physicians turn a completely deaf ear to these warnings. About one doctor out of four will screen potential vasectomy patients for a family history of prostate cancer. The same percentage of doctors will "screen men with vasectomies earlier for prostate cancer than those without the operation" during normal physical exams (Simon et. al., 1998).

Others just haven't quite been convinced yet. Dr. Yosh Taguchi, a Montreal urologist and author of the book <u>Private Parts: An Owner's Guide to the Male Anatomy,</u> has been quoted as stating, "If a causative link is established, I will abandon the procedure without hesitation" (Ross, 1999). I'm glad someone finally wrote an owner's manual for us guys. I hope the doctor gets a chance to read my book too, since that might help convince him to abandon the procedure.

There are also issues for the unborn associated with antisperm antibodies. According to Turek (1999), "Embryo quality is poorer in ICSI cases with antisperm antibodies versus cases without antibodies, suggesting that post-fertilization events may be compromised by the presence of these antibodies." This can lead to the aforementioned "risks of developmental delay and sex chromosome abnormalities in offspring." This has particular implications for men wishing to reestablish their fertility with a vasectomy reversal. Remember, continued presence of significant counts of antisperm antibodies following a vasectomy reversal is a leading cause of infertility for couples where the man has undergone this procedure.

Some of the most interesting and alarming research I found was in the area of "autoimmune orchitis." Now, for those of you unfamiliar with the term "orchitis", it is not a disease of your favorite ornamental plant. Orchids derive their name from the Greek word "orchis", meaning testicle, and are so named because their bulbs resemble the sacks on that odd-ball kid you used to tease mercilessly in the showers of freshman gym class. Not that I would know, of course, but so I've been told. Sorry for the diversion. I thought I needed to add a little humor to an otherwise yucky subject. Why is it so yucky?

Simply put, autoimmune orchitis is a condition in which the body makes antibodies that start attacking the tissues in the testicles, cause degeneration of those tissues. Study in this area goes back to the 1960s, and has primarily been focused in the area of human infertility. But the link to our discussion about vasectomies is remarkable.

In 1999, researchers at the University of Glasgow released a study on this subject, trying to determine causes of the long-term effects of antibodies commonly noted after vasectomies. The researchers performed vasectomies on one side of their subjects, then waited three years and removed both testicles to be examined. The subjects in this study happened to be guinea pigs, the furry rodent kind, not the furry human kind. One can quite easily understand why most men would be unwilling to be subjects in such a test.

What the researchers found was "various degrees of seminiferous tubular degeneration" in the vasectomized side of the animals, including such characteristics present as intraepithelial vesicle formation, loss of germ cells, intraluminal macrophages, and lymphocytic infiltration. This doesn't sound good, does it? The observation was made, "It seems that vasectomy had exacerbated an age-related phenomenon," essentially making the animals, reproductively speaking, old before their time (Aitken, et. al., 1999). Have you ever heard the term "male menopause?" We'll also discuss this in more detail.

The research was unable to determine whether the degeneration of the testis was due to the effects of mechanical damage from the vasectomy procedure itself, the pressure and ruptures that resulted, or the effects of the immune system attack that followed. However, "The results suggest that autoimmune orchitis follows vasectomy" (Aiken, et. al., 1999).

Now, I'm aware that everything wears out and breaks down eventually. I just have no interest in speeding up nature's process, especially in relation to my reproductive anatomy. Goodness knows we all have enough challenges in life already.

Let me remind you that the research in this area has been primarily intended to study and benefit infertility in those attempting to have offspring. However, the links to the problems that follow vasectomy are unmistakable. Ask yourself what would be the effect on your immune system with it engaged in a never-ending fight with a perceived infection multiplying at the rate of 50,000 cells a minute, tens of millions per day. Would that have the possibility of preoccupying and weakening the system? What do you think? Put in a less delicate way, "It's like tying a knot in the barrel of a rifle and being surprised when it blows back in your face" (Carruthers, 1997).

The fact remains that doctors and researchers don't know the full relationship between immune system reactions of the type that vasectomies cause, and the diseases that have been linked to them. Anyone who would tell you different is either fooling himself or trying to fool you. They just plainly don't know but would try to reassure you that vasectomies are perfectly safe anyway, at least for your body.

I was advised long ago to beware of anyone who claims to have a monopoly on truth. This is not a simple matter, and you need to pay attention to your inner guidance. Dr. Malcolm Carruthers calls the results of vasectomy an "immunological time bomb ticking away." What do you think based on what you now know?

Having learned this information because I had to, once again the hard way, I was interested in taking a different and broader view of my pursuit of treatment. I now recognized that the extensive granuloma formation that I had experienced was an autoimmune reaction. And evidently it was happening again.

Two months after my reconstructive surgery, my new MRI films showed that epididymal cysts and hydroceles were forming in my testicles and scrotum, along with what looked like several more granulomas. These cysts persisted regardless of continued conservative treatment with medication, massage, and anything else non-invasive I could think of.

I began noticing several other conditions that gave me warning that my immune system was still under stress, even after the reversal. The Staph infections in my scrotum that I mentioned in a previous chapter served as one indicator. I had never developed that kind of significant infection before, even after other surgeries. I also began to notice frequent sniffles and nasal congestion. Cold sores began developing in my mouth regularly. I experienced skin rashes that I had to treat with hydrocortisone. These types of afflictions were not part of my prior experience, as I had been quite healthy my entire adult life.

Wanting to know more of what was going on inside of me, I went for yet another blood test. This time, it was determined that I had an off-the-scale reading of what is known as sperm IGG antibodies. It seems that the researchers were right that the autoimmune response continues even after a reversal, at least in my case, and the cases of a huge percentage of others.

Since I was also still experiencing a lot of epididymal inflammation, I had to assume that there was continued congestion and maybe a rupture, all of which my MRI had shown as possible at this point. Functionally, this still made walking, standing, sleeping, working, etc., a constant and painful challenge that took its toll on me.

My dilemma became this: how do you strengthen your immune system overall when it is under stress and not increase what is an already overactive autoimmune response to sperm cells that a healthy immune system would naturally fight? Selectivity in immune responses was an issue that was not going to be easy to resolve. There was no such thing as an allergy shot for reactions to sperm.

I discussed this information with my acupuncturist. She proposed an interesting form of treatment, the theory for which goes something like this: The antibodies that produce an autoimmune reaction are looking for injured or perceived disease cells to go after and get overzealous in the process. If you add cells to the body like those the antibodies are trying to destroy, the antibodies then attack the added cells, get used up, and leave the good tissues alone, in this case the tender testes tissues, thereby quieting the autoimmune reaction's destructive tendencies on the body's own cells. There's a lot more to the technical aspect of it than that, but hopefully you get the idea.

She gave me a trial of a supplement called Orchex, the primary ingredient of which was Bovine Orchic Cytosol Extract.

I quickly interpreted this, "So, Diane, you want me to take 88 milligrams a day of bull balls?"

That was the idea. Crazy, but desperation makes you do weird things, and the theory sounded good, anyway. This would make substance number 63 that had been put into my body throughout this process, and I had tried numerous things potentially far more damaging than ground up bull testicles. Besides, I'm sure it's a delicacy in some country, somewhere.

It is with that thought that I offer this story to close this chapter: An American tourist went into a Spanish provincial city for dinner, and asked to be served the specialty of the house. When the dish arrived, he asked what kind of meat it contained.

"Sir, these are cojones," the waiter replied.

"They're what, you say?" exclaimed the tourist.

"They are the testicles of the bull killed in the bull fights today," explained the waiter. "They are the delicacy of our country."

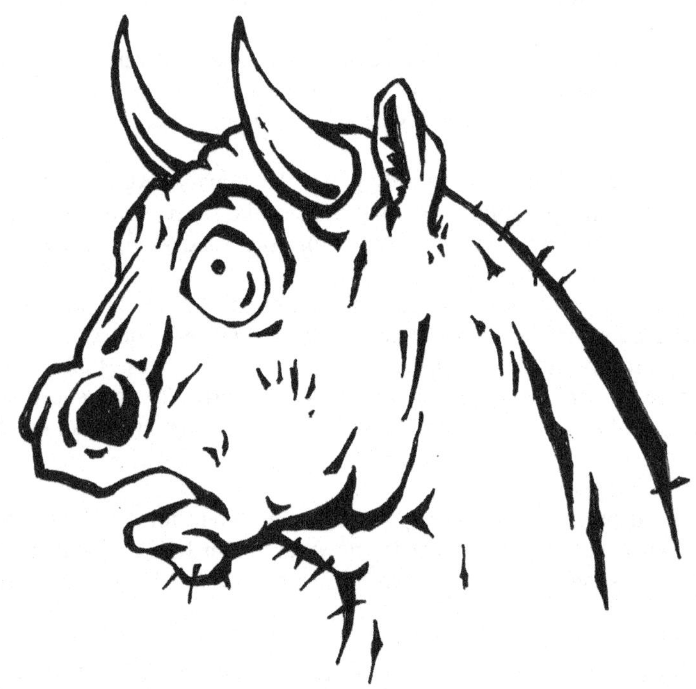

The tourist gulped, but tasted the dish anyway and found it to be delicious. Returning the following evening, he asked for the same dish.

After he finished his meal, the tourist commented to the waiter, "Today's cojones are much smaller than the ones I had yesterday."

"True, sir," said the waiter, "You see, the bull, he does not always lose."

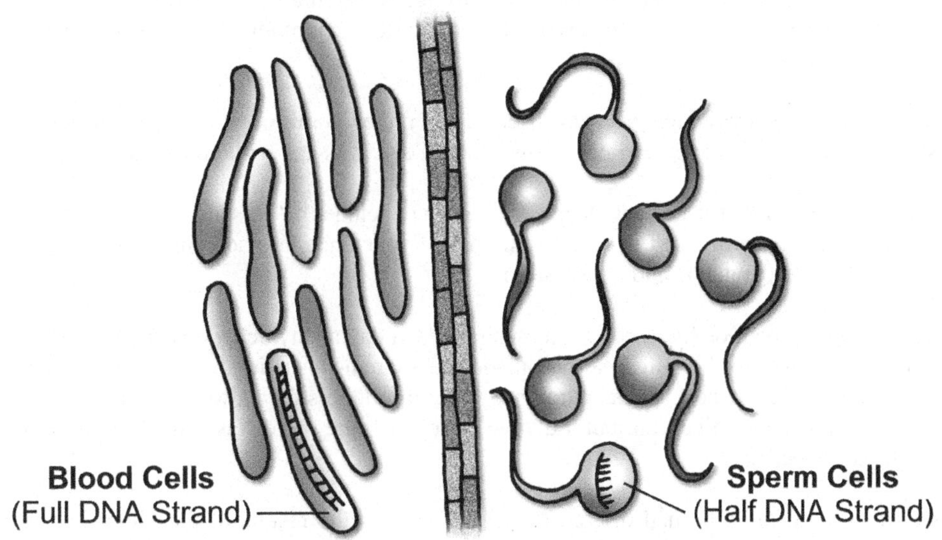

Blood-Testes Barrier Before Vasectomy
(lots of happy little cells where they belong)

Blood-Testes Barrier After Vasectomy

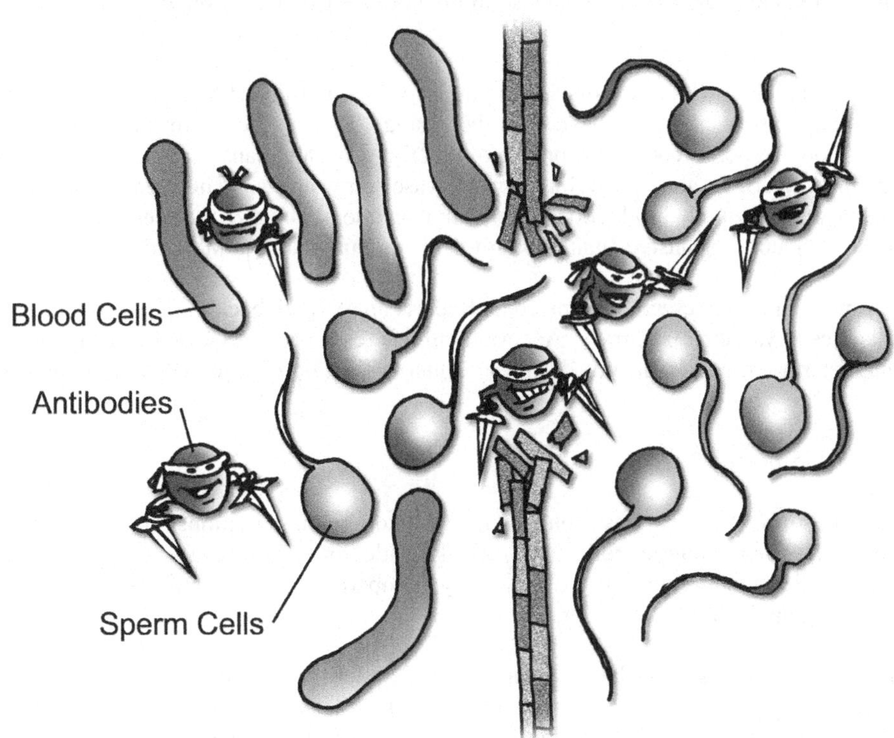

So the picture was becoming clearer to me. Once a man reaches puberty and begins producing sperm cells, his body has formed a natural barrier to keep the sperm cells away from the blood stream and his other tissues. A breach in the barrier causes sperm cells to begin to mix with the blood stream and significant antibody actions begin.

How likely is this to happen? "Vasectomy *does* (emphasis added) result in an immune response to sperm antigens. Sperm and their specific antigens first appear at the time of puberty, long after the immune system has been developed to recognize self and non-self. But the antigens are sequestered behind permeability barriers. Vasectomy results in a breach of these barriers, and an immune response to sperm antigens is initiated" (Kaufman, et. al., 1996). This autoimmune reaction causes inflammation and can cause pain and damage to numerous tissues and organs.

Did you notice that there was no "may happen" in this research article's statement? These reactions will happen, the question is just to what extent the reactions will cause noticeable symptoms. Now I just needed to find the best way to unravel this process for myself.

As I would share my evolving story with friends, when they got through laughing, crying and holding themselves, they would ask, "So, where's the happy ending? How can you end this saga without closure?"

I would assure them that it was my deepest desire to conclude the personal experience aspect of my research and just take testimonials for whatever else I needed to find out. Events thus far had conspired otherwise, leaving me strongly motivated, if not slightly desperate, to find a resolution.

I began taking my beef orchic surprise supplement each day as my acupuncturist had suggested. And each day, I would utter a thankful prayer to the bulls that had made the supreme sacrifice for the benefit of my health. Being born under the sign of Taurus, I felt I had a special empathy. After a little less than a week of this, the aching seemed to let up a notch, not out of the woods yet mind you, but a degree better. Maybe there was something to all this antibody treatment stuff after all, at least I hoped so.

I talked to Phil again, who had offered to help me assess the results of the blood test I had done to check for antisperm antibodies. He felt that looking into treating me for autoimmune orchitis might have some merit at this point. Since I was reluctant to try anti-seizure medication that would act as a general nervous system depressant and mask the nerve pain, he suggested the possibility of some of the immune suppressing medications that were used in the infertility work he did. Evidently, most of these are derived from kidney transplant research, wherein it is very important for the immune system to not have an extreme autoimmune response to the newly introduced kidney tissues and start destroying them. Okay, so far, so good.

In men unable to father children who have low sperm counts or low motility of the sperm they are producing, the problem is due to the type of antibody response we have been discussing. This can be the result of a previous vasectomy that was reversed but the antibody response continues, or due to other injuries and causes. It is commonly accepted that post-reversal sperm counts only return to about two-thirds of pre-vasectomy levels. The medications used by fertility specialists such as Phil will suppress antibody production in general in an attempt to give the sperm a fighting chance, kind of like trying to oust a saboteur. Sounds expensive again, doesn't it? I was sure that I would find out.

Let's go back for a moment to the research in this area. Reports on research back in the 1970's began to document the presence of sperm antibodies in vasectomized men. According to this research as reviewed and summarized by Dr. H. J. Roberts, "The circulating sperm antibodies do not disappear either with time or after vas reanastomosis [vasectomy reversal]."

Sounds like quite a pickle, doesn't it?

It gets even better: "It is of interest that vasectomized men who do not have demonstrable antisperm antibodies in their serum are more likely to show abnormalities reflecting testicular endocrine malfunction.... These pertain to follicle-stimulating hormone (FSH) and lieutenizing hormone (LH) activity "(Roberts, 1993). There's that hormone stuff, again. Surprising how that keeps coming up, isn't it?

My best interpretation of all this was that if your immune system was working correctly, you would have antisperm antibodies after vasectomy and even after a vasectomy reversal. A lack of this type of reaction is an indicator of hormone imbalance that may have far-reaching implications. There is no way to predict how this antibody reaction will affect an individual man, other than to predict the likelihood of some level of reaction. In terms of the effects of these antibodies on the outcome of a vasectomy reversal, "Men with high pre-reversal levels [of antibodies in their blood] would have a low probability of success" (Schwingl, et. al., 2000), that is, a low probability of achieving pregnancy after the surgery.

What is known quite well is how to induce autoimmune orchitis by causing injury to the testicle(s). Numerous research articles speak of inducing "Experimental Autoimmune Orchitis" by causing an artificial trauma to one or both testicles (Sakamoto, et. al., 1995). I wondered about the ethics of such experiments, and was surprised to find they were, in fact, quite common in the literature. For example, researchers have found that by traumatizing one testicle in a subject, autoimmune orchitis (also termed "sympathetic orchiopathia" in this case) will be induced in the other, uninjured testicle within a matter of weeks (Wallace, et. al., 1981). This occurs when antibodies cross the blood-testis barrier, producing an "acute inflammation in the rete testes and epididymis," wherein "antisperm antibody is bound to sperm" within the system (Tung, et. al., 1971). Just to be clear, that is not a good thing and signals the onset of irreversible damage.

Other recent research discusses the autoimmune orchitis response that results from this type of antibody activity, i.e. degeneration of the testicular tissues. Researchers at the University of Virginia and BYU have found that once the "strong blood-testis barrier" is breached, the autoimmune responses will begin. They haven't yet determined how the antibodies act in the degenerative process, but they know there is a relationship: "the precise role of antibody in these autoimmune diseases has not been critically explored. This is an important research problem. Its resolution will influence the future of contraceptive vaccine development… as well as the clarification of the mechanism whereby autoantibody may access ejaculated human spermatozoa to cause infertility (Tung, et. al., 1994)." I wonder if we need a vasectomy vaccine development program to go along with the contraceptive vaccine development.

What is known is that autoimmune orchitis can hurt a lot. Fort example: "Reports of acute orchitis thought to be of autoimmune origin... have been associated with recurrent episodes of acute scrotal swelling and pain. There may be fever and inguinal lymphadenopathy. Unilateral and bilateral [one side and both sides] presentations have been described.... Some cases of autoimmune orchitis may exhibit testicular enlargement first and atrophy [shrinking] thereafter" (Lahita, et. al., 2000).

So what does a guy who has already had a vasectomy do to safeguard his health? The best research I've been able to find says that a man's likelihood of autoimmunity from vasectomy turning into autoimmune orchitis is about one out of four. When other procedures are added to vasectomy, this incidence can go higher. For example: "When vasectomy is added to early thymectomy [removal of the thymus], the risk of autoimmune orchitis increases dramatically from approximately 25% to over 90%, suggesting that local and systemic mechanisms are important in maintaining tolerance [to levels of T cells that react to sperm antigens]" (Lahita, et. al., 2000).

For me, this was turning out to be a perplexing situation with no easy answer. From looking at the statistical data, it appears that men experiencing chronic post-vasectomy testicular pain will most often find relief with a reversal after conservative treatments fail. But most men who have had vasectomies don't want to be fertile again, or to have to undergo major surgery in the process. I can relate to these concerns. They're part of the dilemma. The prospect of unstoppable testicular degeneration was more perplexing yet.

There are those men, like me, who end up with such a convoluted set of complications that it is difficult to determine what to do. What was certain, however, was that the autoimmune reaction I was experiencing was still causing or combining with other symptoms of post-vasectomy pain syndrome to make this situation a real mess. Resolution of this autoimmune reaction seemed to be a top priority, since so many other reactions apparently stem from it. I had the feeling this might be true for others also.

But how? That was the one-hundred-million man question. I was not getting any substantial solutions from my doctors or any of the research I had found thus far. Perhaps this is why so many doctors seemed to clam up or not know about the issue of autoimmune orchitis resulting from vasectomy. It appeared that there was no easy way to deal with this situation and the short-term or long-term effects.

Phil suggested another test, called an immunobead assay, to determine the extent of the antibody reaction I was experiencing before putting me on any other medication. Back to the lab again. I kept telling myself that sooner or later, we had to stumble onto something that would help.

Chapter Seventeen

Here's a Crazy Idea

"Let us begin to get to questions of etiology [cause] so that we can get at the root of these [autoimmune] diseases, rather than being left at the superficial level of just treating the symptoms after the disease has had its destructive effects" (Noel Rose, M.D., American Autoimmune Related Disease Association).

Along this path of mine, I began to wonder why no one had developed a prediction system of post-vasectomy complications since they are apparently so common. After all, there must be some common threads running through all of these maladies that resulted from that simple snip, snip, right? I began asking what seemed like a perfectly logical set of questions.

Is a man's sperm count prior to vasectomy any kind of predictor of the extent to which he might experience a continued inflammatory or immune system response afterwards? After all, it seems simple enough to check for a zero sperm count after a vasectomy. Why not check before to see if there's a correlation to long-term problems? That would guarantee at least two orgasms in the process instead of just one, and who wouldn't go for that?

Later research would prove my hunch correct, as I found that men who have high preoperative sperm counts prior to their vasectomy are more likely to develop "sustained or early high levels of antisperm antibodies" (Schwingl, et. al., 2000). Research showing this particular correlation dates back as far as the 1970's for both animals (Alexander, 1977) and men (Linnet, et. al., 1977), but evidently still isn't important enough to mention at the time of consultation before the procedure. Again, you have to ask yourself why.

How about developing a vaccine for these types of reactions? Actually, that idea has been quite popular as a potential form of contraception in itself, but is also quite problematic. "Contraceptive vaccines to sperm antigens in men might result in an immune response similar to that occurring after vasectomy" (Kaufman, et. al., 1996). Some research had been done in the late 1970's and early 1980's in the area of developing an "antisperm antiserum" to prevent the formation of antibodies after vasectomy.

This all sounded interesting until I found out that in some cases the serum prevented the formation of antibodies following vasectomy, but four out of five of the subjects (Swiss white mice in this case) who had been given high doses of the antisperm antiserum had died during the course of the study (Hofmeyr, et. al., 1984). I'm sure this had the effect of eliminating antibody formation in the deceased subjects, along with all other functions. I got a strong feeling that we were all playing with fire. Dr Robert's comments on the "multiple immunologic responses that occur in the post-vasectomy state" took on a more serious meaning.

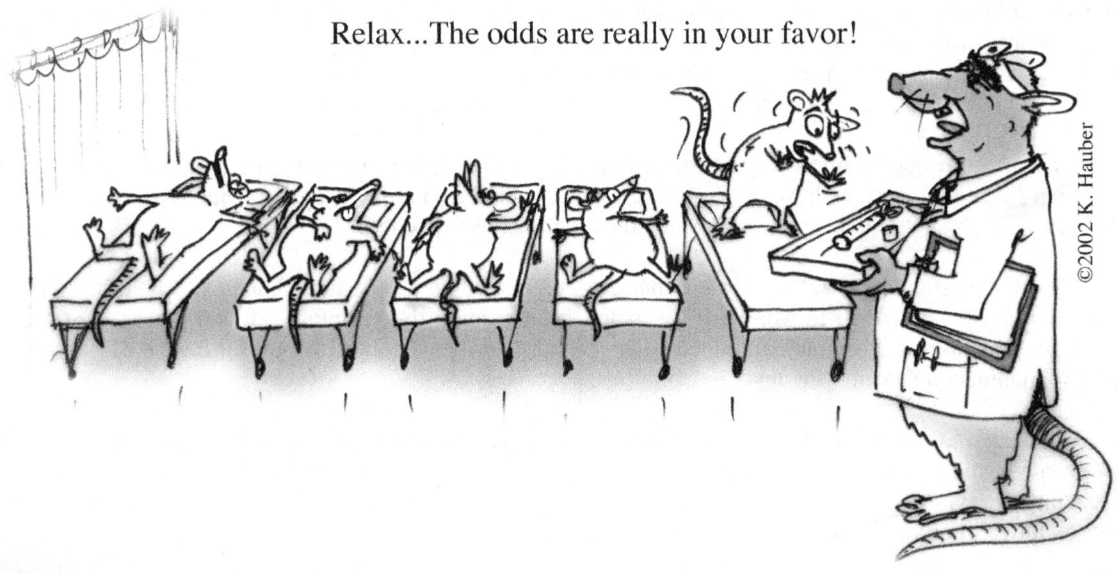

What else is possible? "Studies in my laboratory and in those of my colleagues suggest that vasectomy in animal models and experimentally-induced serum sickness may cause similar changes in several body systems" (Alexander, 1983). Serum sickness occurs when the body starts reacting to circulating foreign particles (like sperm cells) and manifesting numerous negative symptoms. The term "serum sickness," i.e. illness as a result of a vaccine serum, and "immune-complex disease" have been suggested as interchangeable terms.

Another potential downside of the "pre-vasectomy vaccine" idea is the possibility of increased tumor growth. Research by Tung and others has indicated, "Immunologic enhancement of tumor growth could be a major immunopathologic complication of the use of embryonic or sperm antigens in vaccines for contraception" (Anderson, et. al., 1983). Not good.

Later research into development of contraceptive vaccines has had a number of pitfalls. Authors Yee, et. al., (1996) state: "The immunological control of pregnancy is a promising new form of contraception that may be available within the next decade." It's a great idea, right; contraception without surgery. The problem is that researchers have found it quite difficult to come up with a contraceptive vaccine for men or women that does not cause a significant autoimmune response.

What are some examples of the pitfalls, for instance? Well, in one of the experiments discussed by Yee, et. al., (1996), one of the enzymes that was a candidate for a contraceptive vaccine was used to immunize male mice. Of these subjects, 43.8% developed autoimmune orchitis. You remember autoimmune orchitis, it's that nasty degenerative disease of the testicles that occurs after vasectomy. The other major pitfall has been that the contraceptive value of most of the enzymes and antigens tested has been significantly less than that of using a condom or other currently available methods of birth control, even when autoimmune responses are elicited.

Yee, et. al., (1996) outline some sensible basic criteria for what a contraceptive must do, and not do, to be effective: "The initial step is to determine the appropriate antigen for immunization. In addition to the requirements for an antigen that is specific to sperm and nonautoimmunogenic, identifying an antigen that will elicit an immune response that is fully effective for the great majority of participants is critical to the success of a vaccination program." In other words, not only does a contraceptive vaccine need to be effective, but it needs to be safe, i.e. it must not create an autoimmune response in the body, especially if the autoimmune response is irreversible.

Are you beginning to see the same double standard that I am? On one hand it is perfectly OK in the eyes of the medical community to do an invasive procedure on millions of men that has a high likelihood of creating a life-long autoimmune response with untold results. On the other hand, if we are to develop a contraceptive vaccine, it needs to not create an autoimmune reaction if it to be considered safe. Why doesn't this add up? I ask too many questions, don't I?

What about checking hormone levels beforehand as an indicator? How about all these immune system responses? Is there a common predisposition in the immune system of men who have a more severe reaction? Or, alternately, does a naturally strong immune system lead to a higher likelihood of a more severe autoimmune response? "It may be that non-responders [those who don't produce antisperm antibodies after vasectomy] have a genetically programmed low immunological response to sperm antigens. The precise antigens involved in the immune response are still poorly defined" (Schwingl, et. al., 2000). Isn't it worth trying to quantify the reasons behind these observed reactions?

What about trying to find many of the disappearing patients whose results never seemed to get quantified very well? I didn't receive a very enthusiastic response when I started asking these types of questions. I think I was delving into that "dirty little secrets" area again. Maybe another approach was needed.

Then I started thinking again. I know that gets me in trouble all the time, but I can't help it. With all this talk about causal relationships, I had to wonder if we hadn't been treating the symptoms all along instead of the cause. The inflammation, granulomas, cysts, autoimmune response, and epididymal ruptures were all results of one thing: my body continued to manufacture sperm after my vasectomy(ies).

So I began to wonder; if I could stop sperm production, that might reduce or eliminate the other responses and allow for some healing. Then I could have the doctor(s) repair whatever was in need of repair without it blowing out again and reenacting the Battle of the Bulge. This seemed like a plausible idea, but how to do this without removing several of my favorite, albeit troubled, glands?

I happened across another Internet article on a new form of male contraception recently tested by the World Health Organization in numerous trials; good old testosterone. It seems that when you raise the body's testosterone level enough, the pituitary gland thinks the testicles have made enough sperm already as part of that negative feedback cycle we discussed, and adjusts the other hormones to stop sperm production. This is being tested as the male version of the pill, and is claimed to be 99% effective (CNN, 1996). I was already aware of the potential negative effects of long-term testosterone therapy, but I wondered if short-term use might help in this situation. I proposed this idea to Phil, being the fertility specialist that he is, thinking that he might want to try a little fertility work in reverse. That, or he was going to laugh me out of his office upon my next visit.

By now I felt like I was earning my Ph.v degree, doctorate of vasectology that is, what with all the complications, variations on surgeries, and research I was encountering in this little medical sojourn of mine. My internist said I was ready for medical school. Something had to work. I wasn't sure what it was yet, but something had to work.

Everyone was developing an opinion as to what would help my situation. Some wholeheartedly recommended frequent masturbation as the answer to my dilemma. I doubted that this would produce a perfect solution. Please pardon the pun, I just couldn't resist.

Others thought that marijuana was the answer to the pain aspect of the problem. Other than revealing what several of my friends did with a lot of their time in the sixties, this didn't offer much for me either. In my brief attempts at being a pothead earlier in life (I never inhaled, of course) I found myself to be even more useless afterwards than I was now with chronic pain. Besides, now I had kids and that's a hard double standard to explain.

Ironically enough, I decided to seek some further medical opinions about what to do instead of getting out the Vaseline and the rolling papers. My first stop was with a neurologist. After reviewing the medical records with her, I became a little anxious when she pulled out another one of those damned safety pins. What was it with these people? I kept my pants firmly fastened this time, however, and she was only inclined to jab me repeatedly in the back and legs.

This being done, she pronounced that my chronic pain syndrome might never go away, and the best I could plan for was to adapt to what might be a lifelong condition and compensate as best as possible. This was cheery news. According to her, physical therapy might help the back and neck pain I was experiencing, but my best plan was to begin a year or so of various antidepressants to try to control some of the results of the pain. I found the notion of a year of antidepressants to be depressing. Of course there were surgical options also, she added. Thanks for your opinion, doc, I'll try the physical therapy and get back to you on the rest later, probably much later.

I went to see my new urologist next. He thought the idea of testosterone or other hormone therapy had merit, and set me up to have more bodily fluids taken from me once again to start the process of establishing a base level. He didn't have any experience in this particular type of therapy, but could help me do the groundwork. He added that if everything else failed, I could always have my epididymis removed. More surgery still felt like a last resort that could leave me up a creek without a vas, or testicles for that matter.

My next stop was to see an immunologist. This seemed like a likely suspect to deal with what I was experiencing, and in fact I was right. It turned out that the immunologist had considered a vasectomy previously in trying to decide what to do about long-term contraception for himself and his wife. He decided against it though, knowing the possible ramifications on the immune system could be substantial from the retention of all those sperm cells. He had also wondered about the autoimmune responses relative to some family medical history issues for himself.

He had never dealt with a case like mine, but was willing to try. In fact, it reminded him of a friend of his who had experienced a lot of pain since his vasectomy three or four years earlier. Add the friend to the growing list.

Hormone therapy to reduce sperm production and try to let my system heal sounded like a good idea to the immunologist, but short-term was better than long-term due to the potential negative long-term effects of testosterone therapy. Immune system depressing drugs were a less desirable choice according to him because of the incidence of other diseases including various cancers after their use. That could certainly be problematic. The idea of depressing the immune system to lessen autoimmune responses to vasectomy had been tried successfully on monkeys back in the 80's (Curtis, et. al., 1982), but I could find no data on trials for humans. Also, the Curtis, et. al., (1982) study made no mention of increases in long-term incidence of other immune related diseases, or lack thereof, leaving that whole issue to speculation.

He also suggested that several testosterone derivatives might be more suitable and less reactive than regular testosterone. Less reactive worked for me, and we agreed to pursue the matter in conjunction with an internist we both knew who had done a lot of endocrinology work. This had the makings of a plan. According to the immunologist, if the testosterone therapy failed we could always try a course of corticosteroids like Prednisone.

Had I told him about my last experience with Prednisone that left me looking for an AK-47 and a clock tower from which to use it? No, I hadn't told him about that yet, but it was useful information. Low doses might be appropriate he thought. Let's see about Mr. T first, I thought.

Chapter Eighteen

Do You Smoke After Sex?

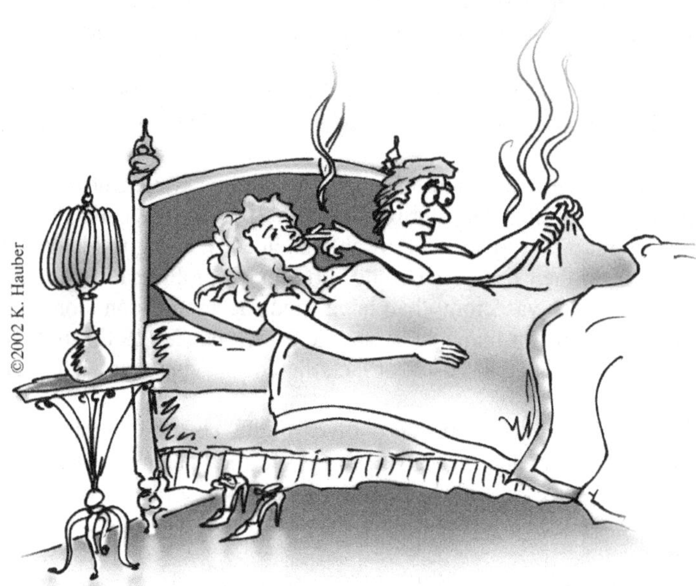

Remember that old joke? The answer of course is, "I don't know, I never looked."   The urologist's corollary to this is, "Do your patients have problems after their vasectomies?" Unfortunately, the answer is often the same; "I don't know, I never looked," or possibly, "I don't want to look."

From the patient's perspective I understand the feeling of not wanting to go back to your urologist, or have anything to do with the breed at all. When you've had problems after a vasectomy the last thing you want to have done is to have someone mash on your aching testicles, which urologists are wont to do quite often. Just making the call to the receptionist for an appointment can feel like a major hurdle.

As a matter of fact, one of the themes that I continually saw in the study literature attempting to quantify post-vasectomy data was a low response rate from previous patients. One has to wonder how much of this was due to problems with upkeep of records or people moving, and how much was due to not wanting to have any further contact between medical science and one's genitals. I had felt that sort of resistance several times throughout my process, and I know of others who felt the same, and I don't blame them a bit.

One study tried to assess these reactions of patients and found some interesting reasons. "Information from 70 men…gave some indication of the reasons, often multiple, for incomplete or non-compliance; these included embarrassment, ambiguous feelings about having more children, inadequate understanding of reproductive physiology and blind faith in the surgeon (Thompson, et. al., 1991)." In another study of 1892 patients, only 3% completed the post-vasectomy instructions for an annual semen analysis (Maatman, et. al., 1997). These are all very human responses to a stressful, sexually-oriented subject.

It would also be a very human response for doctors to not want to look at how much went wrong with the vasectomies they had performed, or to attribute problems to other causes. Even if a doctor was interested in knowing more exact results in terms of complications, this effort can be foiled because "these complications are not necessarily observed by the surgeon, for adverse events can occur months, or even years after a vasectomy is performed. Methods differ, and surgeons may regard their technique and outcomes as satisfactory, but as noted by Peterson and colleagues, definitions of adverse effects are often lacking, with the result that comparisons cannot be made" (Alderman, 1991).

All of these considerations gave me the notion that some type of survey was needed to get a more realistic idea of the true complications and results of all this snipping. The notion that a survey on the Internet might work came to mind. After all, if you are aiming at a target market of guys who are generally well educated and higher income earners, chances are, you might find them online. It would be fascinating to get feedback directly from the horse's mouth, so to speak, about the experience and the long-term results. More on this idea later.

Even when you ask the doctors, and not the patients, you will find higher complication rates. A 1991 study by Alderman in the Journal of Family Practice found an overall complication rate of 10.6%, much higher than the other claims of 2-3% from many sources. There appears to be a growing gap between the advertised promise and actual satisfaction with the delivered product when it comes to vasectomy.

I actually wrote to the AVSC, the Association for Voluntary Surgical Contraception, which acts as a trade organization for the sterilization industry, and asked for information on how the statistics for vasectomy complications were derived and what the specific incidence of a number of complications is claimed to be. A letter came back with a number of brochures on vasectomy attempting to reassure me how safe the procedure was. No direct answers were offered to my direct questions. Perhaps I didn't make myself clear? Or, maybe, there was an attempt to avoid the issue.

According to Dr. Malcolm Carruthers (1997), "Unlike any other operation, however minor, no general medical examination is done beforehand, no central records are kept of how many operations have been performed and counseling is limited to the fact that it is irreversible so be sure you want it done. No inquiries are made about previous histories of mumps or other infections which may damage the testes, or of relevant family histories of heart disease, high blood pressure or diabetes. Any questions about what happens to the sperm are brushed aside with facile answers such as 'They are just absorbed'." This all sounds really familiar.

Dr. Carruthers also observed that "most of the research studies on human vasectomy are unfortunately relatively short term, lasting only two to five years and ceasing before the complications I see 10 to 15 years later arise."

When doctors have been willing to report the complication rates from vasectomy, the results have varied widely. For example, Campbell's Urology (1992), a commonly used textbook for urology students, characterizes complication rates as follows: "Hematoma is the most common complication of vasectomy, with an average incidence of 0.09 to 29 per cent. Infection is surprisingly common with an average rate of 3.4 per cent, but several series report rates from one to 38 per cent.... Long-term effects of vasectomy include vasitis nodosa[chronic inflammation of the vas defrens], chronic testicular pain, testicular function alterations, and epididymal obstruction, and the postulated effect of vasectomy on the cardiovascular system.... Vasitis nodosa has been reported in up to 66 percent of vasectomy specimens in men undergoing vasectomy reversals.... Vasectomy results in violation of the blood-testis barrier producing detectable levels of serum antisperm antibodies in 60 to 80 per cent of men...." Are you noting the growing disparity between the marketing department's claims and the results actually experienced?

There did turn out to be some medical research data that assessed the patient's experience from the patient's point of view. One study by researchers published in the *Journal of Urology* found that only 38.7% of the patients returned the surveys, which consisted of 154 questions; a bit daunting perhaps. It is interesting to note that chronic scrotal pain that lasted an average of five years was the most common complaint in this survey's results (Choe, et. al., 1996). That is a long time to endure chronic scrotal pain, folks.

Actually, these researchers divided the complications studied into early and late categories, i.e. those immediately following surgery and those complication with onset months or years later. The leading early complication was bleeding and hematoma at 12.6%, followed by superficial infection (3.3%) and wound separation (1.1%). Late complications led off with good old chronic scrotal pain at 18.7% (that's nearly one in five men, incidentally), followed by epididymitis at 6.6%, spermatocele (cysts) at 1.6%, and hydroceles (another kind of cyst) at 1.1%. I was amazed at how many of the odds I had beat in experiencing as many of these complications as I already had.

It is notable that this Choe, et. al., (1996) study has been criticized for its findings by certain detractors because the response ratio was so low, saying that those who didn't respond could have been so satisfied that they felt no need to participate. Observing how reluctant most men are to reveal any problem they are having with the function of their genital equipment, I would think exactly the opposite, but let's examine this notion for a moment. If all of the non-responding patients were completely satisfied and had no complications whatsoever, then there would still be 7.2% of the total study population experiencing chronic pain after vasectomy. That's still a lot of sore balls when you extrapolate these results out to the 50 to 100 million vasectomy procedures already done.

How did the men surveyed rate their long-term satisfaction with vasectomy? Of the total population studied, 9.3% were dissatisfied, while another 19.3% were undecided. Chronic pain was the most commonly cited reason for regretting the decision to undergo vasectomy, followed by concerns regarding the possibility of prostate cancer, the incidence of which was not included in this study. I think I can relate to these concerns, knowing what I do now.

Why would these results show so much higher incidence of problems than others had shown? For one thing, according to the researchers, "Chronic scrotal pain is a late complication of vasectomy. Previous series reporting post-vasectomy complications did not mention chronic scrotal pain." It is surprising what you find when you look, ask the right questions, and then look again later.

Another study that followed men for an average of 19 months reported that 27.2% of patients had some pain in the testicles following vasectomy. In 19% of those cases of pain, symptoms persisted for longer than three months. Of the men with persistent pain, 31% needed painkillers for relief. The source of this type of pain is not fully understood, although many physicians believe that in most cases pinched or entrapped nerves probably contribute substantially to the pain (Simon, et. al., 1998).

This is a heck of a pinch when it happens. The pinch was so bad, in fact, that 17 of the patients in the study chose to have the nerves surgically stripped from their spermatic cords rather than continue to endure the pain (Ahmed, et. al., 1997). Speaking of nerves and smoking after sex, most sources will claim that a vasectomy will improve your sex life, as the ad shown near the beginning of this book does. Significant genital pain changes how you feel about having sex. I can make personal testimony to this fact. This is especially true when there has been a nerve injury in the region where the vasectomy is done. It has been noted that, "This operation can damage certain nerves near the vas that are necessary for proper ejaculation" (Roberts, 1993). I don't think I need to describe what this might feel like. Use your imagination. We'll talk more about the nerve subject later, too.

"One recent study suggests that sexual satisfaction among men may be lower after vasectomy" (Sandlow, et. al., 2001). Can you see some reasons now why this might be true? In my case I am beginning to forget what sexual satisfaction is like, since sex has become more of an exercise in pain management than anything else.

So, after looking at all of the data available, where did that low 2-3% complication rate all those doctors were claiming go to? Right out the window. I liken the process of getting accurate information for the average patient contemplating vasectomy to that of going to a car dealer and asking if the make of cars he carries is a good one. What do you expect the car dealer to say? And what do you expect your urologist to say, especially when he has a legal liability in the matter in addition to financial self-interest?

Chapter Nineteen

What is This Doing to My Brain?

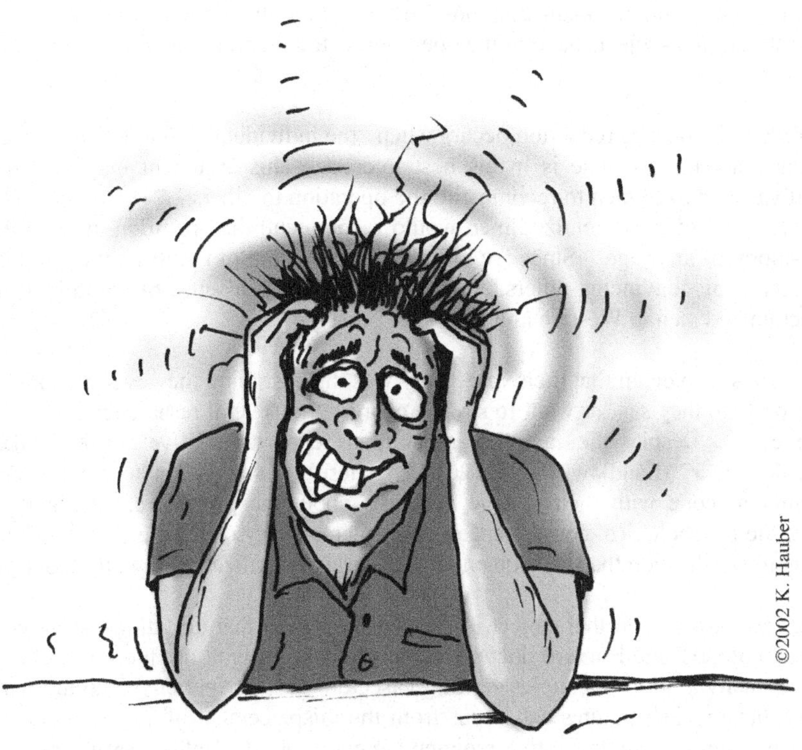

"The removal of his ability to produce the young (or impregnate the mate) he still unconsciously acts to protect must inevitably affect all men on some level, no matter how deeply unconscious" (Wolfers, 1970).

"Most important questions about the psychological effects of vasectomy remain unanswered because of various methodological defects in the published research" (Wiest, et. al., 1974).

"Postoperative increases in coital frequency [that means how often you have sex] – as likely to be a sign of potency anxiety as increased libido – are waived aloft like ball game scores" (Wolfers, 1973).

Hmm.   These statements bring up a few questions, don't they?   I seem to remember hearing the term "methodological defects" before relative to research regarding vasectomies.   Maybe there is some digging to do here also. So let's take a few moments to discuss the "deeply unconscious" psychological aspects of vasectomies.

So far, I have spent a lot of time describing the physical aspects of what can happen, but the mental aspects can be just as significant.   As with many other aspects of vasectomies, the psychological and emotional ramifications of the procedure have been studied for a long time with varying results, often depending on what the researchers were looking for. Since the word "sterilization" tends to bring an emotionally charged response for most people, this deserves examination, without mashing on sore parts this time.

Here's a discussion starter: "A study of vasectomy patients and their wives by Dr. Frederick Zeigler found 'striking adverse changes and reduced marital satisfaction in husband and wife notwithstanding general satisfaction with the procedure itself'" (Bower, 1995). Why would there be adverse changes, you might ask? I know I wondered.

It turns out that Dr. Ziegler, et. al., (way back in 1966) "Confirmed the paradoxical finding that expressed satisfaction with the operation can be concurrent with adverse changes in psychological function." Translation, if you please? This occurs because "vasectomy characteristically poses a threat or challenge to a man's sense of masculinity," leading to a situation in which "high enthusiasm for vasectomy [by the patient and spouse] concurrent with adverse changes is an example of 'dissonance reduction,' in which persons making a difficult decision tend to reassure themselves about it by focusing primarily on the favorable manifestations and ignoring the unfavorable ones." Ziegler, et. al., (1966) concluded that "the investment the subjects have in the operation is too great to allow themselves to have self-doubts about it." Wow!

Stated another way, dissonance reduction occurs when "the individual having taken an irrevocable step has a need to convince himself that what he has done is in his best interest. This argument may also throw some light on the widespread readiness of vasectomized men to recommend the operation to others...." (Wolfers, 1970). This author goes on to note that in one study, "99% of [vasectomized]men would recommend the operation, despite the fact that 5% reported deterioration in the 'harmony of marriage.' Since we look for confirmation of reality in the opinions of others, the need to convince ourselves is served by convincing others. Furthermore, there is a sense of comfort in numbers, and there may well be a need for vasectomized men in Western countries... to proselytize."

So many of the guys who claim that their vasectomy was the best thing they ever did and they've had no ill effects might have more going on than they say, or want to say? According to several researchers, there is more to the story here than meets the naked eye. "Despite the fact that most men report a positive result of their vasectomy, adverse psychological changes do occur" (Sandlow, et. al., 2001). These authors go on to state: "Most men express verbal satisfaction as an attempt to cope with their private concerns about the procedure...and many men experience some difficulty in adjusting to the psychological consequences, and this may vary over time.... It has been shown that men have more difficulty adjusting to sterilization than do women who undergo a sterilization, usually tubal ligation."

What do others have to say on the subject of the psychological manifestations of vasectomy? One of the best summaries is from a group of MIT and Harvard doctors which offers an insight into the sense of urgency that can surround having a vasectomy. "As many as 40% of couples seeking vasectomy have experienced failure with their previous method of nonpermanent birth control. Such failures can occur from the misplacement of a diaphragm, an incorrectly implanted IUD, or noncompliance with an oral contraceptive regimen" (Simon, et. al., 1998). Seems like all it takes is one or two "whoops" pregnancies to have a sense of desperation set in.

The report also discusses the psychological and emotional factors involved. "Some studies have indicated that men with poor self-images, including concerns for their own physical health or sexual ability, are likely to have a difficult time adjusting psychologically to vasectomy. Men who have the operation only for the sake of their partner's health and not because they want the procedure for their own reasons may also have difficulties. Such thoughts on the part of either partner can have devastating consequences on a relationship if they surface only after the procedure has been performed. Openness with each other is imperative in order to make a decision that is clear of any hidden negative apprehensions" (Simon, et. al., 1998).

What might those "hidden negative apprehensions" be? The authors of Simon, et. al., (1998) answer that question in this way: "...it is extremely important for each partner to be as open as possible about any negative feelings they might associate with the procedure. For instance, a woman might believe - incorrectly - that a vasectomy is emasculating, but she might not want to express this idea to her partner. On the other hand, some women may fear that vasectomy may make their partner more attractive to other women and encourage outside affairs."

Other researchers have come up with similar concerns, concluding that data gathered in surveys does not always tell the true depth of impacts the procedure may have. Wolfers, (1970) noted research claiming that "Psychic and emotional effects of vasectomy are much greater than an analysis of such factors as the 'effect on libido,' 'postorgasmal symptoms,' and 'frequency of intercourse' would indicate...." and that "making a man 'safe sexually' (a revealingly aggressive equivalent for infertility) has often resulted in marital infidelity, domestic discord, separation, and divorce." It sounds to me as if nearly all of society's ills are to be attributed to vasectomy, at least according to this research.

Even more shocking is this assessment by Wolfers, (1970): "Sterilizing operations are *never* performed merely as contraceptive measures.... Vasectomy, though often requested as a contraceptive measure, seldom is. It is rather a means for emotionally sick women to castrate their husbands.... The unconscious equating of vasectomy with castration may nevertheless be an unavoidable reality.... The vasectomized man is seen as emasculated...." Wow, again! If this doesn't bring out some really base fears and reactions, nothing will.

Personally, I find it hard to believe that millions of wives are "emotionally sick" and seeking vengeance on their husbands in this Bobbit-esque manner. But one must recognize the fears associated with castration anxiety for men and the natural apprehensions anyone, male or female, has about genital surgery. Coercion is not uncommon, and can come into play. While less aggressive than subversive castration attempts, this is still an indication of problems in the relationship that need to be faced.

According to Dr. Arnold Belker, couples need to be in complete agreement about the procedure: "My first question to a couple sitting across from me is, 'Whose idea was this?'... I have heard a woman say, 'I told him to get this done or don't come near me.' I recommended that they get counseling, not a vasectomy" (Kelleher, 2002). I have received correspondence from numerous men complaining of this type of situation repeatedly.

It's not that men are immune to try some coercive behavior either. Some men "treat the vasectomy as a highly valued pawn in a sub rosa bargaining procedure, so that they reacted postoperatively as though they had made a great sacrifice for the marriage and no longer needed to be so considerate of their wives" (Wolfers, 1970). This notion that the one who makes the physical sacrifices is entitled to certain rewards is a complex psychological issue.

My guess is that these processes may be at work, but often at the unconscious level. This gives rise to yet another factor. Wolfers, (1970) goes on to note that a "still unexplored area [of vasectomy] concerns the stress that may be involved in... the performance of a surgical procedure on one person (husband) for the benefit of another (wife)." These stresses may be exerted on either partner. For example, many people have unthinkingly asked my wife if she feels guilty for my having underwent a vasectomy with the results I experienced. How would we have known?

So what are guy's specific concerns? Ferber, et. al., (1967) adds these to the list of negative apprehensions: "(1) the same sort of feeling one would have before any operation; (2) concern about the effects of the operation on their psychosexual status (e.g., 'I would feel less of a man,' 'it might injure my manhood,' 'it would make me impotent or curb any sexual desire'); (3) projection of fear onto the wife (e.g., 'my wife might leave me because I could no longer have kids'); (4) realistic anxieties about a childless future – especially in connection with the possibility of remarriage; and (5) religious scruples."

These apprehensions may be particularly strong in relation to what men believe others to think or feel about the man having a vasectomy. When asked whether they cared that others knew they had underwent vasectomy, Ferber, et. al., (1967) found that "many subjects flinched and showed tension when asked – even those who said they didn't care. It seems clear that most men assume a loss of status attendant upon sterilization, and while willing to deal with their own internal self-critique, were reluctant to face the disapproval of others. Some of the reported reactions of persons told about the vasectomy were: 'People think it's a form of castration and affects potency.' 'My brother-in-law thought it unmanly. My catholic friends said, 'How could you?'' 'My brother said, 'If I had one, I'd turn into a fairy. In a few years, I wouldn't have any organs left.''" Apparently, even immature and uninformed reactions such as these can cut even deeper than the surgery itself.

Simon, et. al., (1998) take this point further. These doctors from Harvard and MIT go on to say that many men keep their vasectomy secret because they "may believe that the operation is tainted by the stigma of emasculation and knowledge of it [by others] would degrade them in the eyes of their friends and family.... In a few men...problems of poor self-image persist and require counseling. Some men experience depressed and angry emotions similar to mourning over the loss of their reproductive ability.... Their emotional distress most often manifests itself in sexual dysfunction, such as impotence, premature ejaculation, or painful intercourse."

Speaking of subjects such as impotence, a number of studies have attempted to quantify the effects of vasectomy in this delicate area. Some studies attribute impotence after vasectomy to psychological factors (Buchholz, et. al., 1994). Other doctors attribute increased incidence of impotence to hormonal factors in addition to the psychological factors at work.

This is summarized as being part of a male menopause phenomenon related to vasectomy by Dr. Malcolm Carruthers (1997): "Vasectomy makes it more likely that a man will develop the male menopause, and at an earlier age. In a series of over 1,000 cases of the condition...over the past 10 years, 25% had had a vasectomy, about twice the level in the general population. In our global web survey, 35% of men who complete the Andropause Check List reported vasectomy, and at impotence clinics in Australia the rate was reported as 45%."

Here's another big one. "We feel vasectomy does stimulate infantile fears and fantasies of castration, impotence, and concomitant decline in self-esteem.... Most of these men, we feel, successfully cope with these fantasies stimulated by the operation and do not develop overt psychosexual pathology. However, some men fail to cope with their fantasies, and present cases where psychosexual difficulties are traced to and blamed on vasectomy" (Ferber, et. al., 1967).

How many men are experiencing psychological problems as a result of their vasectomies? Again, it depends on who you ask. In Wolfers (1970) study, 12% of vasectomized who were interviewed by psychological professionals following their procedures "signaled some psychological problem arising from the operation, compared with previous findings of 1-3% in pure questionnaire surveys." This raises the ever-relevant question of the motivation of those collecting and assessing the data in any study. I'm reminded of the marked difference in the incidence of chronic pain and other problems reported by doctors who perform vasectomy procedures, being compensated for same, compared to the men on the receiving end who have to live with the results.

"Studies indicate that between 5% and 10% of men have regrets after vasectomy, that men should not make the decision frivolously. Vasectomies may not be right for those who are unsure about having children in the future, whose current relationships are unstable or going through a stressful phase, who are considering the operation just to please their partners, or who are counting on having children later on by storing sperm or surgical reversal of their vasectomies" (Simon, et. al., 1998).

Indeed, another study proved this point when of 860 men who attended a private infertility clinic, 80 were there because of vasectomy-related infertility. Of those 80 men, 91% wanted to have children because of a remarriage. It had been an average of nine years since their vasectomies (Jequier, 1998). This study went on to emphasize the need for up front counseling in this regard due to the pain, expense, and uncertainty involved in trying to conceive after a vasectomy.

According to Simon, et. al., (1998), one should examine "whether recent changes or stresses (an illness, temporary financial crisis, death in the family, or birth of a child) rather than rational, long-term consideration, are influencing a decision about permanent contraception. Vasectomy should not be thought of as a way to cope with short-term problems. Experts recommend that couples wait for a while if they face such situations or that they seek marriage counseling or psychotherapy to be sure that they are not making a decision they will regret later."

Why not just open an account and make a small deposit at the local sperm bank? This might be a good insurance policy if a child was to die or a man was to remarry, right? Well, for one when I asked this question several years ago, I was told the samples don't stay viable for more than a couple of years. Beyond this, "Experts believe that a patient who wants to bank sperm should probably reconsider his decision to have a vasectomy, because such a concern may indicate doubts about giving up his ability to father a child" (Simon, et. al., 1998).

Still want to give vasectomy a try?

What have other studies shown in regard to the psychological effects of vasectomy? "A standard personality disorder test revealed that over 40% of a vasectomy study group experienced personality disturbances between their first testing and that of a year after the operation" (Bower, 1995). All those old jokes and euphemisms about the little head thinking for the big head may have more truth to them than we all want to admit, huh guys?

Of 200 men studied and surveyed by Dias (1983), 56% experienced changes in sexual behavior following their vasectomies. These changes included (in descending order of frequency) decreased sexual desire, decreased frequency of intercourse, poor erections, less intense sensations, more intense sensations, early ejaculation, taking a long time to climax, orgasms with no feeling, and poor lubrication. Was this all in their heads? In regard to behavioral changes, there is research which indicates that "changes related to masculinity tended to result from and not precede the vasectomy" (Sandlow, et. al., 2001). So what is all that false bravado about anyway?

Psychological and physical stress due to vasectomy is not limited to men. Remember, vasectomy is usually performed on men who are in a committed relationship. I like the summary of this notion by W. F. Hendry (1995): "In the complex, rather fragile relationships that exist between men and women, reproduction plays a pivotal role – not only for the self esteem and confidence of the man, but also in the dreams and expectations of the woman. In marriage, initial happiness can turn to sadness and disillusionment if the man's sexual function is impaired or damaged." That pretty well sums it up.

"Other post-sterilization variables among men include decreased feelings of masculinity and concerns about complication or pain after surgery.... Regret is also common among men who find themselves in a new relationship after a separation, divorce, or death of a spouse and for whom desire for children exists in a new relationship" (Sandlow, et. al., 2001). For these and other reasons stated previously, Wolfers (1970) recommends that "histories of pre-existing marital, sexual or psychological instability should be taken as a contraindication [that means don't do it] to vasectomy...." noting that "vasectomy has been instrumental in initiating the sexual and psychological damage" for certain couples.

Most men in developed countries who consider vasectomy do so on a voluntary basis, maybe with some of that loving encouragement and often with some of the high anxiety we discussed previously. The psychological results can be devastating though, when a man is somehow coerced or "persuaded" into undergoing the procedure. Studies in many developing countries have shown high dissatisfaction rates with vasectomy from the patients. For example, "one study in rural Bangladesh found that landless laborers with no previous history of contraceptive use were most likely to accept vasectomy under the conditions operating there at the time ["Recruiters" were employed to persuade men to accept the surgery and incentives were offered]. Half the study population regretted the surgery while among those recruited the rate of regret was almost 95%" (Frances et. al., 1983). Many of the subjects in this study reported numerous physical and psychological ramifications from their vasectomies, as one might expect after being sterilized against one's will.

What I can tell you from my experience is the chronic pain that can result from vasectomies will cause you a significant psychological challenge. This is a challenge that just about anyone is ill prepared for. It is difficult to describe the mental energy required to endure chronic pain, but anyone who has endured it will understand. It took months for me to learn how to be reasonably functional while still experiencing pain. Then I needed to make peace with the fact that there were many times that I was able to do nothing else but breath into the pain I was feeling and let everything else go.

Then there is the effect that occurs when everyone has had enough of you and your "little problem." "Because the symptoms and emotions associated with trauma can be extreme, most of us (and those close to us) will recoil and attempt to repress these intense reactions. Unfortunately, this mutual denial can prevent us from healing. In our culture, there is a lack of tolerance for the emotional vulnerability that traumatized people experience. Little time is allotted for working through emotional events. We are routinely pressured into adjusting too quickly in the aftermath of an overwhelming situation.

"Denial is so common in our culture that it has become a cliché. How often have you heard these words? 'Pull yourself together, it's over now. You should forget about it. Grin and bear it. It's time to get on with your life.'" (Levine, 1997). I have heard these statements a lot from many well-meaning individuals who have no idea of what a chronic pain experience is like. I have found that it takes a lot of fortitude to honor what your body is telling you is needed, and just to let everyone else's opinions be just that, their opinions. This is one of the more challenging aspects that can and will need to be faced by anyone in similar circumstances.

One final thought: Wolfers (1970) observed that many try to justify the use of vasectomy because "the 'birthquake' is the greatest problem facing the world today and that dwelling on reports of possible psychological ill effects of so valuable a contraceptive procedure is not justifiable in the face of such an enormous human calamity." Such arguments "are not valid," according to Wolfers, "even if acceptable on ethical grounds." One has to wonder how a proponent of mass sterilization would feel if the "ill effects" of the procedure were affecting him or one of his loved ones.

Chapter Twenty

Just Cut It Out!

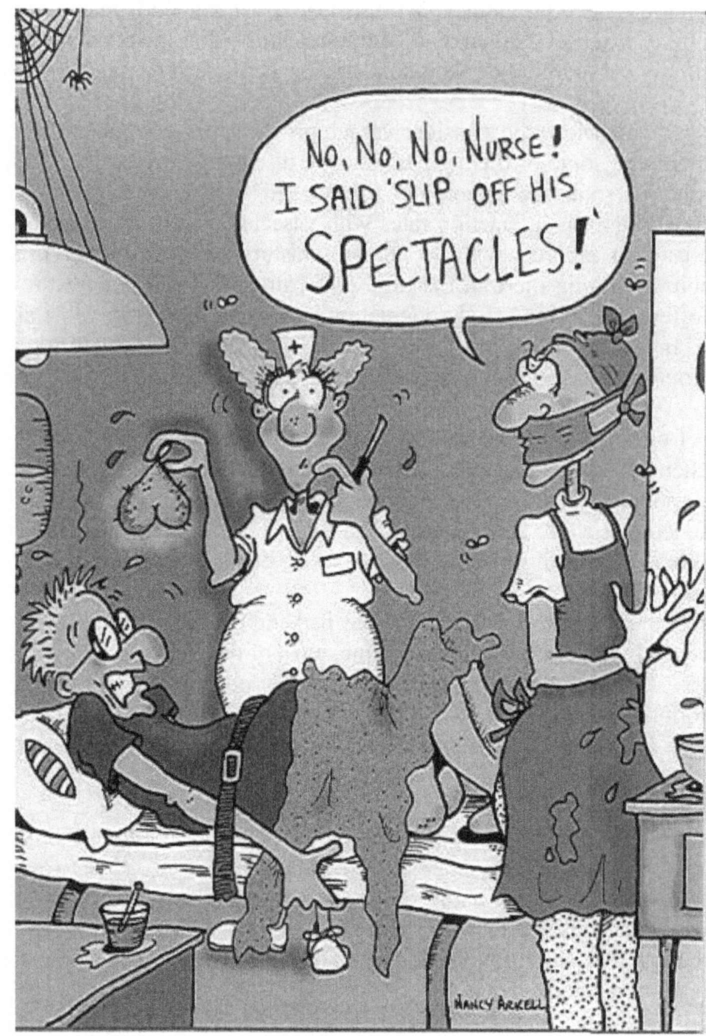

As the months went by, occasionally someone would ask me if I had considered having my beleaguered equipment removed to cut my losses, so to speak. I actually considered this more than once myself beyond the times that the doctors kept offering it as an option like a waitress offers appetizers (turkey nuts?). Finally, I asked my new urologist about this, since I was receiving honest and relatively complete responses from him at the time.

He told me that castration might or might not solve the pain problem I was experiencing because of my surgically acquired nerve damage and the effect it was having on my entire body. That was O.K. since I really wanted to keep the little guys anyway, even if they were so troublesome.

This feeling was reinforced by some subsequent research that demonstrated several problems with the slash and burn approach. For one, there are inherent hormone imbalance problems that result from castration, leaving the castratee dependent on medical treatment for the rest of his life. Also, research has shown a tendency for men to become anemic after their testicles are removed (Fonseca, et. al., 1998). Significant psychological disorders can occur also (Mazeh, et. al., 1997).

117

Why not just cut out the side that hurts the worst and see if that helped? That question is answered well by W. F. Hendry (2000), who offers the following summary on the issue which makes perfect sense to me in light of my experience and the experiences of others I have discussed the issue with: "There is an old adage that a man can 'fire perfectly well on one cylinder', implying that so long as one testicle is preserved, it matters little what happens to the other. Modern immunological techniques have revealed that this is not so. Unilateral [one side] damage to the vas or epididymis can lead to the production of antisperm antibodies in some individuals, and can produce sterility. Sympathetic opthalmia is well recognized with eye injuries: sympathetic orchiopathia, difficult to define exactly, may have a similarly damaging effect on the contralateral [opposite side] organ in the long-term. There can be no excuse for adopting a cavalier attitude to the testicle or its appendages even in the presence of a normal contralateral organ."

There are varying theories for this phenomenon. Some, like Dr. Hendry and also Wallace, et. al., (1981), have advanced the notion that sympathetic orchiopathia is due to the autoimmune response that follows breaking of the blood-testis barrier. Other explanations are based on reactions within the nervous system: "In paired organs, irritation to nerves, such as by physical trauma [like surgery]… in one may lead to changes in the undamaged paired organ through reflex antidromic impulses by way of pathways involving the central nervous system (trophic nerves)" (Wyburn, 1981). Translation: doctors, put away your knives.

The other thing I kept hearing, even from the doctors and nurses I kept encountering was, "you need to write a book about this experience of yours!" My only hesitancy was that writing the story might be viewed as a slam of the medical profession in general, which I did not want to do. It was apparent to me by this time, however, that there was a significant conceptual problem (sorry for the pun again) in most people's minds about vasectomies that deserved some reforming. This included reforming the concept of many of the doctors who recommended the procedure to patients in such a cavalier way. I wasn't quite sure how this might be accomplished, but I had a feeling that a way would reveal itself.

Phil called me one day about two and a half months after my reconstructive surgery. "So are you still hurting all the time?" he asked.

"I'm still just riding the waves of this stuff, Phil" I responded.

"I like your hair-brained scheme," he said, "I want to try you on an injection series of Lupron."
"Please explain what we're talking about doing," I inquired.

Phil explained that Lupron was one of several drugs that act on the pituitary gland to stop sex hormone production altogether. It is often used for male patients about to undergo surgery for prostate cancer and for endometriosis in women. Evidently, the net effect in men is that production of testosterone and sperm ceases or at least substantially diminishes for a period of time, which tends to lessen the aggravating effect that high levels of testosterone have on the prostate gland. In my case the diminished sperm production was the desired effect.

"It's basically chemical castration," Phil summarized.

Gulp. "Uh, Phil, how long does this stuff take to wear off?" I inquired somewhat nervously.

"About a month or two," he reassured, "Come in to see me so we can try this out. Besides, I need to examine you again and redo some antibody tests."

Great, another high-jumping exhibition. At this point I wasn't sure whether more hormones or less hormones was a good thing, but what did I know, I was just the patient, right? I had the sense of taking a temporary position as a eunuch without being cut out for the job. I had also learned to ask very pointed questions after doing some advanced research.

Why Lupron instead of Zoladex (a similar drug), testosterone, or a testosterone derivative? What about side effects? I don't want anything to shrivel up and fall off, after all, or be impotent for the rest of my life. These seemed like legitimate questions and concerns given my experience up to this point. Phil explained that I might experience a decreased libido for a while, but probably not much different than I was experiencing now because of the constant pain. All right, I guess that is no big sacrifice at this point. Hot flashes were a possibility, he added. So now I get to develop empathy for menopausal women too? I was having a tough enough time with the male-oriented issues.

I speculated that the lack of libido might actually help me clean up my thoughts for a while, if not make me a candidate for that monastery up the coast. As for the hot flashes, what could a little steamy heat be compared to chronic pain? Whoops, there I go asking stupid questions again.

When I saw Phil later that week we discussed the various options that had been proposed: testosterone therapy, Lupron and other hormone-eliminating-type drugs, and immune suppressing drugs. I told him that my wife sent her greetings, but if any of this medication made me moody and depressed again she was sending me to live with him until I was better. She wasn't kidding.

Phil laughed, "Good thing I have a guest room."

In case you think this type of stuff comes cheap, it doesn't. For example, the Lupron runs about $300 per injection, and I would need one each month or so for a while.

After considering the various options, I decided to go for the smallest and best quantified hammer first, i.e. the testosterone therapy. It might take longer to achieve the desired effect, but also would be the easiest to stop if I needed to. "Androgel" had just come out a few weeks before, which I could slather on daily instead of having to experience another onslaught of needles once again. No small incentive in my book.

Interestingly, information has begun to emerge about the effects of testosterone therapy, but from a different angle than I was taking. "Extra testosterone will stop a man's sperm production and make his chances for fertility impossible. Even giving testosterone in replacement doses, so that blood levels never are higher than normal, will halt sperm production [yeah!]" (Testosterone-Fertility.com). While this particular author warns of reduced fertility while using testosterone replacement therapy, that was precisely my need and intent.

What were the possible problems I might incur? According to Phil, the aforementioned moodiness was a possibility. It was likely that my testicles would shrink some during the course of treatment since they wouldn't be doing as much work. At that point I didn't care as long as they stayed on, and besides, they could probably use a break by now. I might also experience a lovely breast enlargement in the process.

Oh well, just another opportunity to get in touch with my feminine side.

"Testosterone is a powerful hormone with effects on nearly every body organ" (Bhasin, 2000).

Testosterone therapy turned out to be a relatively simple process compared to the rest of my experience up to that point. Just a little injection of a molasses-like substance in the tush to start things off (needles were phasing me less and less by now), followed by daily application of "Androgel". The Androgel was out of stock at my local pharmacy at the time and turned out to be difficult to get since it had just come out on the market a few weeks before.

I was finally able to fill the prescription after a week. In the days that followed, I waited for my pain to diminish, or my breasts to grow, or some other sign that the stuff was having an effect. I began to notice some interesting side-effects of increased testosterone. For one, my energy level went way up, even with the limited sleep I was getting due to the chronic pain. That was Okay as far as I was concerned, and was far better than dragging my tail all the time.

Conjoined with this energy though, was a certain anxiousness usually reserved for those who drink several fuel-injected, quadruple supercharged lattes to start their day, and I don't drink coffee at all. My wife compared it to living in fear of the Incredible Hulk coming out at any moment: "Stay away from him children. His eyes are glazing over and he's turning green!"

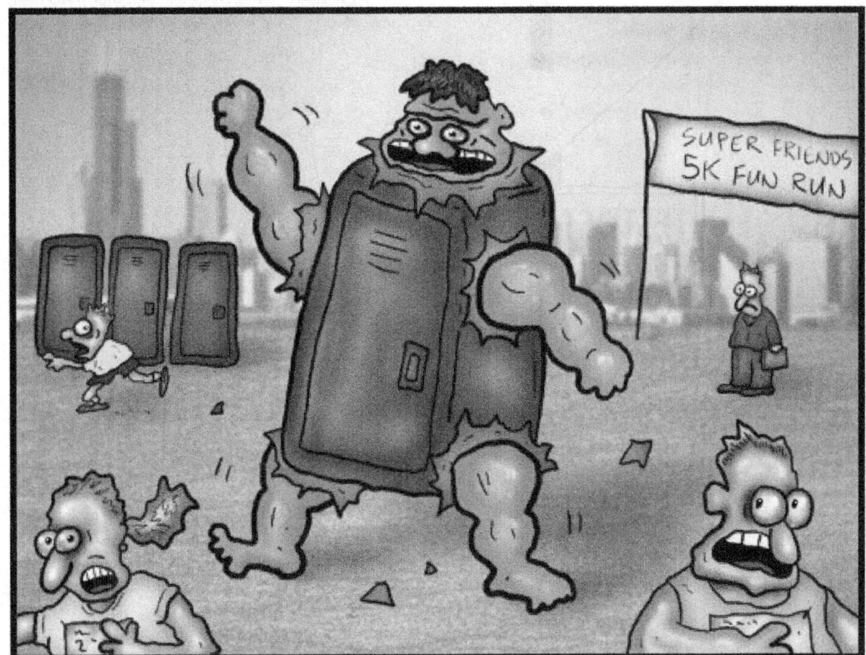

The Port-a-potty was out of toilet paper, and that made Dr. David Banner very angry.

Moods weren't the only thing that became easily excited. I learned what the code phrase in the literature about testosterone therapy means when it says: "May experience increased libido."

Warning: Explicit material approaching at warp(ed) speed.

Yep, that's right. I hadn't sported so many spontaneous erections since I bought my last Olivia Newton-John album, and that was about 1976. Now I knew why so many guys were interested in this Androgel stuff and why it was in short supply! It was a lot like having the sexual energy I had at 15 without the acne or the need to sit through Ms. Penman's English class.

This is how my day would normally unfold: I was typically awakened with pain in my testicles, groin and low back sometime between 1 a.m. and 4 a.m., as had occurred for nearly a year by then. I would then quietly climb into a warm tub and meditate for an hour or two in an attempt to moderate the various stinging and aching sensations I was experiencing.

Since I was now clean, I would slather the prescribed amount of Andro-goo on my abdomen, arms and shoulders and wait for it to dry, intermittently looking like a human directional sign. I could have hired out to hang banners, but in my case it probably would have led to a suit for false advertising, given the prohibitive pain I was experiencing in the peripheral equipment.

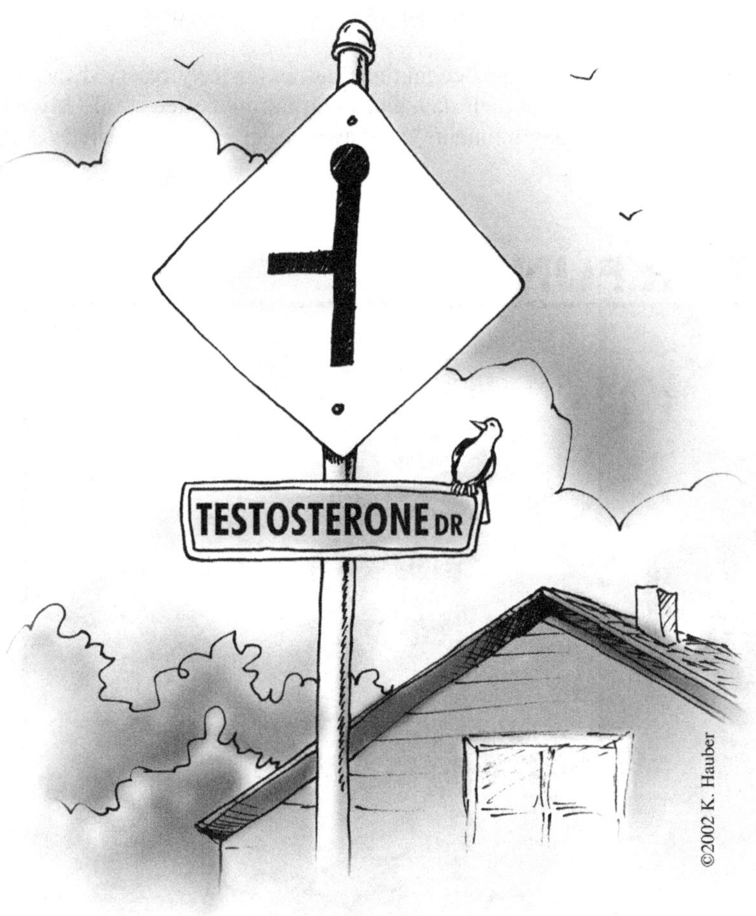

Bet you'll never look at road signs in the same way again, huh?

This provided quite a deterrent to what might otherwise have been an enjoyable experience of new batteries in an old toy. Add to that the prohibition in the medication information telling you not to come in contact with anyone else for several hours while the goo is applied to your skin, lest they get the treatment too. This is generally not too good, especially in the case of women. Why is your voice getting so deep lately, honey? And that body hair? You understand, and so did my wife, giving me a wide berth while working through this new Andro-man role.

So my initial experience with testosterone therapy was that it could leave you all revved up with nowhere to race, metaphorically speaking of course. Phil had said that it would probably take up to six months on the testosterone therapy for my sperm count to diminish. This could make for a long, hard summer, I thought!

Interestingly enough, one piece of information that I did find along the way was that people with autoimmune disorders can benefit from testosterone therapy, at least according to Dr. Carruthers (1997). That was encouraging given all of the negatives I had heard so far. I kept hearing rumors of natural forms of testosterone available, which sounded like a good long-term proposition if this type of therapy needed to continue. Eventually, I was given the name of the herbal supplement Tribulus Terrestris which acts to boost endogenous (inside the body) testosterone production.

A fascinating connection can be made between the autoimmune reactions to vasectomy discussed in previous chapters and testosterone production in the testes. This is explained in detail by Dr. Malcolm Carruthers in his book <u>Maximizing Manhood: Beating the Male Menopause</u> (1997), which I obtained a copy of during the first few months of my testosterone therapy. Dr. Carruthers contends that testosterone levels may initially increase for several years following vasectomy because the body is trying to compensate for the surgical insult that has been received in the vasectomy procedure. However, in the long term, testosterone production by the testes decreases because of the antibody action on the testosterone producing cells in the testicles. This is the same as the autoimmune orchitis effect described previously, and is long-term and degenerative in nature.

In Dr. Carruthers (1997) words: "Logic suggests that if you have antibodies against sperm, you might well develop antibodies against sperm producing cells in the testis, the Steroli [sounds like something out of Pinocchio, doesn't it?], or nurse cells, and indeed this is found in a proportion of cases.

"What was not expected was the finding in other cases of antibodies against the testosterone producing interstitial cell, though this again seems logical. The sperm and testosterone producing cells work together, literally side by side, on the common mission of producing and launching these 'egg-seeking missiles'. Recent research has shown just how closely these functions are linked in many ways, including their own hormonal communications, the so-called paracrine actions. If you suddenly shut down one half of the factory, common sense would indicate that you might have some effect on the other. From my research and that of others, including testicular biopsies from vasectomized men, there is evidence that this indeed is the case."

Some other research I had located supported this idea of vasectomies making men old before their time, at least in terms of their testicular function. Jarow, et. al.,. (1985) stated "We observed quantifiable and significant changes in the human testis after vasectomy, including tubular dilatation, tubular wall thickening, decreased number of spermatids [baby sperm cells, for lack of a better description] and Steroli cells per tubular cross section, and an increased incidence of interstitial fibrosis. All these changes are commonly found in the testes of elderly men, but rarely in middle-aged men."

Sokol (1999) discusses the causes of testicular failure to include orchitis, trauma (as in surgery), drugs, autoimmunity, and granulomatous diseases. As you know by now, these are situations that regularly confront vasectomy patients. I wondered how many men must face the effects of these types of changes with the pain or at least the frustration that is associated with them, and not even realize what is going on, or be in complete denial about the process.

Suddenly, the logic behind this testosterone therapy began to gel in my mind, no pun intended (this time). If vasectomy causes injury and/or an autoimmune reaction that leads to long-term degeneration of the testicles, it stands to reason that many vasectomized men, including me might experience symptoms of decreased testicular function. What might those symptoms be?

According to Dr. Carruthers (1997), symptoms of andropause (male menopause) most often appear 10 to 15 years after vasectomy but typically five years earlier than in comparable non-vasectomized men, which supports the theory that vasectomy accelerates degeneration of testicular functions. Symptoms include depression, irritability, aching and stiffness, a general loss of energy, loss of interest in sex, decreased erectile function, circulatory and heart problems among others. "Especially when there are other causes of testicular failure, such as alcohol or mumps, vasectomy definitely seems to

lower the age at which andropausal symptoms appear." A previous vasectomy was a consistently recurrent factor in Dr. Carruthers' observation of these symptoms in his patients, even if they had no other apparent causes.

I had certainly been experiencing depression, irritability, aching, and low energy for months (just ask my wife). I'm sure living with me was as hard for her as it was for me. This had occurred after years of good health and overall fitness. While I had attributed many of these symptoms to the chronic pain I had been experiencing, this information about the hormonal aspects of vasectomy brought a new factor and possible aggravant to light.

This would also explain why the course of Prednisone I was on previously had made the depression and irritability I was experiencing at the time so much worse. I had learned that corticosteroids like Prednisone, if taken long-term, have a depressing effect on testosterone production. This might also help to explain in part the loss of appetite, weight, and muscle mass I had experienced up to this point. It would appear that my body needed all the Mr. T it could muster to help combat this perceived invasion and maintain a reasonable balance.

One of Dr. Carruthers' patients characterized his experience after vasectomy this way: "I had my vasectomy 10 years ago. It was very painful and I had a lot of bruising. Suddenly, for no apparent reason, five years ago the bottom dropped out of my sex life.... About the same time, quite suddenly my morning erections disappeared and soon the evening one went out of the door with them, especially when I wanted them most.... Also, while I used to really fizz all the time, I became a real slouch, stopped going to parties and started feeling old before my time. Then the circulation in my fingers and toes got quite bad even in mild weather, and my feet started going numb" (Carruthers, 1997).

Just so we're all on the same playing field, erectile dysfunction such as is being spoken of above has been defined as follows: "The persistent inability to achieve or maintain an erection sufficient for satisfactory sexual performance" (Isidori, et. al., 1999). This man's lack of "fizz" would seem to fit into this category. Dias (1983) found that 26 of 200 men he studied after their vasectomies experienced "poor erections." This seems to fit the pattern that is so vehemently denied or ignored by so many doctors.

As an interesting case study to note, Dr. Carruthers started the "fizzless" patient on a regular program of testosterone therapy, and he has felt much better. The patient (a doctor himself) states, "I don't think it's my imagination either, because every five or six months when my [testosterone] implant is running down, my golf gets worse, as does my temper and sex life, and they are only restored by another shot of testosterone." People can use amazingly varied standards to measure quality of life, can't they?

Interestingly enough, testosterone treatment is exactly what Dr. Carruthers often prescribes for his patients with numerous post-vasectomy problems, especially since so many of them exhibit symptoms of andropause. Maybe my intuition about this form of treatment was right after all.

"Particularly in relation to andropause, those who have had vasectomies should not be unduly alarmed, because symptoms generally respond very well to testosterone treatment. However, sometimes higher doses seem needed in this situation and, because the antibody changes are not reversible, treatment may need to be prolonged" (Carruthers, 1997). Even though I didn't consider myself an andropause patient at this point in my life, it appeared that the doctor and I were reaching the same conclusion from different directions.

So how could I make this "prolonged" treatment safe without winding up with an inflamed prostate and the nicest pair of breasts in town? This seemed like a reasonable question.

Well, there are several forms of testosterone therapy available with different formulations and durations. An early form of oral testosterone called methyl testosterone was found to cause multiple maladies including liver damage and increased blood fat levels. Later developments had arrived at formulations that were both safer and longer lasting in effect. Some men have been on these formulations for as long as 50 years with no ill effects according to Dr. Carruthers.

Regular and complete medical work-ups are necessary during the course of this type of hormone therapy according to the doctor. But if properly administered, this type of therapy could be sustained over the long-term with no danger. According to another source, this work up should include "a blood test for testosterone, free testosterone, estradiol, DHEA and prolactin.... All modes of delivery work well... A man may need to experiment with one or two until he decides which type of testosterone is right for him" (Testosterone-Fertility.com). This was encouraging to hear in light of the four- or five-year estimated time frame I was quoted to diminish the autoimmune response my body was having. Hopefully that didn't mean four or five more years of pain while this process went on.

"Prior to beginning testosterone replacement therapy, the man needs to have a baseline urologic exam and PSA blood test. As testosterone stimulates prostate growth and fuels any existing prostate cancer, all men prior to beginning testosterone replacement therapy need to be screened for prostate cancer and prostate enlargement symptoms [Here comes that finger again]. In addition, men with sleep apnea and breast cancer should never receive testosterone for fear of exacerbating either condition. Once a man has his baseline studies and is deemed a good candidate for replacement, he needs his PSA and testosterone levels checked at the 3-month mark. If the blood testosterone increases to a normal level and the PSA increases by less than .4 ng/dl, then therapy can continue safely. While on replacement testosterone, a man should have his PSA checked twice a year rather than once a year" (Testosterone-Fertility.com)

What kind of testosterone was I on anyway, and how was the stuff made? I love Dr. Carruthers' response to the second part of the question: "When asked where the testosterone comes from, doctors sometimes tell patients that it is extracted from Peruvian bull's testicles in the mating season [sounds like the story with the Orchex I was already taking], both to explain the cost of the treatment and maximize the placebo effect, that's a lot of bull really. In actual fact the testosterone is made synthetically from cholesterol, the same raw material as the body uses to produce it. The cost of these preparations at present is usually roughly two to three times that of equivalent oestrogen [sic] preparations used in female HRT [hormone replacement therapy], but hopefully as TRT [testosterone replacement therapy] is used more often, drug companies will be able to reduce this sex hormone discrimination against men" (Carruthers, 1997).

Well, no one ever said I was a cheap date. We'll get into that subject in more depth shortly.

As for the "exactly what was I on" part of the question, I couldn't tell precisely from the packaging information, other than that Androgel was relatively long acting for a topically applied compound, and this seemed to be a good feature. I resolved that I was on the right path and would continue to look into long-term alternatives for hormone therapy and try to find a way to deal with the nerve injury aspect of what I was experiencing also.

At this point, you might be asking yourself the same question I was asking: If a man needs to take testosterone after a vasectomy and reversal to eliminate sperm production because of the negative effects of the vasectomy, why get the vasectomy to begin with? Why not just start with the hormone therapy? He ends up sterile both ways, right? This was one of those no-win questions that I would pose to myself from time to time and cause endless frustration. Other than being the best possible way out of this situation, it didn't make much sense. However, hormone therapy was still a more attractive approach than more surgeries.

When my sperm count was checked again at the end of a month's testosterone therapy, the count had dropped to one third of the prior level. Well at least some form of therapy was achieving the desired effect. I hoped that this trend would continue and alleviate some of the pressure and pain. That kind of relief seemed to be just starting to happen, so I was keeping everything crossed that could be crossed.

The trend did continue. What I noted was that, as my sperm count continued to drop in the ensuing months, the constant aching sensations in my testicles began to subside bit by bit. I still experienced a great deal of pain from the vasectomy sites at the top of the scrotum up into the groin and abdomen as I moved about, but at least some of the pressure and consistent aching was subsiding, which made sleeping somewhat easier. Also, as my own natural testosterone production diminished, being replaced by the testosterone I applied externally each day, my moods stabilized, as did my propensity for spontaneous erections. Easy come, easy go.

Again, science eventually backed me up in what I was attempting, in theory at least. "When the blood levels of testosterone are normal, the brain stops secreting LH [Lieutenizing Hormone]. When the blood levels of testosterone go down, the brain makes LH to stimulate the testes to make more testosterone. Testosterone is required in very high concentrations within the testes for sperm production to occur. So if a man receives outside testosterone, the pituitary gland will 'think' the testes are making enough testosterone and stop stimulating the Leydig cells. When the Leydig cells stop making testosterone, the intra-testicular testosterone drops and sperm production stops" (Testosterone-Fertility.com).

The actual process of getting to a zero sperm count took ten months and eventually required the addition of a progesterone injection as an anti-androgen element in the therapy. This idea came up after I obtained the reports of several World Health Organization trials using various forms of testosterone as a male contraceptive (Meriggiola, et. al., 1996, 1997, & 1998). What was found in these trials is that some men respond quickly to testosterone therapy and go to a zero sperm count, while others are pervasive sperm makers even in the face of a hormonal onslaught. Hopefully, I don't sound like a braggart when I say, evidently, I was in the latter category.

The anti-androgen element in the hormone therapy significantly improved the results of the World Health Organization trials in terms of overall suppression of sperm production (Handelsman, et. al., 1996). In my case, I had reached a very low sperm count by the time we added the progesterone injection and this knocked it down the rest of the way. If I was to do it over again, knowing what I now do, I would start with the progesterone injection as called for in the protocols, then continue the testosterone treatment. I sense this would have given quicker results, but then, who knew? I was still making up the play book as I went.

"The suppressive effect of testosterone is directly related to the dose and duration of treatment. The way testosterone is given, such as shots, pills or creams is not as important [as long as sufficient testosterone levels are maintained]. All types of testosterone supplementation will shut off sperm production.... The interesting side note is that with supplemental testosterone kept in the normal range, there were no side effects such as rage and heart disease [in the World Health Organization trials]" (Testosterone-Fertility.com). Again, I seemed to be a step ahead of medical science and going in the opposite direction, at least in regards to the use of testosterone therapy in relation to treatment of post-vasectomy pain.

My next set of ultrasound tests showed some very interesting results. For one, my testicles had begun to shrink to some extent due to their vacation status. However, the inflammation in the epididymis was diminishing, which confirmed my observation of less aching in the testicles themselves. According to the WHO studies, the testicular atrophy was supposed to go away after cessation of the hormone therapy and normal testicular function was supposed to return. I was betting that they were right.

Concurrent to the hormone therapy, I had embarked upon a program of lymphatic massage. Apparently, this combined with the reduced antibody levels led to an elimination of the hydrocele cysts that had formed previously in my scrotum. My epididymal cysts were unchanged initially, but later went away, and I couldn't argue with this kind of quantifiable progress both in test results and in actual pain response. Just for reference, here's a diagram of what epididymal cysts can look like (the spermatocele/epididymal cyst is the bulge on the left side of the epididymis):

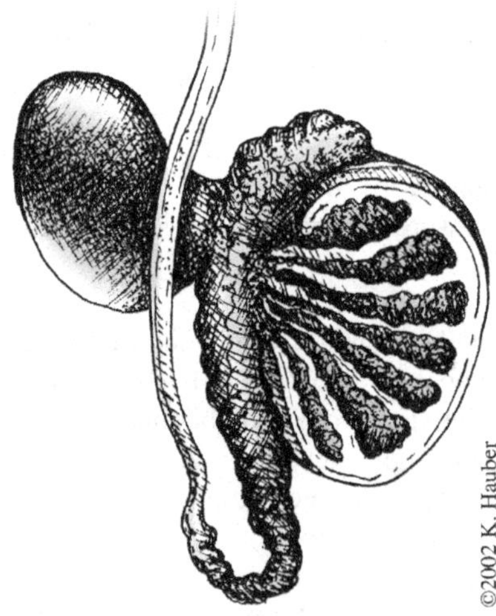

Blood tests showed that my antibody levels had fallen below the detectable level. This was very good news, and gave me good indication that I was headed in the right direction. Previously, the medical data on the subject said that the only way to get rid of the autoimmune response to vasectomy was to remove the source of sperm production, i.e. cut out the testicles. I felt that a new door was opening as an alternative to that approach which was far less damaging in the long run.

After more than a year of this therapy, several of my doctors convinced me to stop for a while to see if my system would "normalize." As I became fertile again, the sensations of my testicles exploding came back, as did the recurrent flu-like symptoms. The hydroceles, epididymal cysts and epididymitis that I had been able to rid myself of previously came back too, as another testicular ultrasound demonstrated. Another Immunobead Assay at Phil's office showed many antibodies being formed in my genital tract.

After several months, I couldn't take it any more, and I went back onto the testosterone therapy, this time using the patch approach. The patches worked well for me in keeping my hormone levels where they were supposed to be, and kept my wife from receiving the therapy. However, the patches left me with nasty rashes that turned into sores that scarred in several places. I felt like I had already collected enough scars on this journey without this addition.

The sensations were like I was always getting over poison oak and this was not a good long-term situation in my estimation, so I opted to have a testosterone implant done as had been recommended to me by several doctors as the "gold standard" for hormone therapy for men. The concept is quite good, except for the fact that putting the implants in is a bit "medieval," as Phil characterized it. Be concerned when your doctor is a bit queasy about the procedure he is about to do for you. Imagine taking a sharpened instrument about the size of a ball point pen and inserting it into the flesh next to your naval and about three inches to the side. I'm not kidding.

Normally, this is done in the abdomen where there is a bit of extra padding for many guys and the implant gets tucked into the extra tissues there. Unfortunately or fortunately, depending on how you look at it, I have always been fairly lean and after my vasectomy experience had even less padding to put the implant into. I was black and blue for weeks afterward the abdominal implant.

I did found this to be a good form of testosterone therapy though, despite the miserable administration. The implants are reputed to create the most even hormone levels, better than shots, patches or gels, and if energy levels are any indicator, I would have to agree. If you ever decide to try this form of therapy, just find a good place to put the implants where you can take being a bit tender for a while.

In the long run, I did go back to using the Androgel instead of the implants since I was running out of places to have the implants put, and didn't want to make long drives every few months to have them done. Also, the implants had a habit of running out prematurely in three to four months instead of six months as projected. This was just too intense. In addition to the Androgel, I occasionally used a new "buccal" tablet that is placed in the gum area of the mouth and gives a 12-hour dose of testosterone if you leave it there. French kissing was out with these in place, but beyond that, these tablets were a good alternative on days I wanted to swim or do something else where the gel would wash off.

Not surprisingly, as time went on not only was my energy level better, but the bursting testicle sensations and the flu-like symptoms diminished again as my sperm count dropped. I was quite convinced that I was going in the right direction, at least for this layer of the situation. Now all I had to do was figure out what to do about that pesky nerve damage layer.

In the meantime, I had a lot of bills to attend to.

Chapter Twenty-Two

I'm Sorry; That's Not a Covered Benefit

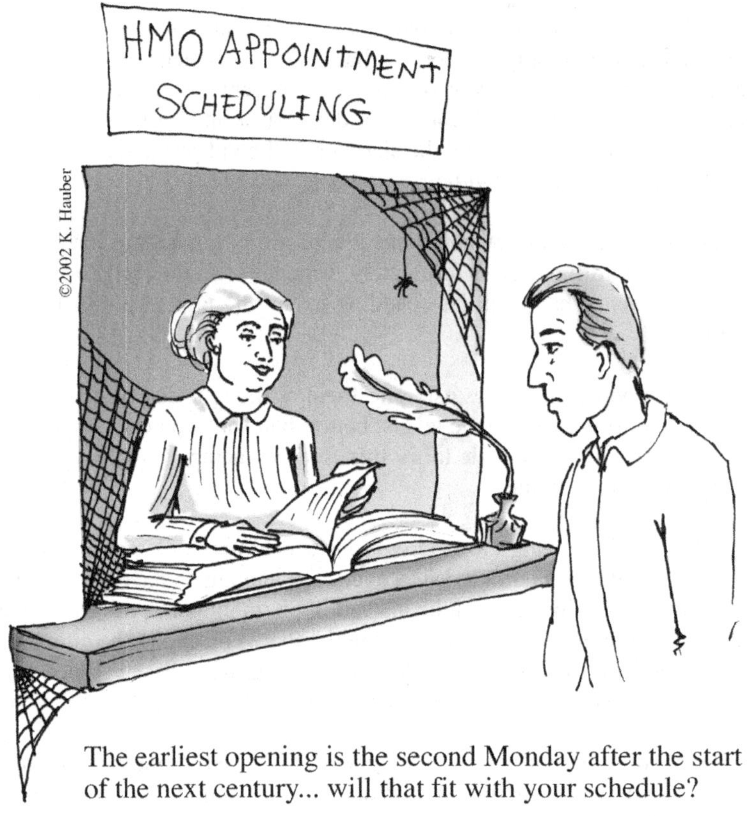

The earliest opening is the second Monday after the start
of the next century... will that fit with your schedule?

HMOs are great. Great, that is, if you just stay healthy and pay your premiums. Great, that is, until you get sick and need some kind of expensive or unusual treatment. HMOs are also great at creating many layers of administration to deny you the benefits of the treatments your doctors recommend, with someone who is essentially an accountant telling you why you don't really need a particular form of treatment to get healthy again.

I recognize that I may be prejudiced by my experience, but I know I am not alone. My perception is that even many of the doctors, physician's assistants, and nurses who work in HMOs don't like the system. The corporations that own HMOs seem to like them, however, and if the HMO isn't profitable enough, then the corporation just divests itself of that particular HMO and moves on to greener pastures. It would seem that the almighty dollar rules in the HMO world, far more than the most beneficial medical choice for the patient. HMOs will often blame their decisions not to treat a patient in a particular way on the medical insurance company.

According to Alan Bonsteel, M.D., there are five basic problems with the typical HMO arrangement in terms of doctor-patient relationships: "First - and this is the real horror story - these programs, and often the physicians working for them, are paid more money when they do less for the patient…. Family physicians like myself often become stuck in the role of 'gatekeeper', limiting access to specialists even when the doctor himself may want the reassurance of a second opinion.

"Second, time pressures on physicians in these programs are extraordinary. In some programs, physicians must see six, seven, or even eight patients an hour in the clinic. With such extreme time pressures, the old Marcus Welby physicians are a thing of the past- there isn't time to get to know the patients, let alone be their counselor and their support.

"Third, in this environment, preventative health goes by the wayside. Managed Care organizations have figured out that their patients come and go, and so they take a short-term attitude. Pap smears, mammograms, prostate-specific antigen blood tests, and counseling patients about their lifestyles become a low priority- even though they should be the highest priority.

"Fourth, 'gag orders' often prevent physicians from telling patients what is going on. Even though the doctors may be prevented by financial reasons from ordering the tests they want, telling the patients the truth can get them fired.

"Finally, managed care disrupts the long-term relationship between the physician and the patient.... Nothing is more important to the physician/patient relationship than trust- and when physicians are explicitly told to hide the truth, trust is the first victim" (Bonsteel, 2000).

That sums it up succinctly. So what should you do if you find yourself in this type of situation? Again, Dr. Bonsteel (2000): "For now, patients must protect themselves and their loved ones by being assertive. If you get turned down the first time in your request to see a specialist or to get the latest or strongest drug available, ask again. It's your life and your health. Do what it takes to get the medical care you deserve.... If all else fails, try the disinfectant of sunshine. Managed care organizations hate bad publicity. A threat to write to your local newspaper, or go on your local radio station, can work wonders."

I hasten to point out that these words are not being put forth by a disgruntled patient, but by a physician familiar with the inner workings of the system. I found the phrase "patients must protect themselves and their loved ones" to be particularly striking.

Likewise, medical insurance companies are great. Great, that is, at finding every possible loophole to deny coverage and delay payment! Great at creating elaborate review and appeal processes in the hopes that they can either wear you down so that you'll stop trying, or die in the process. This is probably a fairly effective strategy, from the insurance company's standpoint, that is.

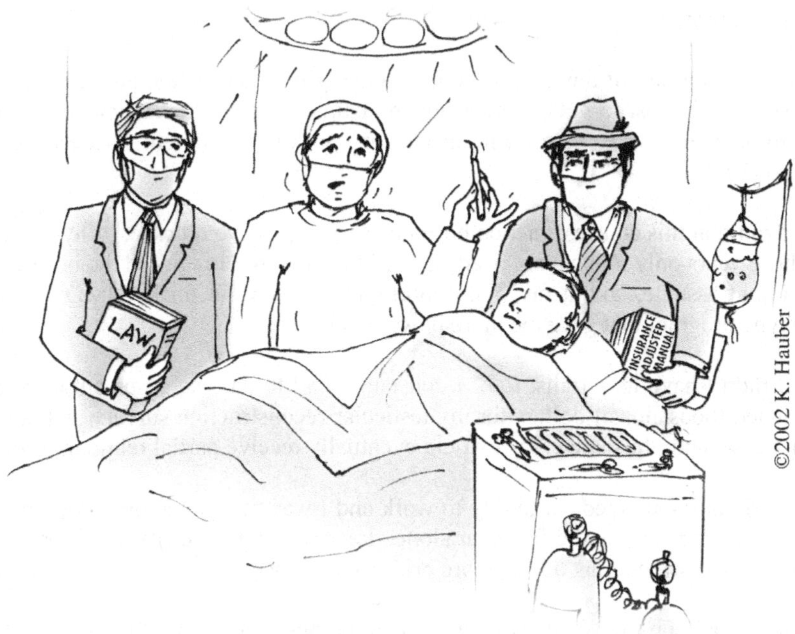

Now, Which one of you would like to make the incision?
- since you both always tell me how to run my practice.

I deal with people's credit reports on a daily basis. I am continually amazed at how many medical bills end up in collection, simply because the insurance company didn't pay the bills when they were obliged to, or delayed so long that the matters were sent to a collection agency. This causes an incredible amount of damage to consumer's credit, and is often very difficult to unravel.

After my own experience, I gained a better understanding as to why perfectly responsible consumers could experience such problems. Tracking and attending to all of the expense and insurance issues surrounding a significant medical condition can become a second full-time job, as I learned.

In my mortgage banking business, I deal with many doctors, none of whom have had anything good to say about HMOs or insurance companies. Most doctors have privately expressed their frustration at having medical decisions taken out of their hands for all but the rare few who are cash patients. The doctor's income has dropped noticeably in many cases over the past few years as reimbursements have been reduced from Medicare and private medical insurance.

Many doctors must now employ entire staffs just to take care of the paperwork and hassles involved in billing for insurance. This is expensive and time consuming. Many of the best specialists will not participate in most insurance plans because of this kind of baloney, and because they are in such demand, they don't have to. It just costs you a lot out-of-pocket to see them.

Enough of that rant for now. Let me tell you a little bit about my personal experience that has made me so jaded toward both HMOs and medical insurance companies. Initially, my medical insurance was through an HMO plan, which, I assumed, worked fine.

It worked fine, that is, until I started needing something exceptional, at which point I found out that HMOs don't think outside the box very well, and the box is pretty damned small to begin with. Howls of protest and angry threats from me were not even enough to affect this intransigent bureaucracy. I eventually engaged in a multi-layered complaint and appeal process that took months. I couldn't help but conclude that this system was quite proficient at dragging an issue out in hopes that I, as the patient, would give up, or not be able to figure out how to navigate its intricacies.

It was amazing to me that I could get full coverage for the initial vasectomy procedure, but getting coverage for any of the treatments needed afterward was like pulling teeth, or in this case pulling testicles. Actually, I probably would have had better luck getting coverage if my teeth were pulled, but then I wouldn't have been able to holler about their policies as well with my teeth missing.

I couldn't get coverage for any of the treatments that actually provided relief, and referrals took weeks or months to be approved. It took six months just to get coverage for the pain and stress management course I took. It was quite obvious to me that I had to be a strong advocate for my needs, and seek the treatment I needed, regardless of my HMO's approval. That's exactly what I did.

However, I found out that this course of action becomes very expensive quickly. Why had I paid all those medical insurance premiums all those years only to have my needs denied the one time I required the benefits? This was more than a little angering, as you might assume, and at my first opportunity I opted out of the HMO system and went back to a preferred provider (PPO) type program that gave me more power to choose.

Not that the PPO didn't have its pitfalls, too. I constantly had to pay expenses out of pocket and then fight for reimbursement. This included thousands of dollars for my testicular reconstruction surgery and numerous other therapies. Talk about rubbing salt in the wound. In some cases I would eventually receive partial reimbursement, in many cases not.

Since this medical situation affected my ability to work and I was paid on commission, my income was dropping. It dropped a lot, in fact; by about one half in the first year alone. I eventually had to file for a partial disability to try to help compensate for some of this loss, surrendering a little more pride in the process.

How much did all this add up to? Well, as I approached the one-year mark of this little drama, the total costs and losses raced past $135,000. Various forms of insurance covered about 36 cents on the dollar when all was said and done. I should have such negotiating skills. Actually, there wasn't much negotiation about it. The usual position was, "That's all we'll pay. Tough!"

The other 64 cents on the dollar was absorbed by me, or in some cases taken as losses by the medical providers. As you might imagine, this became quite stressful. I don't know how doctors can work within this kind of system. I know it seemed highly dysfunctional to me.

This brings us to the subject of cost shifting, a favorite practice in the medical community these days. To illustrate the point, remember how my original urologist said that my reversal surgery would cost about $12,000? Do you get the feeling that this might be another one of those "not exactly" stories? Well, actually the tab for the surgeon and the anesthesiologist added up to about $10,000; bad enough, but not unexpected. Months later I received the hospital bill.

How much did it cost to be near all those "good drugs" for one night? How about $31,000 as a starting bid by the hospital? What!? Quickly doing the math I calculated that out to be nearly $1,300 and hour for the time I was in the hospital. That was without any dancing girls or other services you might expect at that kind of rate. This seemed like a lot given the amount of pain that had been inflicted. I assumed this had to be a mistake and asked for an itemization.

Nope, this was in fact what they calculated the charges to be. The line items included $59 for the very fashionable surgical gown I was given to wear; you know, the kind that always leaves your tush hanging out. Then there was $2,390 an hour or each fraction thereof for the operating room for a total of $14,144 for my four-and-a-half-hours on the table. And I thought the hourly vehicle parking rates were high in Beverly Hills!

Then there was the $273 jock strap they put on me coming out of surgery. At that price, I should have awakened giggling with all kinds of pleasurable sensations occurring, which didn't happen, I can assure you. How about the cost of all the "good drugs?" Glad you asked. The pharmacy portion of the bill came to nearly $1,500, not including the $3,266 for anesthesia. Wow, talk about chutzpah! These folks had balls, or at least had me by mine, quite literally.

The hospital had sent me this bill because my insurance company told them that my coverage had been cancelled, which of course was not the case, but turned out to be a great stalling tactic. I had assumed that the insurance would probably have capped the cost at about $1,800 total based on their contract with the hospital. But since the hospital thought I was now a cash patient, they were ready to kill the fatted calf. Not that the calf was all that fat anymore after the costs already incurred. This added up to nearly a $40,000 calf by the time everything was added in.

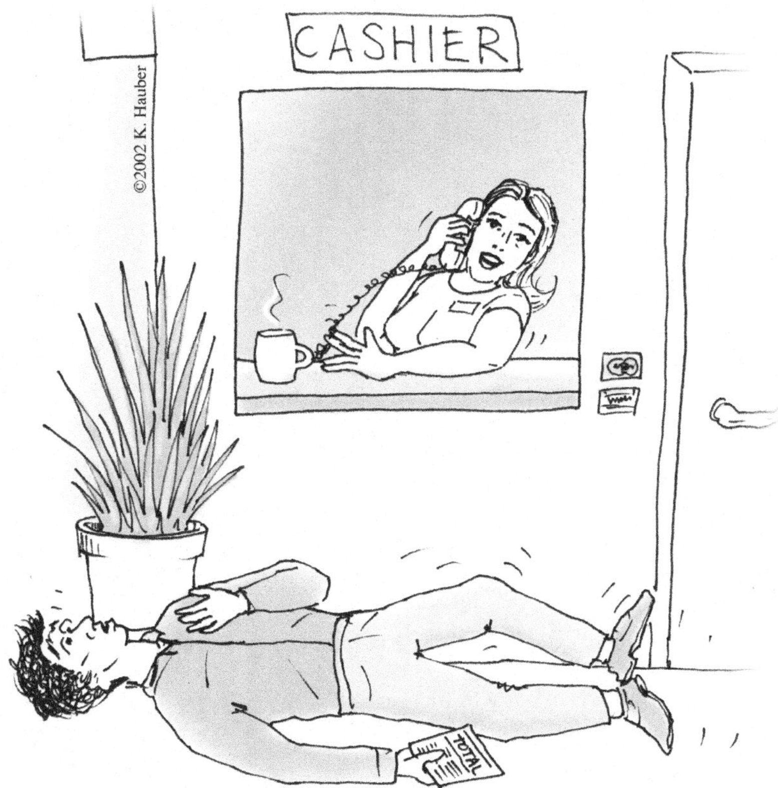

Oh Hi Frank, well... it looks like we have
another cardiac down here in the lobby...

So what happens to the poor guy who ends up in the hospital without insurance or finds that, in fact, his coverage has been cancelled or denied? Well, if he wasn't a poor guy to begin with, which is often the case, he probably will be afterwards because of this type of cost shifting. This is one of the reasons that so many people without (or even with) insurance declare bankruptcy when the bills start rolling in after a major illness.

Evidently, profits need to be made somewhere, and because of the high default rate on many cash patient's bills, the rates charged have gone through the roof. Strangely, receiving the hospital bill didn't cause too much of a gag reflex for me, and I took it in stride along with what had become a long string of amazing experiences associated with this process. I simply made more phone calls, wrote more letters, and forwarded the bill to my attorney.

Lest you think I am the only one who has encountered problems in managing a case of post-vasectomy pain syndrome through an HMO, see what another man wrote on the Prostatitis Web Site/Vasectomy page: "I am a married man, 37 years old with two kids. I had a vasectomy a few years ago and ever since I have not been the same.… I went back to the doctor (an HMO) and was told there was nothing wrong with me.… I have almost constant pain from the general area (a dull burning pain) going up into my pelvis. I cannot wear tight underwear such as briefs.… It has affected my marital duties, as I cannot perform as well with the pain.… The last time I went there [the HMO] I specifically asked to see the doctor who did my vasectomy. He got irritated when I implied that something went wrong and said that to do anything he would have to cut my stomach open and pull my testicles out through the hole. 'You don't want that, do you?' he said. He said I have scar tissue. He went on to say that a lot of people live with pain and so does he."

Sounds to me like this doctor is a good candidate for the vise-grip empathy test! Man, I thought I had encountered some insensitivity along the way: This was a new low. No wonder so many people are hopping mad at what purports to be a medical care system.

Chapter Twenty-Three

Of All the Nerve

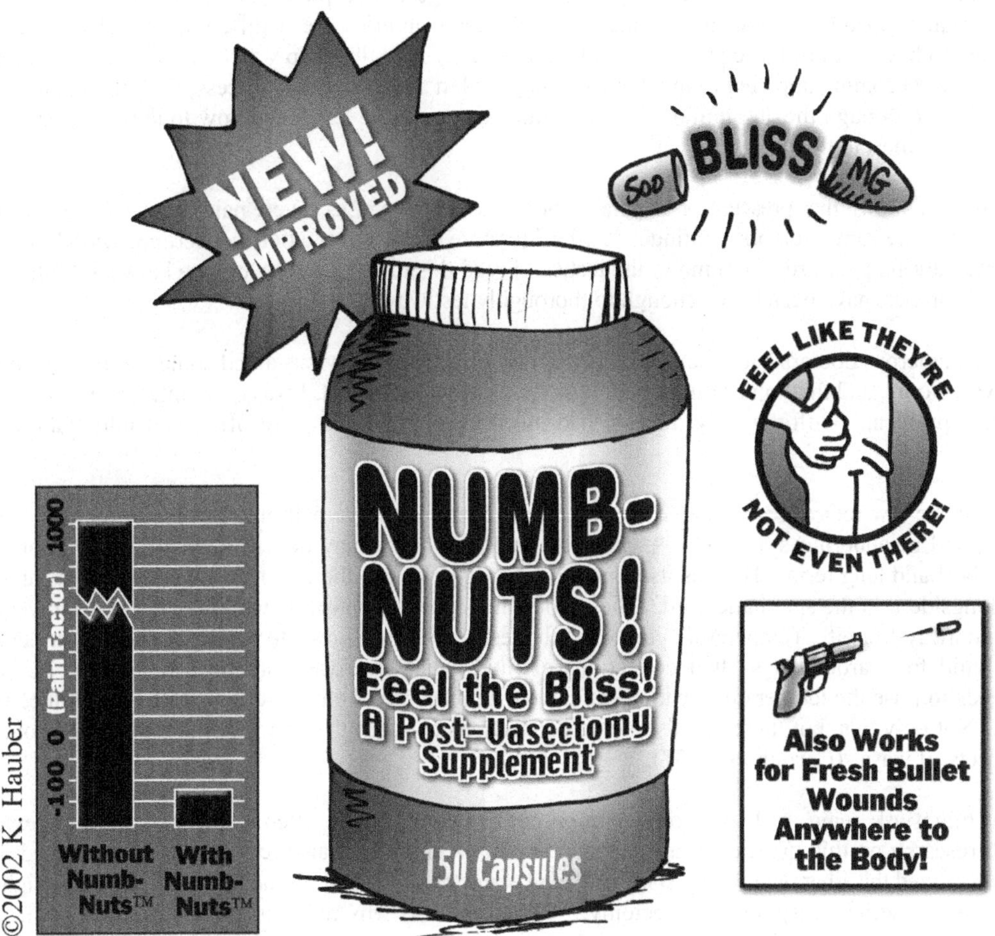

"The most difficult pains to treat are those that result from damage to the peripheral nerves or to the central nervous system itself" (WebMD – Chronic Pain).

"Peripheral nerve injuries are common, and there is no easily available formula for successful treatment" (Lee, et. al., 2000).

"Causes of post-vasectomy pain: A non-meticulous 'rough' surgery where significant amounts of tissue and nerves have been disrupted and/or tied that have caused lingering irritation of the nerves. While this may be one of the more frequent causes of post-vasectomy pain syndrome one can imagine that it would be less common in the patients of experienced vasectomists.... In regards to a rough surgery, this would be the most difficult to treat and to identify as a cause of pain. Possible treatments could include exploration of the area to remove scarred or inflamed tissue, manual manipulation or stimulation of the painful area, or just allowing time to heal.... Time, sometimes 1-2 years, without doing anything at all, may heal the problem" (Vasectomymedical.com).

This last quote is one of the best summaries available of what can result from either inexperience or inappropriate handing of the procedure, and gives emphasis to an often unmentioned fact: when nerves have been insulted by surgery or other processes, going back and creating another insult with another surgery is often questionable at best.

It was becoming increasingly clear to me that there were many things that could go wrong after a vasectomy to cause a man chronic pain. However, one can say broadly that congestion, ruptures, and autoimmune responses fall into one category and require specific treatment approaches, while nerve injuries are a different animal altogether. If you are unlucky enough to have both of these problems, as I have, you are in really deep water, and the cumulative effect is almost unbearable. It was becoming apparent to me that I was engaged in an un-layering process; first through the congestions and rupturing level, then through the autoimmune and inflammatory response level, and now to the nerve damage level, which was probably the hardest to treat.

"It is well known that pressure or trauma to the testis of man causes severe pain" (Peterson, et. al., 1973). There's a revelation! But the same authors continue: "…the literature lacks information concerning neural activity in afferent testicular nerves during pressure or trauma to the testis." I read this to mean that everyone knows it hurts a lot, but neither subjects nor researchers have been brave enough to thoroughly test why.

Since numerous doctors had discussed the fact that I had apparently sustained some form of nerve damage during my original vasectomy, and that injury might be long-term or even permanent, I was quite interested in finding a solution to this part of the problem. Unfortunately, no one had much encouraging news to offer, and information resources were scarce.

One of the few references available on the subject discusses nerve pain due to vasectomy in the context of other complications and neighboring structures: "…after the operation there may be a variety of complications, which can be divided into short and long term. The vas itself may be damaged, as can the fine blood vessels, nerves and lymph vessels which run alongside it in the spermatic cord. These nourish the testis, control its temperature to within very critical limits and drain fluid away from it. Temperature control of the testis has been shown to be impaired after vasectomy, as has the drainage of fluid from around it so that collections of fluid called hydrocele are formed in some cases. This 'water jacketing' tends to raise the temperature, which can have a harmful effect on the testes' ability to produce both sperm and testosterone. Not only this, but there are also nerve connections between the two testes and damage to one can affect the other in a variety of ways "(Carruthers, 1997).

You might ask again, as I did, how common is this nerve damage after vasectomy, and how extensive? There wasn't much research on this question from recent years, but a study by Pabst, et. al., (1979) published in *Fertility and Sterility* characterized this phenomenon by stating, "On average, about half of all the nerves in the near neighborhood of the vas deferens were resected [cut] during vasectomy." Perhaps that is why many guys hurt as much as they do after their vasectomies, despite their doctor's assertions to the contrary. My suspicion was that more extensive damage beyond the local area of the surgery is necessary to cause chronic pain.

The researchers in the Pabst, et. al., (1979) study were actually trying to determine the extent of the effect vasectomy had on ejaculatory function. In particular, they were examining reasons for low sperm counts after reversal. This also relates to our prior discussion about vasectomy reversals and the problems encountered with low pregnancy rates following those procedures. "If during vasectomy the nerves to the proximal [testicular] part of the vas and the epididymis are resected [cut], even a perfectly restored continuity after vasovasostomy will be a functional failure because the denervated parts of the vas cannot perform a coordinated, rapid, powerful contraction during emission…. Vasectomy can disrupt the nerve supply to that part of the vas deferens between the point of vasectomy and the epididymis…. Additional nerves are probably destroyed by grasping or clamping, or after scar formation" (Pabst, et. al., 1979). The parts of the system that are affected by damage to the nerves contain approximately two-thirds of the stored sperm that would normally be ejaculated (Frances, et. al., 1983), which can significantly affect post reversal sperm counts compared to pre-vasectomy counts.

Other research backs up this view. "Many epididymal changes are found [after vasectomy]…. An absence of muscular contraction post-vasectomy [has been demonstrated]. Nerves posterior to the vasectomy site appear to undergo degradation and, in some cases, do not appear to return after vasectomy reversal" (Kaufman, et. al., 1996). Also, "Studies make it clear that epididymal dilatation and granuloma formation are common [following vasectomy]. Insufficient attention has been given to the possible role of denervation in producing these changes…. Denervation of the epididymis in the rat results in spermatazoal accumulation, particularly in the cauda…. Impaired innervation, and consequently reduction of contraction of the cauda epididymis at ejaculation, may partly explain poor fertility after successful recanalization"

(McDonald, 1996). Other research backs up this view showing vasectomy to cause "a marked reduction in the noradrenergic innervation of the muscle coat" following vasectomy (Dixon, et. al., 1987). Simply put, the nerves get cut, the muscle stops working, and it is difficult to impossible to regenerate.

If the damage to the nerves from the surgery is severe enough, the body will form traumatic neuromas around the injured nerves in an attempt to reconnect the severed nerve tissues. This occurs in conjunction with scar tissue formation in the testes, which is often extensive due to the autoimmune response discussed previously. In 20% to 30% of cases, neuromas which form are of the painful type (Olsson, undated). This is what happened in my case.

This nifty diagram gives some idea of the many nerve systems in the region, along with showing some of the lymphatic tissues that were discussed in previous chapters:

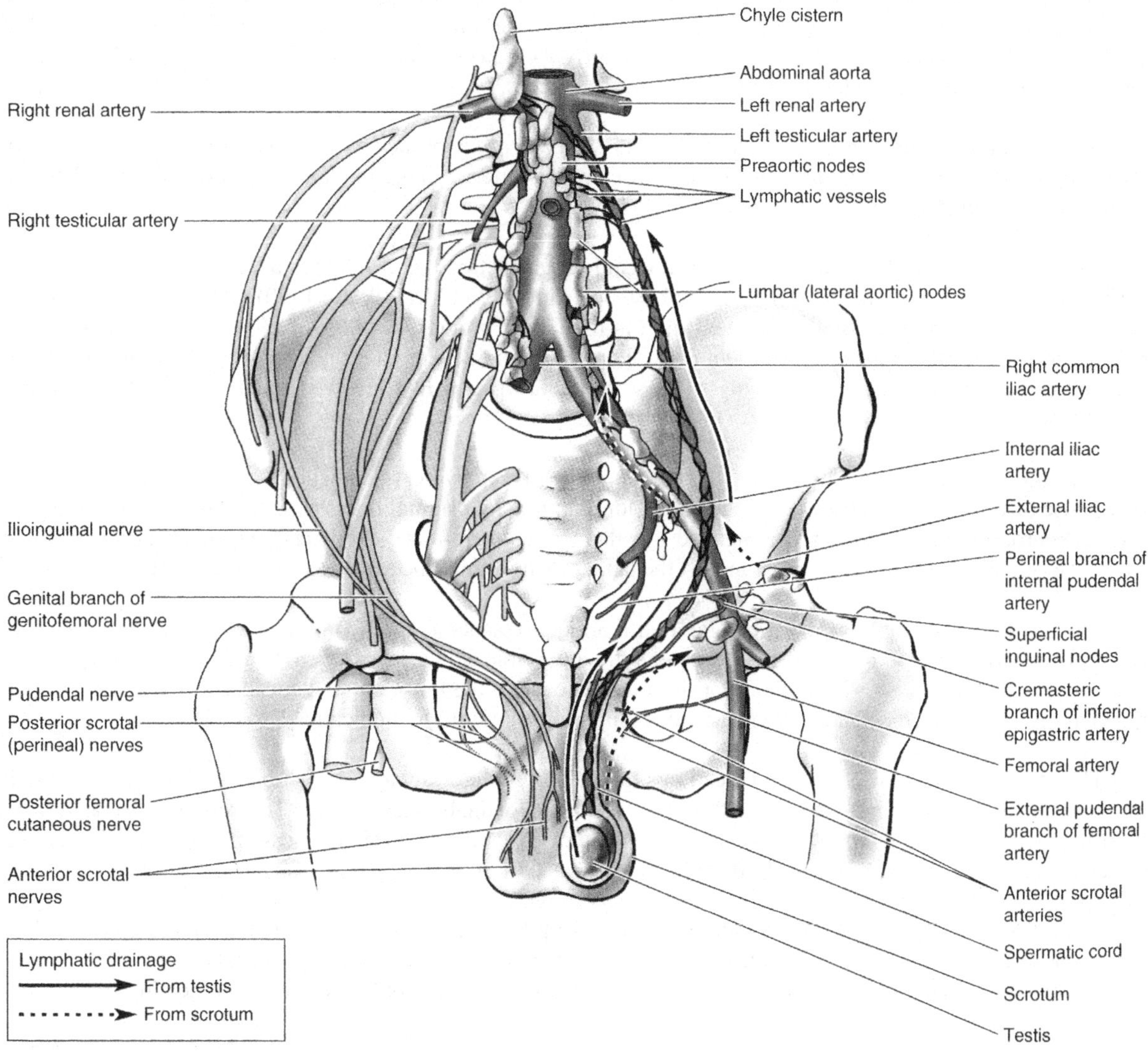

There is interplay to be considered between autoimmune reactions, scar tissue formation, and nerve entrapments that cause pain. McDonald (1996) reports that: "Interstitial fibrosis [scar tissue] frequently surrounded and distorted nerves… post-vasectomy pain [was attributed] to obstruction and dilatation of the reproductive tract with fibrosis involving nerves, particularly in the cauda and ductus [vas] deferens."

Several researchers seem to have a good handle on why this post-vasectomy pain problem occurs: "The main cause of chronic testicular pain following vasectomy may be related to sensitization developing at the dorsal [back] horn of the spinal cord. This form of pathological pain develops after an injury [like surgery] to an area [and] is associated with the frequent transmission of impulses along small unmyelinated C- [nerve] fibers. These induce a state of sensitization in the dorsal horn receiving the impulses, after which normally innocuous mechanical stimuli [like walking or sitting] may be perceived as being painful. The duration of these central changes may greatly outlast the duration of the sensitizing impulses, and it is thought that they may produce long-term pain" (McConaghy, et. al., 1996). This is one of the best summaries I am aware of about the nerve pain aspect of post-vasectomy pain syndrome, which considers a wider source of the pain response than just in the genitals. This type of systemic pain response is more in line with what various pain specialists I had seen discussed, with the recognition that each of us is one complete organism and not just a collection of subsystems.

Unfortunately, even with this knowledge, damage to the peripheral nerves of the hypogastric plexus, which go to the testicles and abdomen, and the nerves of the sacral plexus, which supply the scrotum and other external tissues (and erectile function for that matter) are not the best-studied or easiest nerve injuries to resolve. Recent research literature states: "The management of peripheral nerve injury continues to be a major clinical challenge" (Flores, et. al., 2000). It appears that why these kinds of pain syndromes occur is fairly well understood, but a solution to the problem is much more difficult. This seemed to mirror what I was getting from the doctors.

What could be done? Well, there was always the wait and see approach, which could take years and still might not ever show any improvement. Then there were drugs, which were offered to me in copious quantities and varieties, most of which my body reacted to strongly and negatively.

Speaking of strong medications, the World Health Organization has developed a "Three-Step Analgesic Ladder" to describe the increasing increments of pain control by medication (WebM.D./WHO 1990). At the base are pain relievers such as acetaminophen and ibuprofen. The next rung in the ladder progresses to medications such as Vicodin, Lora, and acetaminophen with codeine for more persistent pain. For even more severe pain the next step is an opiod (narcotic) such as Morphine or Fentanyl. I recognized many of these as being drugs I had received, often repeatedly during my post-vasectomy process.

Then there is the "beyond the ladder" approach to pain caused by nerve damage or cancer. The approaches for this include the use of tricyclic antidepressants such as the Imipramine my original doctor had tried out on me, anticonvulsants such as the Neurontin that had been recommended by others, and "membrane stabilizers" which are oral versions of local anesthetics. Evidently, I had raced right up and off the ladder by now and I needed to consider these options.

I had looked at the option of various long-term antidepressants as the neurologist had suggested. In reading the material on these drugs, I found that swollen testicles were a possible side effect, which would be counterproductive given what I was trying to accomplish. This, plus my prior experience with the Imipramine that caused several key normal bodily sensations to disappear raised considerable resistance in my mind about these medications.

Then there was the anti-seizure medication suggested by several doctors, which had a whole raft of possible side effects, including that nagging impotence and the sudden and unexplainable death stuff. This too, sounded as if it would be counterproductive. I wondered about the potential effectiveness of oral anesthesia medications, given the increasingly low effectiveness I had experienced with injections of local anesthesia throughout my numerous surgeries.

At best, any of these medications would only cover up the pain symptoms, as had been attempted before by my original urologist leading to disastrous results that put me in the hospital with bleeding intestines. I wasn't anxious for a repeat performance. None of the medications offered an actual cure, nor would they facilitate healing of the underlying injuries.

Several types of nerve blocks with local anesthesia could be tried, again. My painful prior attempts at these types of interventions left me highly suspect of anyone approaching my privates with a loaded needle. The likelihood with any type of anesthesia was that the effect would be temporary and also only act to partly cover up the pain.

I had found reference to a research article about a form of local anesthesia injection into the area of the perineum and prostate (yep, that's correct, right into the old crotch) that had been effective in relieving pain in six of eight (brave) patients upon whom this had been performed (Zorn, et. al., 1994). The article didn't mention if these men's testicular pain was due to vasectomy, but the likelihood seemed high. I didn't get a very enthusiastic response from my doctors about the prospects of this working well for me, but it did bring up some valuable information.

The authors of Zorn, et. al., (1994) stated that their research showed that a significant portion of nerve signals, i.e. pain signals, from the testicles travel through the pelvic plexuses, in addition to the signals that are normally routed through the spermatic cord plexus. They saw this as an explanation for why testicular pain often follows prostate surgery.

I looked at it this way: If you are driving down the street to a particular destination, and the street is blocked off, you probably won't choose to stop and die there, but are more likely to find a detour and get yourself to your destination. Evidently, the nervous system works in much the same way. So I began searching for a more permanent way to create a Berlin Wall in my body that pain signals dared not cross.

Then, I began finding a number of research articles on surgical denervation (nerve stripping) of the spermatic cords to treat chronic testicular pain that was unresponsive to other treatment. I had sworn this surgery off initially, as I had sworn off so many other severe treatments that I had eventually ended up undergoing. But long-term pain makes your mind a little weird, actually a lot weird, and I figured I could always say no after a look-see and before the doctor got out the sharpening stone. The research was interesting, quoting high success rates for pain relief, but not mentioning much about the long-term effects on quality of life, sexual function, etc. Plus, the surgeons who did this type of work looked to be few and far between, with a few doctors authoring articles in the U.S., and a number of others in Great Britain.

I wanted to undergo another surgery about as much as I wanted, well, about as much as I wanted to have my testicles cut on again, but if this approach avoided removing key pieces and left everything else pain-free, it could fit into my plan. Naturally, I was concerned and wondered whether nerve-stripping of the cords would leave me with more than just numb nuts, a moniker that had been used in reference to me numerous times throughout my life already.

My research into nerve-related treatments coincided with a referral to yet another urologist. This time I went to Stanford University Medical Center, which had a reputation for solving the most unsolvable of medical problems. After reviewing my medical records and doing an exam that gave me yet another opportunity to do my rendition of "Twist and Shout", I had another of those frank doctor-patient discussions. So, what were my options at this point?

According to the doctor, when pain has continued on one side this long, he would often consider an inguinal orchiectomy, i.e. cutting into the groin and removing the testicle and cord. But when pain occurs on both sides, the removal of one testicle alone is unlikely to give relief, and the removal of both testicles requires hormone and other treatments for life, and this was undesirable. I quickly expressed that I agreed with him and that removing one or both of my testicles wasn't a good idea and I wasn't open to it. Why did these doctors always lead off with this option? Was this supposed to make the other options sound more attractive?

Next! The doctor had treated a dozen or so men, several of whom had experienced post-vasectomy pain as severe as mine. He had achieved good success with surgical nerve stripping of the spermatic cord, with a success rate of 90% or better.

Yes, but could these men get an erection afterward and enjoy sex? No change according to the doctor since the penis and the testicles are on different nerve paths. That sounded like saying your next door neighbor to your condo can set up a crystal meth factory and it won't affect you a bit. Aren't all these parts connected somewhere along the line? I'd had several surgeries by now intending to reunite the pieces and create everyone one big happy family again.

Could he put me in touch with someone who had success with this treatment? No, he couldn't give out names. I remained skeptical. What other complications were possible? Well, if there is a continued pain source, the pain can find other pathways eventually, and I could end up back where I started. That wasn't very encouraging, but it echoed my other research.

What else? The surgery to take out a section of the nerve is done in the inguinal area of the groin, and it can damage the blood supply to the testicle(s). This can lead to testicular atrophy (shrinkage and dysfunction) and potential need for removal of the (by then) diminutive testes. This sounded like what Phil had talked about in regard to an epididymectomy. So what did he think was causing the pain I continued to experience? The cysts that had formed in my scrotum again on both sides were a possible symptom or aggravant, but neuropathy (nerve damage) was the likely culprit given the symptoms. The way to test this was to do another spermatic cord nerve block with local anesthesia.

Had I described my last experience with a nerve block? That was not something I was interested in repeating. Not to worry, according to him, this block would be done higher up in the inguinal areas where the surgery was contemplated, not near the penis where the last block was done. I was still quite skeptical. He wanted to refer me to the pain clinic to set this up while I gave this whole course of action consideration. Fine.

What about the continued autoimmune response? The doctor confirmed what my research had told me; two out of three men, or more, will experience a permanent autoimmune reaction after vasectomy that won't stop even after a reversal. According to him, there's no way to resolve it. You can perform various procedures with the sperm to attempt inducing pregnancy, but as for the reaction in a man's body, once the cat is out of the bag, so to speak, it's out. I tried to assess the situation as best I could. I was still experiencing constant, significant pain and a continued inflammatory response after a year and five different invasive procedures. What, other than a claimed 90% success rate, would make me think that another surgery would succeed, this time removing pieces where there was no possibility of putting them back? The reality of this "path of no return" gave me cause to pause.

Besides, even if the surgery was successful, the pain could come back later due to inflammation, autoimmune reactions, and whatever other sources of pain that remained after the denervation procedure. This still felt like quite a quandary. Eventually, I discussed the possibility of nerve-stripping again with yet another doctor who had helped to pioneer the technique. What I found out was fascinating. According to him, post-vasectomy pain syndrome can cause Reflex Sympathetic Dystrophy(RSD)-like symptoms in which all of the tissues on and around the spermatic cords can contribute to the pain response and become conduits of pain signals. This syndrome has several other synonymous names including causalgia, and Complex Regional Pain Syndrome Type II. The basic idea with all of these terms is that trauma to the peripheral nerves in some part of the body causes a pain cycle to start that sensitizes the central nervous system in the spinal cord also.

For this reason, when the procedure is done not only are the nerves removed, but typically the vas deferens, cremaster muscle, veins, and sometimes even lymph vessels are also stripped away. If these structures are not removed, there is a higher likelihood of continued pain, at least according to the doctor. I considered the trouble that I had experienced with many of these structures thus far, particularly the rupturing and autoimmune results of having my vas tied off, and decided that this didn't sound like the best of ideas for me, even though the doctor was claiming 75% or better pain relief on the 27 or so men he had operated on thus far.

I was reminded of a quote in one of the research articles I had obtained: "Various operations advocated in the literature for non-responders [to conservative measures of pain relief] included epididymectomy, scrotal orchiectomy [castration through the scrotum] and inguinal orchiectomy [castration through the groin], all of which have a significant failure rate" (Choa, et. al., 1992). I decided to take the conservative approach instead of running headlong into a scalpel again. Sticking with the testosterone treatment for the time being seemed wise. How long might that need to go on? Well, according to the immunologist and the endocrinologist I was consulting with, six months seemed like a good starting point. Weighing that against the possibility of months to recover from yet another unsuccessful surgery didn't seem so bad.

How long might it take for the autoimmune response to go away, assuming I could reach a zero sperm count and stop the aggravating influence of all those pesky little cells? According to my immunologist, the inflammation might take months to diminish, and the antibodies might take four or five years to go away after the precipitating cause went away. Four or five years, you say? This was looking like a longer process all the time.

I did eventually see the folks at the Stanford Pain Clinic on referral from the urologist in the same hospital. My initial appointment was with one of the young doctors there who turned out to be a very cool and understanding guy I came to know as Dr. Steve. When I explained what I was experiencing and gave him copies of the medical records, I noted the stunned and bewildered expression I had become accustomed to seeing emanate from the faces of so many medical people already. "Ouch" he exclaimed several times as I recounted what I had experienced so far. Ouch is right!

After an exam to confirm all this he disappeared for 20 minutes or so. I was beginning to wonder what was up when he returned accompanied by the senior doctor at the Pain Clinic. The senior doctor confirmed that he had seen other patients with similar symptoms as a result of vasectomy, and that further surgery was in all likelihood inadvisable. Thank you, God! Finally, I felt like I was being heard and understood by these guys. They suggested a series of nerve blocks with local anesthesia to assess my body's reaction to the possibility of long-term non-addictive pain medication. More nerve blocks? I really hadn't liked the pain and drama involved in any of my prior blocks, which I made quite clear to them. Not to worry, they wanted to take a different approach. This sounded fine in concept, but I intended to do a lot of research before any of these moves were made.

A different approach in my case started with what is known as an Intravenous Lidocaine Infusion, which is basically a test where they hook you up to an I.V., pump you full of local anesthesia, then see how your body reacts and how it affects your pain level. Since this was supposed to take about an hour to do, I brought a good book to read during the test. Once the I.V. was in and the pumping began, I immediately started feeling like I had the world's biggest fraternity party going on in my head. So much for the good book. Part way through this little adventure, Dr. Steve came to pay me a visit.

"How are you doing?" he asked.

"I'm flying right now, Steve. Wanna join me? It's easy. Just strap in, hook up an I.V., and away you go!"

Unfortunately, he had rounds to make and more patients to see. But he did comment that the initial effect is a lot like that of nitrous oxide. I hadn't had any dental surgery in quite a while, so I wasn't readily able to relate to this, but it did give me an insight as to what medical students might do in their labs when they are bored on weekends. The lidocaine infusion was effective in knocking down my pain level substantially, and my whole body hurt somewhat less for a few days after. So far, so good.

The next procedure was less fun to administer. This was what is known as a Superior Hypogastric Nerve Block, wherein a doctor takes some more of those damnable long needles and sticks them into your body on either side of your sacrum. With the guidance of an x-ray machine the needles are then inserted down into the interior of the pelvis to the nerve plexus that is to be numbed with local anesthesia. Here's another one of those nifty diagrams to give you an idea of what this little procedure was going after (the superior hypogastric plexus) and all of the other goodies in the neighborhood:

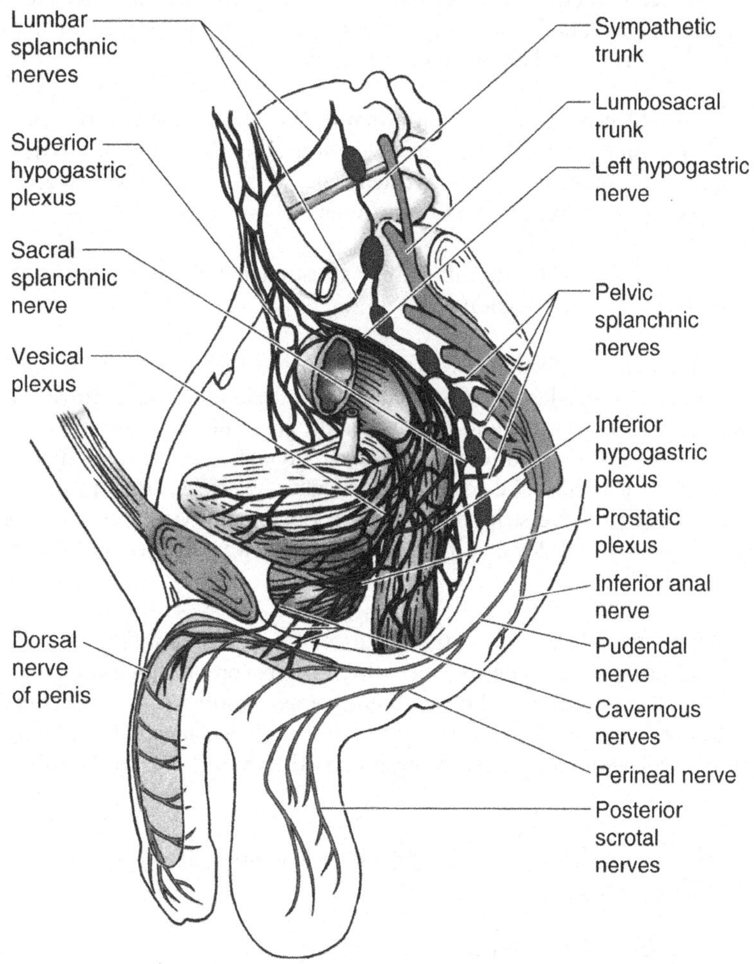

When I arrived in the operating room to have this done, I found that Dr. Steve was nowhere to be seen, and one of the junior doctors on the staff was to do the needling with the senior doctor whom I had met previously supervising the procedure. This was OK in concept, save the fact that the junior doctor had a problem getting the initial needle where it belonged, and started grinding it around to try to relocate it while it was in me. This was more than a little painful, and I got to do a lot of that deep breathing practice again. When my pulse dropped in half to 32 and alarms started going off, the senior doctor asked me if I was in pain. No shit, my toes just usually curl up for no reason!

"I think you're in the right spot, because I can feel what you're doing all the way down in my groin!" I exclaimed. I was beginning to understand how people died during "simple" procedures. Was this modern medicine or voodoo?

At that point they started pumping me up with medication to give my heart a "squeeze" and bring my heart rate back up since I was close to passing out. This "squeeze" was not exactly the kind of hug I was used to. When this didn't work the first time, they did it again. Then came the narcotic sedation, which I had specifically refused, so I wouldn't continue to feel the prying of the needle. I'd been in enough recovery rooms by now to know that if you have been sedated, they hold you a lot longer before you can leave, and I was hoping for a fast food approach to surgery. This was not meant to be.

The remainder of the nerve block process only took a few more minutes after this little drama was done and then the senior doctor said, "OK, all finished." Well that was one more rigorous procedure under my belt, quite literally.

"How long should I expect this to last?" I asked hopefully.

"From six hours up to several days," he projected.

"Up to several days" turned into one hour of blissful relief before the pain started to return, and it returned in a big way within just a few hours after the irritation from the procedure. My wife and I determined that we should have found a by-the-hour hotel while we had the chance and enjoyed ourselves.

The upshot of these several procedures at Stanford was that one of the doctors wrote me a prescription for a membrane stabilizer medication he thought might help me. Upon leaving the clinic, my wife asked what the medication was called. I looked at the paper the prescription was written on. "Fe....," I tried to make out the writing. I turned the paper sideways and then upside down. It didn't look much different.

"Flu...., Fri...., oh Fukitol. That's it: Fukitol! I think I just named my own medication. And if it makes me feel anything like that lidocaine infusion did, it's a great name."

My wife agreed that this was a perfectly appropriate response at this stage. One thing of which I was sure: it was time for another hiatus from medical procedures! In subsequent discussions with Dr. Steve, he clarified that the name of the medication being prescribed was Flecanide, and that he would gradually increase my dosage to avoid the frat party sensation I had experienced earlier. That seemed like a good idea. No one was able to predict how long I might need to try this new medication, or how much it might take to achieve the desired effect. But, in his opinion, it was worth a try. Besides, in his experience, even after a nerve stripping surgery is done, pain will often come back in the long run, and it will come back in an "angry" form when it does, so trying medications was a better option. Angry nerves did not sound good in this case.

His first recommendation, though, was that I try a course of Neurontin initially, and if that didn't work well, bring in the Flecanide as the second string. Considering the other options previously presented, like more surgeries with potentially greater side effects and complications, the Neurontin seemed worth a try. Besides, by this time I had enough of my physicians cast their votes in favor of the Neurontin to wear down my resistance. My pharmacist was more than a little apprehensive about the strong medications that were being proposed to me. I was getting that sense of playing with fire again.

This situation reminded me of the story of the guy who came home from his doctor's appointment looking very worried. His wife asked what was wrong.

"The doctor told me I have to take one of these pills each day for the rest of my life!" he explained in a distressed manner.

His wife replied, "So what! Lots of people have to take medication their whole life."

"I know," he said, "but he only gave me four pills!"

For me, the Neurontin turned out to have as many side effects as most of the other medications I'd tried. As the dosage increased I lost my appetite again along with bowel and bladder pressure sensations. When my anxiety level increased so much that I didn't sleep for several nights, I determined it was time to stop the chemical experimentation. Dr. Steve agreed, but had a few other tricks up his sleeve.

Believe it or not, those tricks included repeating the superior hypogastric nerve block some months later. The premise for this was that if you can break the pain cycle enough times, the pain levels can actually start to diminish. This time though, he would use a long-acting anesthesia to get a greater effect. That was the theory at least. The application was more like a circus.

When I arrived at the hospital and checked in, I noticed the outpatient surgery center was quite busy. They must have been offering a special. The crowded conditions led to a three hour wait. The admitting nurse greeted me in a very friendly manner and then spent the next 20 minutes telling me how attractive she found me, finishing by telling me how she wanted me to father 100 children for her. I told her that she needed to look a little further down the chart at the reason I was there. The course of the conversation changed after that.

An hour or so later I was brought to the preoperative area and allowed to change into one of those highly fashionable and highly over-priced hospital gowns. Then after four more stabs attempting to find my elusive veins, my I.V. was hooked up (Is this a karmic thing, or what?) while my new nurse friend stayed nearby.

While I waited, my wife joined me and we played hang man to pass the time. At one point a doctor with a thick Norwegian accent came into the pre-op room and began talking to the man in the bed next to me. He flipped through the chart quickly, and then said, "So, remind me, what are we cutting off today?"

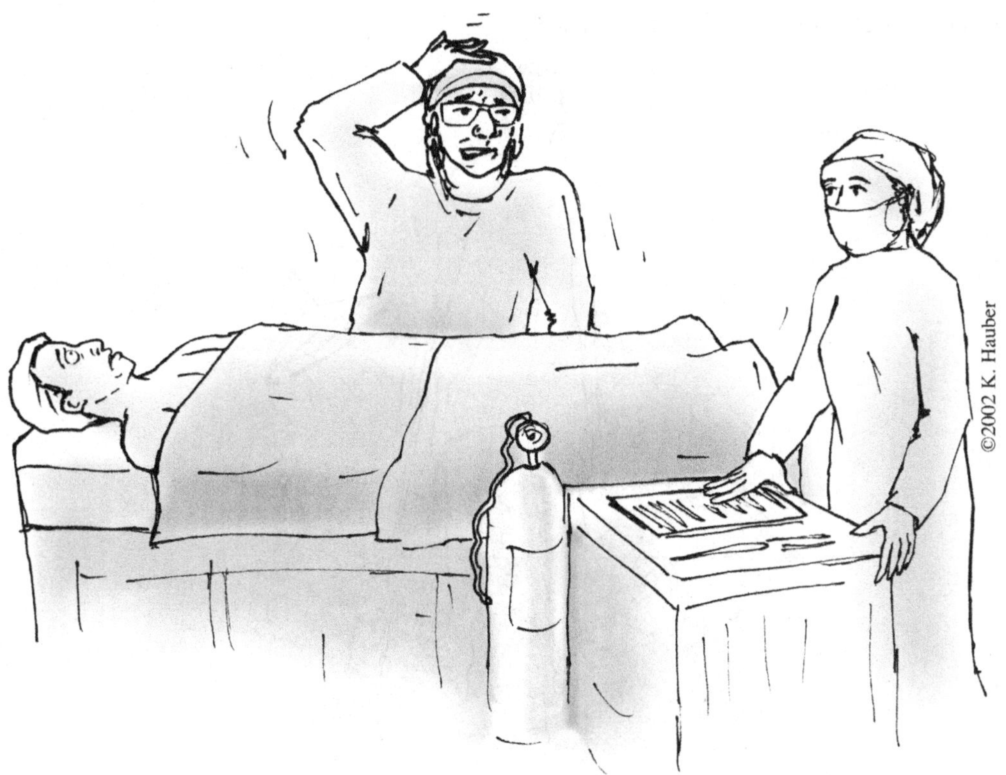

So, remind me... What are we cutting off today?

I was speechless. My wife and I looked at each other with that deer-in-the-headlights expression and both nearly bolted simultaneously. "What are we cutting off today?" I'll bet the man was glad the doctor asked. Given my experience thus far with surgery, this was not inspiring any confidence. And the fun wasn't over yet.

When I was finally wheeled into the operating room, I found that Dr. Steve was, once again, nowhere in sight. No big deal, I was learning to be my own advocate quite well by then. The same lady junior doctor with her own thick accent that had done my block before was there. She remembered me from the last procedure in one of those "Oh, you're here again" ways. I wasn't sure if that was a good thing or not. As she loaded up the needles, I asked what anesthetic agent she was using this time.

"I'm using 10cc. of Marcaine," she replied.

"No, you are supposed to use Chirocaine as a long-acting agent. That was the whole point of doing this procedure again," I insisted.

She started flipping through charts and rummaging through cabinets while I lay there, sunny-side up on the operating table. I was about to order out for pizza since it was taking quite a while and I wasn't allowed to eat anything all day because of the pending surgery. My experience has been that there is not much that pepperoni and mushrooms won't fix.

"We don't have any Chirocaine in the operating room," she finally confessed.

By then I had received some sedation through my I.V., or I probably would have gotten up off the table and walked out. The head surgeon came in and the two doctors spent a fair amount of time deciding on a suitable substitute. They finally settled on a substance called Carbocaine. Cabocaine, Chirocaine, what's the difference? This situation must have shaken up the lady doctor a bit, because as she tentatively stuck the first needle in with the guidance of the operating x-ray, she hit a nerve.

"Wow, my leg feels like it's on fire!" I exclaimed.

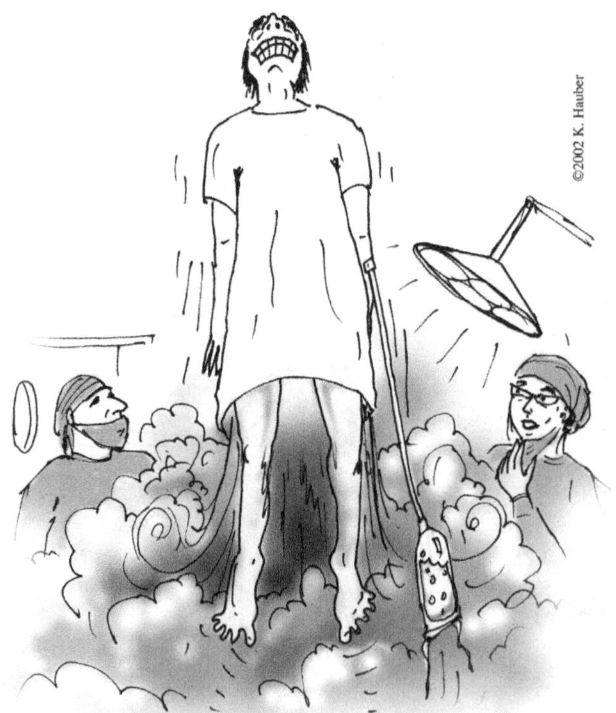

Oh, Dear... Did that cause you pain?

Oops. This on fire sensation progressed to numbness in my inner leg that lasted for five or six hours, making walking afterwards a Pinocchio-like experience. By the time I was released from the recovery room several hours later, I was ready to blaze out of there and never look back, save the wobbly legs that wouldn't let me blaze anywhere. The block itself was effective for about eight hours before the pain came back with a vengeance. This just seemed like an awful lot of drama to go through for eight hours of relief.

Dr. Steve and I subsequently agreed that more nerve blocks might not be in my best interest at this point, but he had even more ideas that he wanted to try out on me. I could hardly wait.

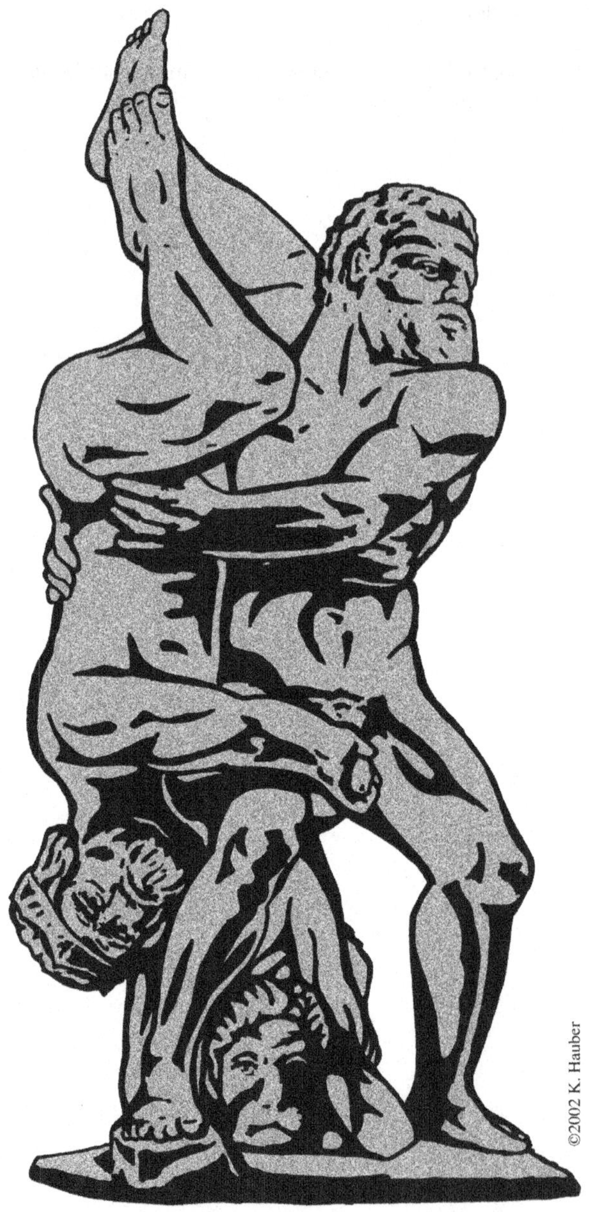

Oh yeah? Vasectomy This!

Actually, the original title of this sculpture is "Hercules and Diomedes," by Vincenzo dei Rossi. Carved in the 16th century, it depicts Hercules throwing Diomedes into the trough of Diomedes' own man-eating mares. I just happen to like my title better. The Italian Renaissance sculptors certainly had a flair for "gripping" drama, didn't they?

When I began to have problems after my vasectomy and friends and acquaintances became aware of it, I was amazed to start hearing about how many of them had numerous problems associated with their vasectomies too. Sometimes the men themselves who would confide in me such simple things as their pants didn't feel comfortable any more or that they get sore testicles a lot now.

Others spoke of shooting pains in the groin periodically. One female friend stated simply that for something that was not supposed to have changed their sex life at all, it was in fact different, and not for the better. I didn't pry into what that meant, but it wasn't a positive review.

Another friend of mine called to say that he heard I wasn't feeling well, and expressed his sympathies. He felt in a particularly empathetic position since he experienced periodic severe episodes of epididymitis.

Really? Had he had a vasectomy, I asked? It turned out that his recurrent epididymitis started three years after his vasectomy, and would send him to bed with pain and fevers for days at a time when it occurred. His doctor had told him that if this pattern continued he would need to have his epididymides removed. His doctor never mentioned anything about congestive epididymitis, post-vasectomy pain syndrome, or any other term of the type for this condition. Coincidence, or misdiagnosis and misinformation? You make the call.

I spoke with a friend of a friend who had his original vasectomy done many years ago. The doctor told him he was fine to resume normal sexual activity shortly after the procedure. Then he conceived his third child. There's another nail in the coffin for the low failure rate argument. So he had his vasectomy done over again and this time ended up with chronic pain, especially during sex. Along with this he would get periods of itching in places that it was difficult to scratch in public. This continued for several years until he finally went to a university hospital where he was told there was nothing more that could be done for him. It took a number of years for the more severe pain and other symptoms to subside. Decades later, he still gets a good shot of pain when he sits down too abruptly. In his words, he found out that this simple procedure wasn't simple at all.

I connected with yet another friend of a friend who told me that he would experience pain so severe at times after his vasectomy that it would drop him to his knees. After much protesting to his insurance company, he had a reversal done which resolved the pain. After this, he and his wife had tried to have another child only to find that his sperm cells were not motile enough to impregnate an egg, even with the help of a fertility specialist. Evidently no one had told him about the autoimmune aspect of vasectomies persisting even after reversal. So I sent him some of the research I had gathered in hopes that it might help his situation.

Then I heard from a college buddy who told me that he had experienced chronic pain and severe headaches since his vasectomy a year and a half earlier. His doctor had told him that he was one-in-a-million also. By my count I think we're up to at least five, six, seven and eight in a million aren't we? No one had ever mentioned the possibility of any of these complications to these men before their vasectomy procedures were done.

I wasn't alone in my observations. Remember Richard Barcham, the guy in Australia who had the same kind of pain experience after his vasectomy as I had, which put him in the hospital also? Barcham said, "In speaking with other men-and I've now spoken with quite a few of my friends, acquaintances, and other men that I know about my problem, I've been struck by the rate at which men report relatively long-term complications for vasectomy"(Radio National, 1997).

Numerous postings on Internet sites by men in long-term pain after their vasectomies served to further my conviction that I was not alone, and in fact, much of the information needed to properly diagnose and treat these problems is swept under the carpet. One man that I corresponded with had suffered with post-vasectomy pain for nearly ten years, had undergone numerous surgeries, including eventual castration, and still was in constant pain. At the time he was planning to have a permanent anesthesia device surgically implanted in his spine. He had lost his physical therapy practice, and this pain syndrome had irreparably changed his life.

Another man I corresponded with had experienced post-vasectomy pain for over five years. He was finally being taken off active military duty and being referred to a pain specialist. His comment: "I'm 28 and this is not how I want to live my life!"

I read about another case in which a man experienced cardiac arrest during his vasectomy. I knew the procedure could be stressful, but wow! The article concluded, "The surgeon should be able to provide basic life support during out patient vasectomy" (Lamberg, et. al., 1996). So let's do our pre-surgery equipment review: Anesthesia, check; scalpel, check; sutures, check; cauterizing tool, check; CPR certification, check; defibrillator, check!

All this feedback furthered my resolve to question the statistics regarding low post-vasectomy complication rates that are commonly quoted. First question is this: If 6, 18, 27 or 33 percent, or more, of men who have vasectomies end up with some form of chronic pain (depending on who's figures you believe), how could the complication rate be less than three percent? This bit of curiosity led to the information I shared with you in previous chapters. Quite obviously, the problem is much more widespread than much of the medical community is aware of or willing to reveal.

If I were to attribute the injury I sustained to anything more than just a slip of the scalpel, it would be the hurried pace at which modern medicine is forced to be practiced. Certainly my original urologist was well-trained, and used one of the techniques widely promoted for minimizing complications. I'm convinced that in his mind he was and is a caring professional trying to do the best he could for me and for his other patients. Something simply went wrong, both in the carrying out of the actual procedure, and in the addressing of disclosure issues which I expressed concerns about but he chose not to reveal.

However, it is also my observation that my original urologist and many other doctors can't take the time to slow down for exceptional cases and still maintain profitable practices, whether they had a hand in creating these exceptional cases or not. Increased pressures of expectations from patients, the financial squeeze associated with insurance coverage and reimbursements, along with an expectation to keep up with the latest technology and methods which don't come cheaply, have all conspired to push medical providers for more while they earn less for their time and investment.

This leaves precious little time to focus on problematic cases, especially when they fall outside the doctor's scope of prior experience or the area the doctor has chosen to focus on for his or her practice. Combine this with a natural human tendency to avoid difficulty and anything leading to possible litigation and you've got quite a tough situation. This seems to be where I landed. I was going to have to force my way out.

Nonetheless, to be responsible practitioners, medical providers need to find a way to allow the space needed for every patient to be heard, their needs validated, and treatment options explored. This is not easy and will require rethinking many of the basic economic forces at work in the system today.

Likewise, if HMOs and medical insurance companies would quit playing the "starve them out" games with both patients and medical providers and stop trying to practice medicine for those providers, they would have a lot less need for large legal departments. The whole system needs to open up more to alternative modes of treatment beyond the narrow Western medical model and allow everyone to have a valid area of expertise, including patients who should be able to choose what works best for them whether the HMO has a contract with the provider or not.

That was a good rant wasn't it? But isn't there a lot of good common sense in these ideas? Isn't it better to deal with some very basic issues such as these than to continue to support a system that is out of control and unsustainable? Add in the problems of access to a system that is so expensive now that a huge portion of the population can't afford to receive medical treatment, and if they do need to receive treatment it can be ruinous for them financially.

Full disclosure of the risks involved in any treatment is one key change that is needed, particularly in relationship to vasectomies. Not one man that I have met who has had a vasectomy ever had his doctor fully disclose verbally or in writing that chronic pain or expected immune system responses are known complications of the procedure despite decades of research in these areas. This is irresponsible. If patients receive adequate disclosure of what is to be done to them, and the risks involved, they are much less likely to be inclined to sue their doctor when something goes awry.

We'll discuss the legal aspects of vasectomies in more detail shortly, but in the meantime, given all of this evidence, including my experience and the painful and problematic experiences of others discussed so far, it is worthwhile to discuss some of the myths propagated about vasectomies and the facts that are the realities behind those myths:

Myth Number One:

A vasectomy is a safe, simple surgical procedure with few known complications and a high rate of satisfaction.

Fact: Performing a vasectomy may be simple from the surgeon's point of view, but the effects on a man's body are by no means simple. The possible complications are numerous, up to and including death from resulting infections. Documented associations also exist for complications that include chronic testicular pain, lifelong autoimmune responses, hormonal changes, serious bleeding and swelling, formation of several types of cysts, chronic inflammatory responses, kidney stones, and psychological impairments, to name just a few.

"Fear of life-threatening sequelae [results] have dominated the literature on vasectomy in the 1990s.... Most reviews on vasectomy and health, including the most recent by Linnet (1993), Hendry (1994), and a large survey by Coulson, et. al.,. (1993), mention that a number of men suffer chronic local pain or discomfort, attributed to epididymal distension and sperm granuloma formation.... There is a growing body of reports of local morbidity [disease, pain] following the procedure" (McDonald, 1996).

In addition, nerve injuries can occur during the vasectomy procedure, which can magnify the extent of the pain experienced to an extreme, leaving you feeling like you have been kicked in the testicles or, alternately like they are being torn off, all the time. I know of what I speak in this regard, and know that I am not alone.

Myth Number Two:

A man's body is unchanged after a vasectomy, save his newly acquired sterile state.

Fact: Any doctors who tell you that there are no physiological changes in a man after vasectomy are either completely unfamiliar with the medical findings on the subject, or are ignoring the decades of documented research on the issue in their own medical journals, or are just plain lying to you. For example, Jarvis, et. al., (1989) reports that: "Scrotal sonograms were obtained in 31 men before and after vasectomy to determine the effect of the surgery on the sonographic appearance of the testis and epididymis. The sonographic appearance of the testis was unchanged after vasectomy. However in 14 men (45%), there were persistent changes in the epididymis. These consisted of enlargement (14 patients)[45%], development of cysts (11 patients)[35%], and an inhomogeneous echo pattern (five patients)[16%]. The presence of these sonographic changes was unrelated to symptoms [of pain]."

Apparently, even if you don't feel any different afterward, there are still significant changes going on. The possible long-term results of these changes have not been defined well enough to offer the type of blanket reassurances given by many medical practitioners. In fact, much of the evidence is to the contrary, as you are starting to see by now.

One problem that is nearly universal is significant scar tissue formation as a result of the vasectomy procedure. Scar tissue formation increases with the time interval after the procedure. Shiraishi, et. al., (2002) state: "Interstistial fibrosis (scar tissue) contributes to the irreversible damage of vasectomized testes." This type of scar tissue formation can also entrap nerves causing the types of pain sensations previously mentioned.

Myth Number Three:

A doctor will use the best, most current technique possible in performing a vasectomy.

Fact: A doctor is likely use the technique he or she is most accustomed to using even if there is evidence that there are problems associated with that technique. In the typical vasectomy procedure, the doctor snips each vas and ties all four of the newly created ends off, trying his best to hide them from each other. Post-surgical complications like bleeding and swelling can be minimized using the no-scalpel vasectomy technique in which a single smaller incision is made to access both vas deferens. However, less than half of all doctors use this technique currently. Even fewer doctors use or will even offer the open-ended vasectomy technique, which has repeatedly been shown to result in a lower incidence of chronic post-vasectomy pain.

Myth Number Four:

Sperm cells are just reabsorbed into the body with no resulting problems.

Fact: A man's body continues to manufacture sperm at the rate of 50,000 cells per minute after the vasectomy. Days, months, or years later sperm can build up pressure and congestion in the delicate epididymis portion of the testicles, causing the structures there to rupture, known as a "blowout" in the trade. This can be quite unpleasant, take my word. This congestion and rupturing process can lead to a condition commonly referred to as Post-Vasectomy Pain Syndrome (PVPS), congestive epididymitis, Post-Vasectomy Syndrome(PVS), or Chronic Post-vasectomy Testicular Pain(CPTP), which your doctor likely forgot to tell you about before the procedure was done, if your doctor was aware of it at all. Silber (1980) says that "all vasectomized patients have 'congestive' epididymitis." Silber also concludes that a "percentage of vasectomized men are going to experience some pain no matter what technique is used," and that "it would be inappropriate for us to suppose that one can perform vasectomies without the risk of some scrotal discomfort." It is just a matter of when and how symptoms may manifest. In fact, this condition is diagnosed many times as recurrent infectious epididymitis when

146

that may not be the case at all. Even the government is willing to admit that a diagnosis of epididymitis is more common in men after vasectomy. Research has shown that one-third or more of vasectomized men will experience some level of chronic testicular pain as a result of their procedures.

Researchers expect reports of post-vasectomy pain syndrome to occur more frequently as the population of vasectomized men ages. Post-vasectomy pain syndrome can be minimized by the use of the open-ended vasectomy procedure, in which the testicular ends of the vas are left open, and only the upper ends are sealed off. Surgical treatments for persistent post-vasectomy pain when conservative methods fail include vasectomy reversal, removal of the testicle(s) altogether (orchiectomy), removal of the epididymis portion of the testicle(s) (epididymectomy), and stripping of the nerves from the spermatic cord(s). None of these procedures can guarantee a resolution of pain. All variations of the vasectomy procedure put men at risk of the autoimmune responses described below, since sperm cells are retained in the body and released into the blood stream.

Myth Number Five:

Sperm granulomas are a rare, easily resolved complication of vasectomy.

Fact: Ruptures or leaks in the epididymis or vas will typically lead to the formation of sperm granulomas, which are a reaction of the immune system trying to isolate what it considers to be a foreign body, i.e. sperm cells where they weren't naturally intended to be, namely, outside of the vas and epididymis. "Extravasated spermatozoa in all mammals elicit formation of a sperm granuloma, a mass of degenerating spermatozoa surrounded by macrophages and chronic inflammatory cells. Histologically, sperm granulomas resemble those of tuberculosis. Degenerating spermatozoa release fatty acids similar to the mycolic acid produced by tubercle bacilli…. It seems that, after some time, spermatozoa are no longer able to drain freely into the initial granuloma, and the intraluminal pressure [in the vas] again rises and forms a new granuloma closer to the testis. Vasectomy leads to a mixture of tubular dilatation and single or multiple sperm granuloma formation" (McDonald, 1996).

Chronic inflammation that results in the affected tissues leads to granuloma formation in 60% of patients, with some estimates higher; up to 97% of patients in one study developed sperm granulomas (McDonald, 1996). Silber (1980) states simply that a "sperm granuloma is an inevitable and unavoidable consequence of vasectomy." Sperm granulomas can be quite painful (again, take my word) and may need to be removed surgically. A related inflammatory phenomenon is known as vasitis nodosa, which has been shown to occur, often concurrently with sperm granulomas, in 66% or more of vasectomized men. Vasitis nodosa has been noted for having benign tumor-like characteristics, which must be carefully determined, so as not to lead to the inadvertent hasty removal of a testicle that is not, in fact, malignant.

Vasitis nodosa and granulomas can have an effect on your sex life too. "For more than 20 years, symptomatic [painful] granulomas at the vasectomy site have been reported (Schmidt, 1966; Livingston, 1971; Schmidt and Morris, 1973), often presenting as a tender nodule (Schmidt, 1979). Pain is usually localized, worsens during sexual excitement, may be severe at ejaculation, and may continue as an ache. It has even been mistaken for renal colic according to Schmidt (1979), who found nerves adjacent to some sperm granulomas and attributed their stimulation to (1) the inflammatory process, (2) the bolus of sperm reaching the granuloma at ejaculation, and (3) compression due to muscle contraction at ejaculation" (McDonald, 1996).

These effects can make you old before your time, sexually speaking at least. "Granuloma formation in the caput epididymis occurs as a late event and is associated with degenerative changes in the testis" (McDonald, 1996). This furthers the discussion of vasectomy as a cause of autoimmune orchitis, i.e. a degenerative process in the testis.

Myth Number Six:

Some men will have a slight allergic reaction to their own sperm.

Fact: Doctors familiar with the research on the subject expect that sperm retained in the body will create an autoimmune reaction wherein antisperm antibodies form en mass to attack the continual supply of sperm cells being produced in the testes. They might even admit this if pressed and acknowledge that it happens in up to three men out of four. Some studies have shown antibody reactions in as many as 86% of vasectomy patients (Gupta, et. al., 1975). The extent of the impact from this autoimmune reaction is not fully known, and it is currently not possible to predict how a particular individual will react. Research has also indicated links between vasectomy and the long-term incidence of numerous immune system-related diseases, including various forms of cancer and degeneration of testicular tissues.

Very little is known about how to treat this autoimmune response, and further research shows that it does not stop, even after a vasectomy reversal, which is in itself a highly unpleasant procedure. Unfortunately, I can also attest to this first hand. Ironically, medical science can help you mitigate the autoimmune response on the sperm themselves so that you may be able to father a child, something which you were probably trying to avoid with a vasectomy to begin with. But there is very little that medicine can do to effectively stop your body from making war on itself once this reaction has begun.

Although a vast majority of urologists are aware of the potential immune system-related problems associated with vasectomy, they keep right on doing the procedures anyway. In one survey, 92% of the responding urologists knew of the studies linking vasectomy to prostate cancer. However, 94% of these urologists claimed that this evidence made little or no difference to them in their practice of performing the procedures (Sandlow, et. al., 1996). "Don't confuse me with facts, my mind is made up." Or, maybe old habits die hard, especially when they are profitable old habits. As we have discussed previously, the facts of the research surrounding this issue are often not disclosed to the patient before the procedure or even after the patient develops problems.

Myth Number Seven:

Your medical insurance will cover you fully for any illness.

Fact: Insurance coverage for these types of problems is generally non-existent or minimal, particularly through many HMOs. Complications of vasectomy are regarded as rare, and anything "outside the box" will be difficult to get coverage for. You might have no problem getting coverage for enough narcotic pain medication to turn you into an addict, or at least create a dependency, but not be able to get coverage for therapies that really provide relief for your condition without damaging your health more than the actual illness. It is quite rare for vasectomy reversals to be covered by medical insurers. You will have to kick and scream about the part of your body that you are least likely to make a public fuss over to get adequate coverage. You might even need to resort to legal action.

Myth Number Eight:

Vasectomy is a sure-fire method of contraception.

Fact: Unintended pregnancy after vasectomy occurs with regularity, at much higher percentages than is often quoted, for a variety of reasons. Even if failure (recanalization) does not occur, a man can still have occasional sperm in his ejaculate for no explainable reason.

Myth Number Nine:

Vasectomies are easily reversed should a man wish to father more children.

Fact: "The results of reconstructive surgery in several published series were good with respect to restoring the continuity of the dissected vas, and sperm again appeared in the ejaculate in up to 83% of patients. In contrast to the anatomical success, the functional results (that is, the postoperative conception rates) were rather low in most series: 14% to 55%. Two major reasons were discussed for this discrepancy. Agglutinating autoantibodies appeared after vasectomy and were [negatively]correlated with the pregnancy rate after vasovasostomy…[and] the destruction of the nerve supply to the vas deferens during vasectomy" (Pabst, et. al., 1979). As we have already noted, the presence of sperm antibodies is quite difficult to eradicate, and nerve damage may never heal.

Myth Number Ten:

Your doctor will disclose all of the relevant facts to you before the procedure.

Fact: Many doctors, including many urologists are not fully acquainted with these facts, or disregard them as being theory or conjecture. They will tell you that these occurrences are one-in-a-million or that links to numerous other diseases are just rumors. Having lived with many of these maladies, and then having read over 200 research articles discussing the problems associated with vasectomy, let me assure you these complications are a very real experience. I now have found many friends and acquaintances that could tell you the same.

Consider this quote by R.F. Raspa in the (1993) *Journal of the American Family Physician*: "Family physicians should be aware of the potential effects and complications of vasectomy so they can appropriately counsel patients seeking sterilization. Vasectomy produces anatomic, hormonal and immunologic changes and…has been reputed to be associated with atherosclerosis [hardening of the arteries], prostate cancer, testicular cancer and urolithiasis [kidney stones]. Complications of vasectomy include overt failure, occasional sperm in the ejaculate, hematoma [bruising], bleeding, infection, sperm granuloma, congestive epididymitis [a synonym for post-vasectomy pain syndrome], antisperm antibody formation and psychogenic impotence."

Putting all this in a laundry list format, vasectomy has been linked in research and case histories by numerous doctors and researchers to dozens of potential maladies, including:

- Life long autoimmune (allergic) responses

- Decreased testicular function including changes in testosterone production

- Chronic testicular pain (a.k.a. neuralgia, testalgia, causalgia, or orchialgia)

- Chronic inflammation

- Scrotal and epididymal cyst formation including granuloma, spermatocele, and hydrocele cysts.

- Epididymitis (infectious and non-infectious)

- Prostatitis

- Prostate cancer

- Testicular cancer

- Vasitis nodosa

- Erectile dysfunction/impotence

- Circulatory problems including phlebitis

- Rheumatoid arthritis

- Pulmonary embolism

- Lupus

- Arteriosclerosis (hardening of the arteries leading to heart disease)

- Autoimmune orchitis (degeneration of the testicles)

- Staph infections including infections of the heart valves

- Gangrene and other serious infections

- Loss of libido

- Lung cancer

- Non-Hodgkin's lymphoma

- Multiple myeloma

- Personality disturbances

- Diabetes

- Multiple sclerosis

- Some types of hepatitis

- Adrenal gland malfunction

- Narcolepsy

- Migraine and other related headaches

- Hypoglycemia

- Generalized lymph node enlargement

- Liver dysfunction

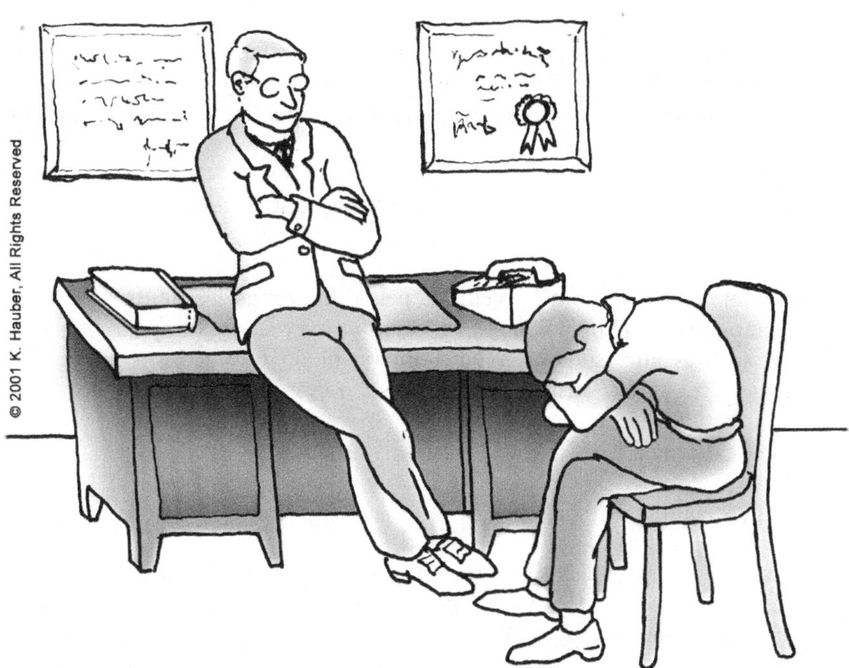

*Come on, it's no big deal. **There are no more than three** dozen serious diseases that can come of this simple and safe procedure.*

Let's take a practical approach to this. Can all of these observations and all of the research associated with them be wrong? What if this is a correct association in only half the cases, or only one-fourth of the cases? Given the number of men involved is over 100 million, isn't this a cause for concern?

The reaction of the medical community in general has been to acknowledge that there may be numerous problems of this sort, but they don't know why, or what the "biological mechanism" is that causes these diseases, so they will keep doing vasectomies by the millions until they do know one way or the other. How's that for a Readers Digest-type summary? Ready to schedule your snip?

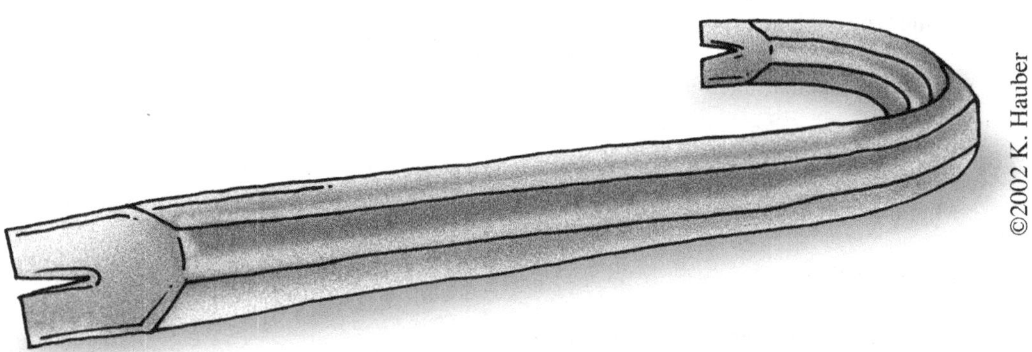

Life is weird, and if you think this story has been weird so far, well, you're right. But there's more. I swear to you that what I am about to discuss really happened, as much as I would like to have experienced otherwise.

I continued to consult with the Pain Clinic folks at Stanford Hospital. After all, this is one of if not the leading medical facility on the West Coast, right? Amid the various examinations, nerve blocks, and medications Dr. Steve was trying out on me, he noticed that my body was carrying a lot of tension after having been in constant pain for a year and a half or so.

"This gets a little weird," Dr Steve said to me one day (so what else is new?), "but I want you to try having pelvic floor releases done."

So what's a pelvic floor release, anyway? Well, the pelvic floor muscles run from your pubic bone to your tail bone and serve a variety of purposes including holding up all of your internal organs, your genitals, etc. When the pelvic floor muscles are bound up, such as after surgery or other injury, blood flow tends to be restricted and this slows or completely hinders the healing process. This seemed to make sense so far.

"So how is this 'release' accomplished, Steve" I asked.

"That's the part that gets a little weird," he said.

Evidently the best way to facilitate this type of release is from the inside, with a gloved finger up the old tail pipe, bent in a "come hither" fashion, and then essentially prying into the muscles and tissues until they finally cry uncle and release, or until the patient cries uncle and leaves. Huh?

"You're sure this is supposed to help?" I inquired hesitantly in my best "what the *%&# are you talking about?" tone.

Dr. Steve told me that he'd had good luck with this approach in similar circumstances, namely in men with chronic pelvic pain following prostate surgery, so he suggested I give it a try. Well, yes, everything in the area was consistently sore, but was this really the best way to facilitate healing? Probing of this sort was not a pleasant thing for me, but I was still just desperate enough to be willing to give it a try.

I wasn't the only one who had received this recommendation. Many men experience what is known as "chronic pelvic pain syndrome" after having undergone prostate surgery or when experiencing prostatitis. Several medical researchers have concluded, and a variety of studies have indicated, that myofascial release of pelvic floor muscles conjoined with progressive relaxation training is helpful in alleviating these painful symptoms over time (Gower, 2002). Dr. Steve felt that my situation was similar enough to justify this type of therapy.

The therapist who ended up doing this pelvic floor release therapy in my case was a charming young lady named Laura who helped to make the best of what was a very uncomfortable situation. There I sat, or laid actually, in a birthing-like position while this prying went on, trying all the time to carry on a civil conversation while waves of hot pain would run through my body. I'm sure the view from her end of the conversation must have been difficult to go home and talk about. How would you even recognize your patients on the street, I wondered?

The funny thing was, after this unpleasant invasion, I would spend a day or two with the sensation of having been in prison, and then I would actually move a bit easier for a period of time. The pain in my testicles didn't go away, but the rest of my body felt a little less tense. That was OK, but how could I get this benefit without an eight hour round trip drive that tended to make the pain worse.

"Well, I could show your wife how to do this," Laura offered one day.

"But she has nails," I quickly remembered. "Besides, after all the indignities that have occurred since my vasectomy, I'm not sure our relationship is ready for that."

"Well, you can do this yourself with an instrument called a Crystal Wand," said Laura.

This sounded like it was meant to be used in some pagan ritual. I still think that isn't far from the truth. Actually, the Crystal Wand is an S-shaped contraption that allows you to reach places you normally wouldn't be able to, or necessarily want to for that matter.

"How do I get one of these 'Crystal Wands' and how do I use it without causing permanent damage?" I asked. "This kind of stuff is not my forte, you know."

"You'll have to go to one of those stores without any windows to find one, or you might be able to find one on the Internet," she stated in a matter-of-fact manner.

Great, now I get to peruse the porn shops trying to find some exotic sex tool on the recommendations of my doctor and therapist. The folks back home would never believe it.

I live in a very conservative, cute little town, which happens to be void of such windowless stores, and I surely didn't want to order that kind of item over the Internet. I already received enough weird SPAM as it was without adding that to my Internet profile. If you don't believe me, just do a few Internet searches on the words testicle, vasectomy, or painful ejaculation and see what starts showing up in your in box.

I would try to find this little toy when I traveled for various doctor appointments out of town. I found one shop in a backwater little town on my way home one night and asked the attendant about the Crystal Wand.

"Crystal wand? What the hell is that? People around here are so unsophisticated, I could never sell something like that!" he stated emphatically, and began rummaging through his catalogues trying to find one. Well, if this guy thought I was kinky, at least he thought I was sophisticated about it.

So now I was not only looking for a sex tool, but an exotic sex tool to stick up my own tail for therapeutic purposes. I stood there for several minutes that dragged on like hours, praying that no one that I knew would walk in while he searched for my prize. Then I realized that if anyone I knew walked in, my excuse was much better than theirs would be! I guess my request was just too sophisticated for that little town, because he couldn't find anything resembling a Crystal Wand. There were lots of wands of other varieties, big ones in fact, in various colors, but not the one I needed.

I finally ended up finding this little item in a shop in San Francisco (where else?) that Laura recommended I check with. Was this beyond weird by now, or what? The sales person felt compelled to instruct me about how to clean and care for my new instrument while I fidgeted and looked for an opportunity to head for the door.

"Is this what I've been looking for?" I asked Laura upon my next visit pulling the Crystal Wand out of my bag.

She seemed surprised that I had actually been able to find one, as if no patient had ever demonstrated that much tenacity, or lack of good sense, before. I wasn't sure exactly where I stood in that regard.

All of this little pry and stretch routine didn't turn out to offer enough progress to satisfy Dr. Steve, though. So he wanted to add "trigger point" injections to the process of the pelvic floor releases. This involved a series of quite fiery injections into my crotch while the prying was going on in a further attempt to get the muscles to relax and the pain to go away. But regardless of how much anesthesia was pumped in from any direction, the pain would persist. Have I stretched your imagination yet? Hang on; it gets better!

"If this doesn't work," Dr. Steve stated one day, "we can always try Botox."

"What the heck is Botox," I queried.

"Actually it is a weakened strain of the botulism virus that is injected into selective muscles to make them relax for up to months at a time," he responded. "Botox is used a lot by plastic surgeons to make wrinkles relax and smooth out, for example."

"So let me see if I understand, you are talking about injecting what was once a deadly virus into various parts of my genitalia to try and get those parts to relax," I observed. "Not that I wouldn't like to get the wrinkles out, but you know there are muscles down there I might like to call on to work once in a while when the opportunity avails itself."

"Well it doesn't sound so good when you put it that way," he said, "but my aim is usually pretty good."

"I think I'll pass on the deadly viruses for now, thank you," I affirmed, "let's just stick with the fire-down-under anesthetics for now."

I told you this was going to be weird, didn't I? Even Fellini would have had a hard time putting this stuff in one of his movies.

Eventually I found a therapist in my area named David who knew how to do pelvic floor muscle myofascial release work from the outside and didn't use any of the fiery injections. This seemed much more in tune with what my body was willing to tolerate. So we adopted a slow, patient approach to this work, with far less drama involved.

"Tell me what the sensation you feel is like," David asked one day.

"It feels like a little man with large hands is hanging from my testicles all the time and squeezing them while he tries to tear them off," I replied, being as vividly accurate as possible.

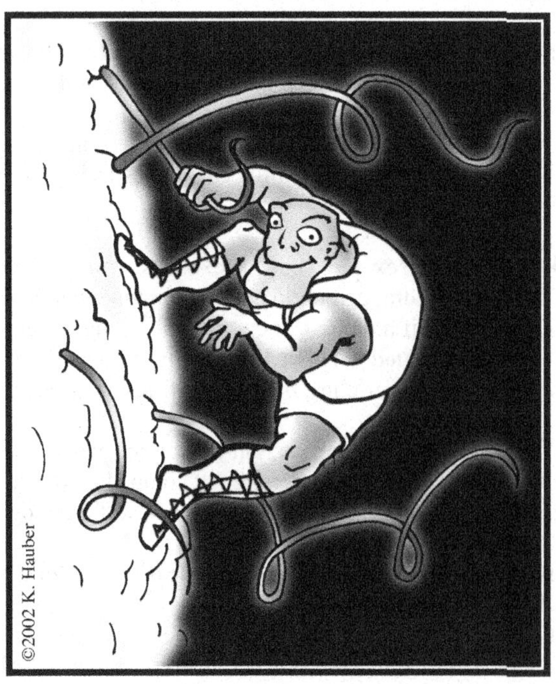

"Ah, Testicle Gremlins," David concluded.

That was the most accurate image I'd heard yet, but getting that little guy to let go was turning out to be quite a chore.

By this time I'd learned that I would make the world's worst drug addict, what with how negatively my body responded to so many of the more than 150 medications that had been offered and tried out on me. I had surely figured out how to read the warning information in the medication package inserts, and learned to ask lots of questions in that regard.

What I learned throughout the months that all this new "adventurous" therapy occurred was that I could find some reasonably effective ways to mitigate the spread of pain throughout my body for a period of time, often at a significant price, but the actual center of the nerve pain wouldn't go away and was much more difficult to treat. This was the core issue that no one had a very good suggestion about. So the search for the "magic bullet" continued, while I continued to adapt and experiment. What else was there to do?

Interesting proposals were made along the way in regards to what that magic bullet might be. I eventually underwent a new form of MRI known as Neurography which gives a highly accurate mapping of any problems with nerves. I was looking for a specific neuroma or other problem that could be resolved in a conventional manner. What the study showed instead was that I had nerve damage and inflammation that went from my testicles all the way up though my groin on both sides. This was not what I had hoped to find out, and I couldn't help but look at the images and think, "Boy, am I ever screwed!"

Months later, when I returned to UCLA to see the head of the urology department, and to Stanford for a consultation with the head of the pain clinic there, I wanted to discuss what had been termed "neurogenic inflammation" that was evidenced in the Neurography study, which simply means that the nerves get aggravated and it won't let up. Various experimental studies have tried to test the viability of Amazonian herbs and other therapies to treat this neurogenic inflammation.

The response I received at UCLA and Stanford was quite different from what I expected. The head urologist at UCLA told me that I had done everything he would have recommended and he had no further ideas for me, end of story. I had greater hopes for my Stanford visit, but the head of the pain clinic there told me straight away that my nerve damage was permanent, and that it might never heal. This was less than encouraging.

All that could be offered to me were various ways to try to block the pain signals in my spinal cord. This would be most effectively accomplished by a "spinal cord stimulator" which is essentially a hockey puck-size device that would be surgically implanted in my butt and controlled with a magnetic device. This implant would have to be removed surgically every five years or so to change the batteries. No screwdriver with a trap door was available here unfortunately. And I would likely set off metal detectors and have to explain to airport personnel why my butt had metal in it.

Wires would then be implanted into my spinal cord to create an electrical interference to block the pain signals. However, when I turn the device on, it might turn me on, giving me constant erections. Kristen looked scared when the doctor mentioned this. Later she told me she wondered how she might get any rest if this were the case, i.e. I wasn't in pain any more and I had a constant erection. It seemed as if medical science really had come up with that Orgasmatron after all.

When I shared this tidbit with several of my male friends, in unison they shouted "Where do I get one of these spinal stimulators?" Just shows you the different perspectives men and women can have. I'd wanted to think that this device would help me put my best foot forward, but I felt that would be inaccurate in so many ways. All that aside, this was not the magic bullet I had anticipated.

Part IV

Where Do We Go From Here?

Chapter Twenty-Six

Extra, Extra

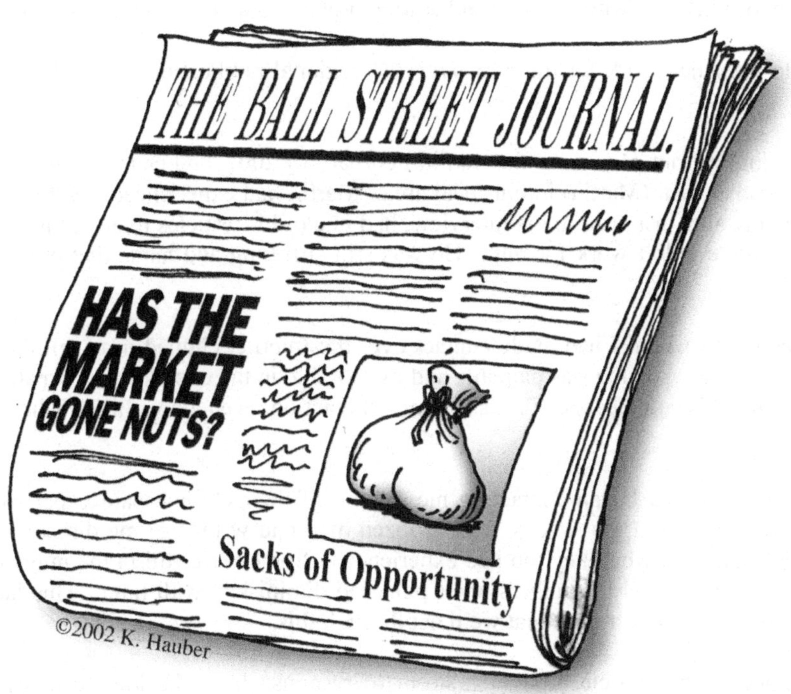

In case you haven't noticed by now, this is a very difficult subject to read about (and to write about for that matter). As a matter of fact, this is probably one of the more difficult subjects you could choose to communicate about with anyone, male or female. Interestingly, I have found that it is often easier for a man's spouse to discuss this subject than the man himself.

Many men seem to have a reaction like, "Whoa! Way too much to think about! Way too painful!" I have found this to be true often even among men who are experiencing pain or other symptoms following their vasectomies, whom you would think would be very motivated to learn as much as possible. Often their wives or even other female relatives have been willing to communicate openly about the subject, but the men just can't bring themselves to discuss the situation. In some ways this is understandable given the devastation this situation causes in a man's life, yet it is a very important subject and needs to be discussed and made widely known. This apparently is where I come in.

It became obvious to me that no one could or would speak about this issue like someone experiencing it first hand. My notes became more of a book as I continued to write and I started communicating with other men who were experiencing the same type of predicament over the Internet and in person.

Out of this process the www.dontfixit.org website was born. I didn't know what to expect in this effort other than to open the lines of communication for anyone willing to enter the discussion. Soon, dozens of men and their family members wrote to the web site telling their stories of pain, complications, and all the associated dramas. Within a year the site was receiving an average of over 700 visits per day. I consistently received messages of gratitude and praise for bringing this issue to light in this way. While this in itself was gratifying, I became more convinced than ever that vasectomy was causing a disaster phenomenon with far reaching implications that had been consistently and successfully swept under the carpet in the past. It was time for a more thorough house cleaning.

While at the pool during one of my mid-day swims, a friend questioned what was going on with me, since he had noticed my posture, workout habits, and general demeanor were different. I told him the story frankly.

156

"I'm so glad you told me," he said, "my girlfriend has been wanting me to get a vasectomy myself."

I knew he had done some publishing and editing work himself, so I offered him a copy of the manuscript of this book, with the anticipation that it would be to his benefit and mine. That's just how it worked out. Not only did Stacey (yes, that is a man's name too) help me with the flow and editing process, but he also made me another offer one day.

"You know I do freelance work for the *New Times* (a regional publication)," he began, "so what if we worked together on a piece."

This idea turned into a front page story that ran in February of 2001, and caused quite a stir. The article featured stories of about me and another man (Martin) in our local area. Martin had experienced severe pain, infections, and other reactions since his vasectomy and, just prior to his interview, had one of his testicles removed in an attempt to alleviate the pain. Even removing a testicle didn't work for him. He was still suffering and made that evident in his interview with Stacey.

Several other men with whom I had made contact over the Internet chimed in to tell their stories as part of this article in the *New Times*. The shock value was palpable and memorable in the expressions of many who read the story. "I had no idea that anything like this could happen," was a common reaction, even among those who had vasectomies without complications.

Other men in my local area began contacting me, telling of their chronic pain experiences of varying severity following their vasectomies. Within a few weeks, over a dozen men had written to me directly or through the web site, expressing their empathy because of what they too had experienced. Some were still in the midst of their pain experience or other complications, while fortunately for others, their pain had diminished with time. This latter group often offered supportive words, trying to assure the rest of us that we'd get through this.

As might be expected, this article brought a storm of response from the local urology community, citing the purported rarity of these kinds of problems associated with the procedure. Curiously, one of the patients who was still in pain and who had contacted me was, in fact, a patient of a doctor who was quoted in the article as saying that he hadn't had a patient turn up with post-vasectomy pain in years. It's funny how that might happen, isn't it?

In their response to the editor that followed, a group of local urologists quoted a medical text book confirming the facts I had asserted in the initial article regarding autoimmune responses after the procedure, saying that an expected 60% to 80% of men will become autoimmune after vasectomy, but then tried to say that they just didn't consider this fact to be a big deal. That was quite obvious since they weren't willing to inform their patients about it beforehand. One of the doctors posted a message on the web site objecting to the article, but also saying that he planned on revising his informed consent practices with his patients. That was fine as far as I was concerned; baby steps are OK.

I started to send the article out as far and wide as I could. Before long it caught the eye of the health editor for *USA Today*, John Morgan, who had been referred by a friend. He and I eventually put together an article for *USA Today*. Now, if you haven't noticed how *USA Today* articles work, they are kind of like the fast food for the mind approach to journalism. They also insisted on an identifiable celebrity as part of this article. If you think that getting a regular guy to talk about his testicles publicly is difficult, just try finding a celebrity who's willing to do so.

John eventually got Night Court's Harry Anderson to do an interview about his vasectomy. The only problem was, Harry was one of those "no problem" guys who portrayed the procedure as no big deal. In fact, he wanted to talk more about his new magic shop than he did his vasectomy. Even the title of the article took this bent: "Magician's Vasectomy Makes Fertility Disappear." Buried deep in the article for those willing to read that far was my story and the reference to the www.dontfixit.org website. They say that no publicity is bad publicity, so I took what I could get.

The next event was an e-mail from CBS News in Los Angeles. A friend of mine used to date an executive at CBS, and she told the executive that he had to do the story. I should have hired her as my agent. Anyway, the assignment was eventually passed to a producer in Los Angeles named Rodney Foster, who contacted me wanting to cover the story. This was interesting. It seems that Rodney underwent a vasectomy himself a number of years before. At one point he started having some adverse reactions: low energy, lethargy, etc. He decided to have a reversal done and ended up with chronic pain afterwards. He had the reversal repeated again later with satisfactory results. Needless to say, he had a sympathetic ear to my story and the stories of the other men I put him in touch with.

The final version of the CBS story focused on the saga of Rob Morrison, who had to have his reversal repeated four times (!) before he had relief of his chronic pain symptoms, having fought his HMO, doctors, and medical insurance companies every step of the way. Numerous men later told me that this story alerted them to the possibilities of treating the chronic pain they were experiencing following their vasectomies.

Since video and TV appeared to be an effective method of communicating the issue, I went to work interviewing post-vasectomy pain patients myself in an effort to produce a documentary and infomercial on the subject, with the intent of using those features both on the website and for media distribution. Most of the men I interviewed were quite willing to tell their stories, including a doctor friend of mine who had experienced chronic pain for several years following his vasectomy in the early 80's. By the way, his vasectomy had been done by a partner of my original urologist. The one-in-a-million myth was surely beginning to unravel.

I organized and sponsored a first-ever "Healing From Vasectomy Workshop" for couples experiencing this problem in the spring of 2002. Those attending came literally from all over the country, and each had exhausted the medical model in search of a cure. Each had felt hopeless and desperate facing the prospect of pain with no end in sight. We focused on medical and alternative therapies to deal with the problem of chronic post-vasectomy pain, and on how the wives and partners were affected by this situation; an approach which had never been taken, to my knowledge. Afterward, one of the wives wrote to me and said that the workshop had probably saved her marriage, which helped me to know that I was on the right track.

The local media was eager to cover this story by now, and I was invited to make numerous appearances on TV and radio in the area, much to the chagrin of a number of urologists, who protested bitterly in letters to the editor columns, but failed to step into the spotlight as I and the other men who had endured pain at their hands told our stories. I was a guest on a call-in radio show one day discussing the potential perils of vasectomy which made the host squirm in his chair.

One of the callers to the show was a man named Duane. It seems that Duane had his vasectomy back in 1957. Being the man's man that he was, he didn't see any reason to take it easy after the surgery, so he proceeded to pick up and deliver two trucks full of concrete! Because of this, his stitches tore out which led to some dramatic swelling and bruising. Then, about the time the swelling and bruising went away weeks later, Duane began getting spontaneous erections that lasted for about two years. I asked him if he thought this was a problem, which he did (I assumed his wife might have been happy about this). Amazingly though, he contended that all this talk about long-term problems due to vasectomy was "a bunch of crap."

Dr. Lou Zaninovich came out with his book about this time, titled <u>Vasectomy–Before and After</u>. In his book he states, "I completed the writing of this book several months ago but was still hesitant to print it as it lists all the negatives about vasectomy. I felt I could be criticized for not balancing it with the positives. What really made me decide to go to print was the urging from patients who regretted having their vasectomy. A typical example is the story of one patient: Mr. Kevin Hauber.... Kevin had a vasectomy and had such serious problems afterwards that he felt duty bound to warn other men so he wrote a book.... I have read his book and discussed his problems with him. He is dismayed that despite his full enquiries about the possible risks, he was not informed of the potential danger of vasectomy. The result is quite a saga that makes very interesting reading and I commend his book to you" (Zaninovich, 2002).

Validation is nice when it happens. I was sensing a slight change in the tide (finally, I might add).

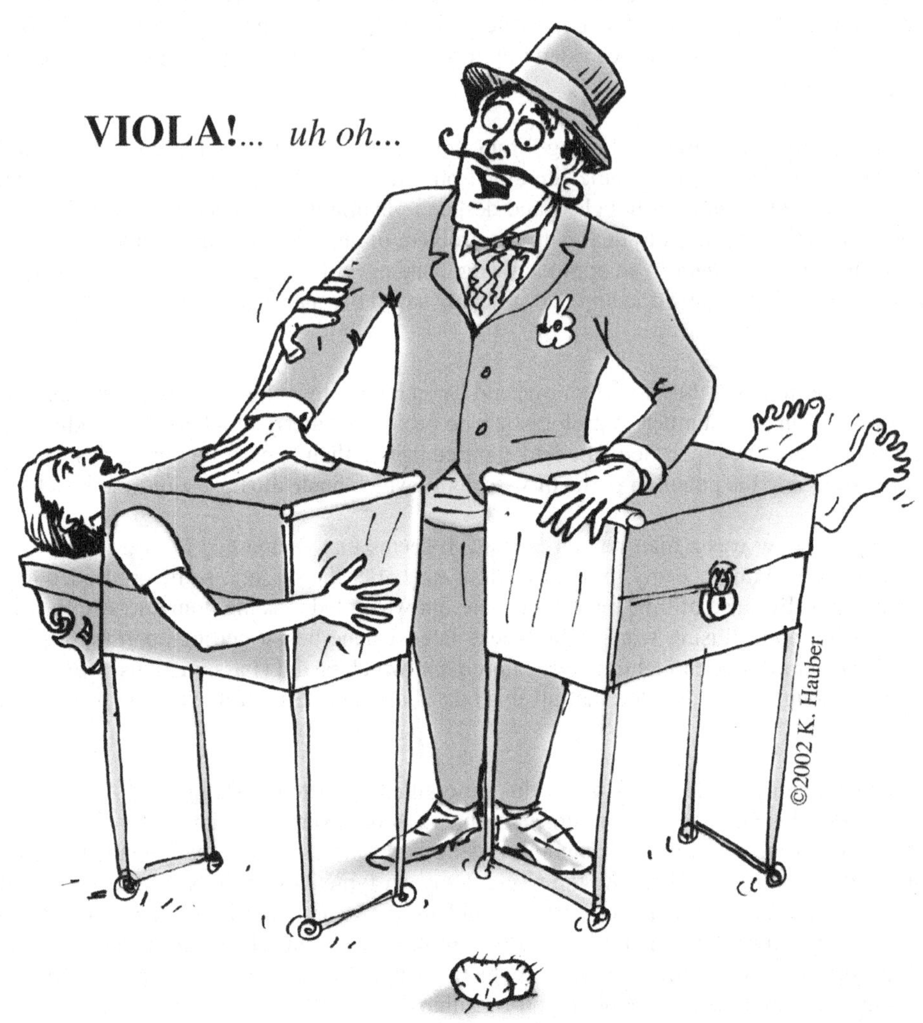

"I tell my friends, 'I will personally kick the shit out of you if you have a vasectomy. Yes, it's your life but I will not let you get one. You do not have free choice in the matter while I am around. You will be physically stopped from going to the clinic to get a vasectomy'" (Simon, post-vasectomy pain patient, and a good friend).

"Primum est non nocere"

This is translated to mean, "First of all, do no harm," and has been the motto of the medical profession for thousands of years.

To this I would add the motto, "Second of all, tell your patient the truth."

In the book of Genesis there is a passage wherein Abraham commands one of his servants to find a wife for Abraham's son Isaac: "So the servant put his hand under the thigh of Abraham his master and swore to him concerning this matter" (Gen. 24: 9 NRSV). Guess what was under Abraham's thigh? In the ancient world of Greece and the Middle East, when one man swore an oath to another, he would do so while holding the other man's testicles. This provided the root of the modern word "testimonial." One has to wonder what this practice might do to enhance the truth-telling process in modern American courtrooms, but that is another speculative matter.

The ancients were obviously less uptight about sexuality issues than we are in this day and age, but such a practice demonstrated an implicit trust that truth was being expressed when a man made himself vulnerable in this way. The practice of a man allowing his testicles to be operated on today in an elective procedure should require no less a level of trust and truth. As you can see by now, this is often not the case.

Patients need to be told the truth, in advance, of the potential consequences and complications they face in considering a medical procedure. This includes the facts that would make them want to go ahead *and those facts that would make them think twice!* To exclude the latter is simply deceptive salesmanship and is totally inappropriate to any professional setting.

Christiane Northrup, M.D., makes the following observation in one of her best selling books when asked if doctors are taught in medical school to withhold the truth: "There was indeed an unspoken belief among our teachers in medical school that patients (and family and friends) were not really able to handle the truth, and that this belief resulted in many things being left unsaid.... I and everybody else [in the medical profession] had been socialized in a thousand nonverbal ways to talk with my patients in a certain way, and that this way left out a lot of the truth of their experience and mine. Of course there was no "Don't Talk to Patients 101" course, I said, but I'd learned by example that a hand on the doorknob, the sight of a doctor racing from bed to bed on rounds, conveyed a world of information to patients about what they could and couldn't expect in the way of communication and contact with their physician" (Northrup, 2001). This is where the change must begin.

First, let's consider the prohibitions. Here's a good plan as outlined by David and Helen Wolfers in *Family Planning Perspectives* way back in 1973: "No pressure, however light or however subtle should be exerted on any man to undergo it [vasectomy]. Men should not be told it is the most marvelous present they can give to their wives. They should not be told it is reversible in a substantial proportion of cases. They should *not* be told that more than 70 percent of men report increased libido after vasectomy, nor that more than 20 percent report improved general health. They should not be told that vasectomy can make marriage more stable and harmonious. They should *not* be told the operation was ever used for rejuvenation, and if they show signs of wanting vasectomy as their contribution to the solution of the world's problems, they should be discouraged from undergoing it." That is a good start for the "shouldn't" list.

Now for the "should" list. The Wolfers continue this way: "The decision to undergo such a procedure is a momentous step in a man or woman's life. Those contemplating it are entitled to the fullest and most factual information regarding the procedure itself as well as alternative means of achieving their objectives. They are entitled to access to informed and unbiased counsel from professional sources who will be influenced by no considerations whatever but the interest of their clients. They are entitled to freedom from blandishments, advertisements and half-truths of those with other interests to serve." I couldn't have said it better myself.

Now, let's get down to some specifics: Doctors, tell your patients the truth that in considering a vasectomy, the procedure is quite likely to result in a life-long autoimmune reaction. Medical science does not know or fully understand the extent and implications of autoimmune reactions, and the manifestations for the individual are not predictable at this time. Tell them of the many studies that show correlation between vasectomies and a significant rise in long-term complications and diseases. Present that, if you like, along with conflicting evidence showing no correlation, and then relate the fact that at this point, you just don't know for sure.

In this context, relay the fact that, for all intents and purposes, vasectomies are still an experimental procedure. Even though they have been done for decades, thorough research on the long-term effects on a man's body is still under way by the World Health Organization and many others.

Let your patients know that research indicates that changes in hormone levels in the body typically follow vasectomy. Let them know that the long-term effects of this are still being studied.

Make sure you tell of the strong chance that the patient will develop a chronic inflammatory response, such as a spermatic granuloma or vasitis nodosa in his genitals following the vasectomy procedure. You can use the words of Dr. Stanwood Schmidt (1979) who, in discussing this response stated: "Spermatic granulomas are specialized abscesses which frequently occur at the site of vasectomy…. Spermatic granulomas are often symptomatic and may cause agonizing pain." Let your patient decide if he really wants to take that risk.

Tell them the truth about the incidence of chronic pain that results from vasectomy, and about the highly unpleasant measures often needed to deal with that condition. Explain to them how their quality of life can be negatively affected by such a condition. Tell them also of the alternative techniques available such as open-ended vasectomy that lessen the chances of experiencing chronic pain.

In the words of Dr. Stanley Myers, et. al., (1997), "Most urologists will encounter a significant number of patients with the post-vasectomy pain syndrome during their career." Take the time to become thoroughly familiar with this syndrome and the treatment methods for it.

Inform them of the limited resources available to help them, should they experience this kind of condition, and do so before you start cutting and snipping. This is not the kind of stuff you want to have patients finding out the hard way, after the fact.

Counsel your patients thoroughly about vasectomy failures and state conclusively that there is no guarantee that the procedure will be permanently effective as a means of contraception. Let them know that, essentially, in choosing to have a vasectomy, they are establishing a long-term relationship with you and other medical providers that may require numerous future follow-up visits for potential conditions such as epididymitis and possible future surgical invasions for such conditions as sperm granulomas, hydroceles, and spermatocele cysts, among others.

Remind your patients that medicine is a business, after all, and what is most profitable and expedient for medical providers and insurance companies may not be in the patient's best interest. Let them know that medical treatment decisions today are as often driven by dollars as by valid medical necessity.

Let them know also that if they have problems later on, or change their minds for any reason, they are likely to find a very expensive, painful, and time-consuming process on their hands for which they will receive little or no support from most medical insurance companies.

For goodness sake, don't take the attitude that was expressed to me by my original urologist when I asked him why we hadn't discussed post-vasectomy pain syndrome before. His response, "I'd heard about it, but didn't believe it could be this bad." Believe it. It can happen, and does, with surprising regularity.

The pain and suffering of one person is an unfortunate thing to be sure, and is very trying to experience. I freely recognize this. I am not so ego-involved as to believe that everyone would care about the pain I have experienced. But I have observed that most people care deeply about the pain and problems that they and their loved ones experience. If I had found I was alone or unique in my complications from a vasectomy I would have never written this book. As you can see, however, there is a remarkable amount of evidence that suggests I am not alone in the negative consequences.

What went wrong in my case was probably more extensive and immediate than most. This allowed me to immediately see the "causal" link between my surgery and what I was experiencing. Unfortunately, it appears there are many, many others who have experienced similar problems over the long term without having the benefit of making that link, or the information as to what to do about it.

As was mentioned earlier, I believe most men will undergo a vasectomy thinking it to be the best way to secure that their family doesn't burgeon beyond their capacity to love and provide for them. I know this was my original intention and the stated intention of many others with whom I have spoken.

It is very difficult to be a good father, husband and provider when you are sick all of the time and in pain. I have been amazed at the body of evidence which shows that these types of life altering consequences are not uncommon. I was also amazed at how this information is either not known or not freely shared by most professionals who perform vasectomy procedures.

My post-vasectomy pain and complications occurred after what I felt had been an adequate amount of research into how to eliminate complications before I had the initial procedure. I trusted my doctor to tell me the truth in my inquiries. This didn't happen, and in fact his reassurances led me into a false sense of security about what I was doing. I thought I was making an informed choice. After the procedure went awry, I began my medical research in the face of what I was told was a one-in-a-million medical situation. In the process, I found compelling evidence that not only am I not alone in the results I experienced, but that the medical community is largely unaware, or in some cases blatantly ignore or hide the problems that often result from doing mass numbers of vasectomy procedures. I found this to be an issue that not only affects me, but many of my friends, and in fact millions of men worldwide.

The problem evidently has been that many affected men are reluctant to speak out on this issue or are plainly unaware of the underlying cause of their problem or condition. Dr. Ian Banks (2001) states: "Despite their health problems, men remain under-informed about health issues, take excessive risks and are reluctant to seek help." That sums up much of my observation. As a group, we men often let our doctors do the thinking for us, even if we might sense something isn't right for our bodies. What's the solution? Start paying attention to your body and the messages it gives you; they occur for a reason!

While some of us have had severe repercussions from our vasectomies, others haven't experienced any apparent symptoms yet, and are quite content with what their vasectomies have done for them. Then I came along to be the loud mouth about this issue. Actually, I consider it to be more like being the grain of sand that causes the irritation for the oyster to form a pearl. I am sure a better means can be found. In the meantime, the truth needs to be told.

Do I think there is some kind of mass conspiracy regarding this issue? No, probably not, though certainly mass ignorance and misinformation does exist. My experience indicates that most doctors are either unaware of or ignore the potential consequences of what they are doing in performing these procedures en mass. Actually, I perceive an underlying intention of most doctors to provide a truly beneficial service to their patients. The method is just ill advised, and methods can be changed.

As for the individual doctors and organizations who are aware of the facts outlined here, but who do not make plain disclosure of them, this indicates a distinct lack of social conscience. Aside from this, a tremendous liability is created, and not just a legal liability either. Imagine the reaction against the medical establishment all the medical research is made widely known. When the personal pain, anger, cost and, in fact, potential loss of life that will result in the long run from these procedures is tallied, the sum is staggering.

You may say, "Well, I dispute this report," or "I disagree with that bit of evidence."

Do you dispute all of it? How can you? This information was written by numerous medical professionals over the past four decades! Are they all out to lunch, or do their conclusions just not suit your purposes? Medical research is evolving, just like we are in our understanding of the miracles of these bodies we have been given. So what if a fraction of the research done so far is improved upon in the future? So what if there is conflicting evidence now? *What if even a small fraction of the research presented here, in fact, turns out to be correct?* There is still compelling evidence to change the current practices employed in performing mass surgical sterilization due to adverse health consequences. When a situation affects millions of people, it is an issue that impacts our society overall.

Truly, the only thing that can be said to be "simple" about vasectomies is the procedure itself, with all of the associated benefits for doctors and insurance companies. Any insistence that the procedure has no effect on a man ignores a great deal of basic biological facts which research has repeatedly demonstrated. The truth is that no doctor can look inside your body to determine how the processes there will be altered by a particular procedure; no one, regardless of how accomplished a doctor he or she is.

The long-term effects of performing millions of vasectomies are not fully quantified yet. In my humble opinion, and in the opinions of many others who have researched the subject extensively, many of the current indicators and studies suggest caution.

So the dilemma remains: In the face of all of the evidence that says that vasectomies are not such a great idea, what can be done to allow for a normal, spontaneous sex life and still avoid exponential population growth? I am speaking out as a man who had a strong enough belief in this issue to willingly have myself operated on the first time. We do have needs, both personally and at a societal level, to wisely control our population and still freely express our personal passions and experience intimacy.

Let's be frank for a moment and discuss the reasons why you would want a vasectomy to begin with. Picture yourself in this scenario: It's 3 a.m,, the house is quiet, the kids are all asleep, and you awaken in a passionate mood. You roll over, embrace your wife, freely touch each other and join in union. No worries involved; just pure primal drives. No need to fumble for a condom, wait to put in the diaphragm, etc. It's purely the little head thinking for the big head, which is what we men do best.

In my case the only additional factor is a little reassurance, "Don't worry honey, you won't feel a thing."

Isn't this the kind of vision that brings most guys to be willing to undergo vasectomy to begin with? Isn't that the kind of freedom that we would all, men and women, desire to result from the process? It only takes one or two "whoops" experiences, though, with a missed period or an unexpected pregnancy to force the left side of our brain into gear in a less hormone-driven moment and consider long-term contraception options. This might also have something to do with the house becoming so crowded that you and your wife never get a chance to touch each other, but that's another form of birth control that historically has only limited success.

For thousands of years the only answer for males was to remove a man's testicles, thereby, permanently resolving the fertility issue, but often creating many other problems. Given the unattractiveness of this option in the modern world and an understandable resistance to it, modern medicine has come up with the "simple" but poorly understood procedure of vasectomy and offered it up as our procreative salvation.

Consider this: Medical science would not advocate that you stop the natural flow of anything else that was intended to exit your body, be it breath, or urine, or moving your bowels, among many processes. The effects of blocking up the body's need to eliminate something are well documented. So why would it make sense to block the natural outflow of millions of sperm cells, and why wouldn't you expect to have a reaction?

The problem is that we are trying to interrupt one of the most natural processes we possess as physical beings. There is nothing more basic to life than procreation. It is at the core of what makes us human, and is in fact, what allows our continued existence on this planet.

I envision doctors who take a critical look at the data here uttering a Dr. Frankenstein-like, "I've created a monster!" response. I hope so. But I'm sure that was not their original intent.

Is it a human tendency to try to justify past behavior? Absolutely, and last I checked, most doctors are still human. So, in recognizing that humanness, there are several things that you, as the potential patient, need to do.

My first recommendation would be that you, as a patient, take charge of and responsibility for your own health and the decisions about what will be done to your body. Don't allow someone else's agenda to determine your choices, regardless of the authority you perceive them to hold. It is your body, and you get to live with the results, not them.

Taking responsibility for your health also means having and seeing a doctor for regular check-ups, more so as you age. I know the prospect of personal questions and gloved fingers up your tailpipe is unpleasant, but get over it. Believe me, there's worse (see Lindholm, "Why Men Avoid the Doctor." as listed in the Bibliography). Such examinations are important for your overall physical health.

In terms of some of the specific issues we have discussed in this text, you would be well advised to start doing a regular testicular self-exam if you don't do so already. You can find an outline for how to do this in the next chapter. You'll only be self-conscious about it the first dozen or so times. Again, consider the potential negative consequences of not doing it.

As a man, one observation I share with you is the consistent theme among medical providers that keeping the pipes clear is beneficial to your long-term health. Whether this means having your chosen form of sexual activity once a week, once a day, or once an hour is more of a matter of preference and convenience. The basic message is quite consistent: Use it or lose it. In this light, it is hard to believe that a vasectomy would be beneficial to your plumbing in the long run.

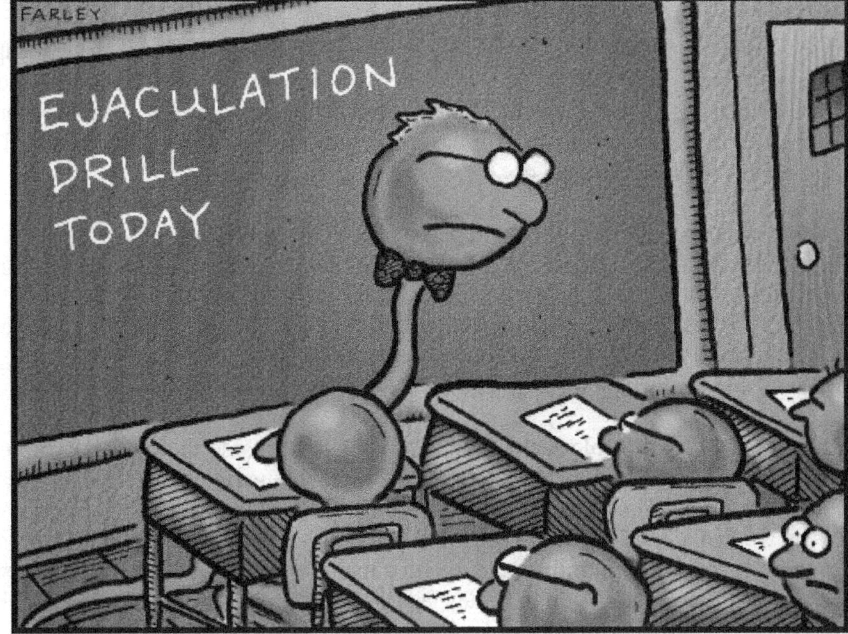

Sperm School

Speaking of vasectomy, expect the procedure to be sold to you with an "Everybody Needs Milk"-like campaign. But, just like those who are lactose-intolerant have found, be aware that the reactions can be significant.

Next, do your homework. Thoroughly research all forms of contraception available to you and the inherent risks of each. Go beyond what your doctor tells you. Most doctors are wonderful, caring individuals who truly wish the best for their patients but are often pressed for time to such an extent that giving you all the relevant facts is impossible.

If you think my presentation of the material here has been extreme, find out for yourself. Do your own homework and reach your own conclusions. It is my fervent hope that no one will ever have to experience what I (and many others) have as the result of a vasectomy. Anything that can be done to help prevent this is worthwhile.

What other contraceptive methods should you consider? This one is up to you, and you probably know more about the subject than I do, although I'm learning fast. Several friends observed that my experience with vasectomy made a great case for a lifetime of oral sex. I encouraged them to go home that evening and try that argument out, wishing them the best of luck.

I know people who actually claim that abstinence works for them. I'm not sure how, but that is the claim. Given everything I have found out about the negative effects of long-term retention of sperm in the body, I wonder about the health ramifications of this choice.

Others still practice the withdrawal method. Aside from the dangers of wanting to go "just a little bit longer" with this method, there is the issue that all those little sperm cells get active and can start flowing even before ejaculation. I have a friend who used the withdrawal method before the birth of several of his kids, and now calls it the "pull and pray" method.

The rhythm method deserves mention. There's an old joke that goes like this: What do you call people who use the rhythm method for birth control? Answer: Parents. Actually, the science of this method has become a bit more refined over the years and is explained and advocated by a number of sources, including the Couple to Couple League (www.ccli.org). This organization claims a high success rate for their recommended natural method of contraception.

Other than these somewhat roulette-oriented methods, you are left with either the option of creating a barrier or a chemical reaction so all those little sperm and egg cells don't do their dance. On the barrier front, I've never been a big fan of condoms, finding that no amount of ribbing or rainbow striping makes up for good old skin to skin. After the experience I've had though, I would gladly wear five layers thick rather than have a vasectomy.

The female versions of the barrier approach most commonly used are the diaphragm and cervical cap, which are reasonably effective if used properly. Several years ago, I heard about a female version of the condom, also termed the pouch (makes you sound like you're making love to a marsupial, doesn't it?) that has been developed and was also supposed to help prevent the spread of sexually transmitted diseases. I haven't heard much about this lately, but it definitely falls into the try-to-build-a-better-mousetrap category.

Tubal ligation for women is quite popular and this method has both its proponents and detractors. There have been studies that show a correlation between tubal ligation and a four to five times increased incidence of hysterectomy in the five years following ligation (Hillis, et. al., 1998). It would appear that both men and women just aren't meant to be plugged up indefinitely. Obviously, I'm less intimately acquainted with the negative aspects of tubal ligation than I am with the negative effects of vasectomy, but if you'd like to find out more on the subject, check out www.tubal.org which is the web site of the Coalition for Post-Tubal Women. You'll be fascinated with the content on this doctor-hosted site.

There is a new method being developed to block the fallopian tubes from inside the uterus so as not to cause a surgery that invades the abdominal cavity. Early studies have promoted this as a superior method of female sterilization (Kerin, et. al., 2001), but I would be curious about the long-term results. My concern centers around the long-term retention of reproductive cells in the woman's body and the results that will have. I realize a woman only produces one or at most several eggs per month versus the hundreds of millions of sperm a man produces each day. Even considering that, if I were a woman, I'm not sure that I would want my body to be a beta site for such an experiment, but, undoubtedly, some will choose to allow it.

The publicized problems associated with long-term hormone therapy (i.e. the pill or the patch) for women are well known. According to health provider claims, pregnancies that occur while women are on the pill are most often due to misuse, a claim that is hard to make with a vasectomy unless a man doesn't wait for the all clear signal. It is commonly proposed that as a woman ages, other contraceptive choices start to become more attractive because of the increased health risks of long-term hormone therapy.

A pointed, and I feel accurate, summary of the effects of the pill for women is offered by Dr. Yosh Taguchi (1996): "The contraceptive pill may make pragmatic sense – it is, after all, 99.9% effective – but it is so unsafe and unfair to women that I wonder why the women's movement has not made a bigger issue of it. When the pill was developed, it was tested on a vast number of female volunteers. It was then judged safe over many thousands of menstrual cycles, implying that women could take the pill indefinitely. What was not clearly spelled out was that there was a difference between five thousand women testing the pill for three cycles and fifty women testing it for a lifetime, even though the two groups represented comparable numbers of menstrual cycles. Clots in the veins, strokes and death caused by the pill came as a total surprise to the medical profession fifteen to seventeen years after the pill was put on the market. It can be stated today that the pill was never properly tested over time. It is argued that since complications occur in fewer than one in a thousand women on the pill, its use is justifiable [sounds like a familiar argument, doesn't it]. This may be so, except for the one woman who happens to be the unlucky statistic. Young women must decide whether the one-in-a-thousand chance of a clot to the lungs or the threefold increased risk of stroke is worth it. The actual death rate attributable to the pill is 1.5 per 100,000 women between the ages of twenty and thirty-five. Women not taking the pill have a death rate from a blood clot in the lung or brain of 0.2 per 100,000. Thus the pill increases the risk 7.5 times. Women over forty increase their chance of heart attack five times by taking the pill. Consequently, most concerned physicians will not allow women over forty, especially if they are overweight, smoke, have high blood pressure, or are diabetic, to take the pill. The risks are simply not acceptable."

This is a perspective which I appreciate and with which I heartily concur. However, given what has been revealed about vasectomies and the negative long-term health effects that procedure can have on a man, why wouldn't the same criteria for evaluation be applied to vasectomies as is applied in Dr. Taguchi's statement about the use of the pill by women? Why the double-standard?

Testosterone treatment for men as contraception is being developed with mixed results thus far (Zhengwei, et. al., 1998). There are long-term risks associated with this also (i.e. prostate cancer and testicular atrophy, among others), just as there are risks in hormone therapy for women. Other hormone treatments are being tested and developed for men to allow us to participate even more in the contraceptive process. Notably, the use of testosterone plus progesterone to increase the effectiveness of contraceptive regimens is being studied repeatedly (McLachlan, et. al., 2002). This is actually identical to the method I eventually arrived at for stopping my own sperm production in an effort to treat the autoimmune responses I have experienced as a result of my vasectomy.

Along the same lines, the Chinese have been working on a nifty plan of giving a man one type of hormone (progestin, a female hormone) to stop sperm production. They then put long-acting testosterone pellets in the scrotum or elsewhere to balance out the hormones and maintain the sex drive the guy wanted to keep from the beginning (www.Discoveryhealth.com, August 1, 2000). Another approach being developed uses drugs to alter the proteins that allow sperm to swim vigorously and to penetrate an egg (www.msnbc.com). The interesting thing about this approach is that it is being tested for both men and women as a pre-intercourse and a post-intercourse contraceptive method. However, this is still highly experimental and even farther away from ready availability than any hormonal method for men.

All of these efforts may provide other contraceptive options, but the core issue to remember is that long-term alteration of hormone levels in men or women has significant health consequences, as does surgical alteration of the reproductive system in both sexes. You will have to decide if you want to be a part of that experimentation process that either proves or disproves the claims by doctors and drug companies of no ill effects for any given treatment.

There are also numerous foams and gels to complement the chemical action of some of these other methods. Add to that the IUD, for which researchers still lack a complete understanding of why it works after decades of use, and only know that it is reasonably effective in it's barrier/chemical action. IUDs earned a particularly bad rap when they were first introduced years ago, with many women experiencing significant health consequences due to their use. The basic premise of the IUD is to create a long-term inflammatory reaction in the cervix by introducing the constant presence of a chemical (usually metallic), which makes an inhospitable environment for achieving pregnancy. Let's see, another situation wherein an inflammatory response is created in the genitals but with claims of no negative effects. Where have I heard this before?

On the experimental front for men is a contraceptive method undergoing clinical trials in India called Reversible Inhibition of Spermatazoa Under Guidance (say that 10 times fast), or more simply, RISUG. The concept is novel. Instead of cutting the vas, a fluid with the consistency of honey is injected into the vas (under local anesthesia, I hope). After a few minutes the fluid coalesces into a soft plug.

Here's the interesting part: "The plug is loose enough that sperm is still allowed to pass through the vas, but the plug is polarized and carries a negative and positive charge. The charges in the plug disrupt the negative charge on the membrane of the sperm, which renders it incapable of fertilization. The study in India has shown that it has been 100 percent effective for as long as 12 years, and researchers feel that its effectiveness should continue for decades. Toxicology studies have shown the RISUG fluid to be safe and non-toxic, and there have been no problems reported with any part of the procedure" (Williams, 2002).

Notice the phrase, "no problems reported." I think I've heard that before too, but the idea at least has the possibility of reducing such phenomenon as epididymal blowouts, continued autoimmune responses to sperm in the bloodstream, and injuries from overzealous surgical methods. I wonder if you could get the same type of polarity by attaching a AAA battery to you scrotum? Who's up for a clinical trial of that? It would be a great ad for the Energizer Bunny (Still Going!).

Ah, but I digress. Williams continues: "What makes RISUG even more exciting is that the effects can be reversed in about 10 to 15 minutes by, once again, exposing the vas and then injecting sodium bicarbonate [baking soda] to ash the plug out of the vas and down the urethra." A 100 percent success rate is claimed once again for the reversal technique. I still take the attitude of "Looks dangerous; You go first!" but then, I may be just a bit jaded about medical claims by now. By the way, the RISUG procedure costs the patient the equivalent of $10 US. Our health care system could probably take a few examples from them.

Another novel concept mentioned by Williams (2002) is actually a revival of an old one developed during periods of drought and famine in the 1930s in India. Tests have shown that if a man sits in a shallow bath at 116 degrees (Fahrenheit, that is), "immersing the testes only for 45 minutes a day for three weeks [he] would be temporarily sterile for a period of six months." The process is purported to be repeatable for 20 years or more. This may not be as much fun as sitting in a hot tub with your honey, and I'm not at all clear on what the long-term hormonal effects might be, but it beats needles and scalpels in the privates all to heck, wouldn't you agree? Imagine, you could sit around with the guys, catch the game, and knock back a few cold ones, all while insuring sterility. Hey, I think I just came up with an idea for a new sports bar! Maybe I'll get to use that "Great Balls of Fire!" title after all.

There are many more aspects of contraceptive methods to discuss, with each method having its own risks and benefits, but the basic message seems to be the same: If you want to play, you have to be ready to pay. There are also issues to consider about the variance between the use of any contraceptive method under ideal conditions and those encountered in the hormone-charged real world with regular use.

A good summary of the effectiveness of various forms of contraception can be found on the Internet at www.discoveryhealth.com. Look for His Health, then Effectiveness of Contraceptives In Preventing Pregnancy And STDs. I might take issue with some of the more cavalier statistics given about vasectomies, but at least you can assess the relative risks of various methods. There's also a good article titled "Proper Use of A Condom" in case you don't happen to be proficient in this art form.

It is apparent, to me at least, that the safest forms of contraception in regard to long-term health for both men and women are found in the various forms of barriers available when used properly. If this is a downer for an individual because of personal preferences in sexual practice, then the choice becomes either altering one's sexual habits, or accepting the substantially increased risks of other forms of contraception.

Fortunately, we still live in a country where you are free to make decisions for yourself about what will be done to your body. Exercise this freedom and make your own choice. This is not the case everywhere around the world, where the regard for human life is often viewed quite differently.

To quote government sources again, "All contraceptive methods carry some risks as well as their recognized benefits. When making decisions about contraception, each individual or couple must be informed about and weigh the various risks and benefits in light of their particular circumstances and the risks associated with pregnancy"(National Institute of Health, 1996). Do yourself a favor and get familiar with those risks before they bite you in the…well, you know what I mean.

If, knowing this information, you decide to go ahead and have a vasectomy, I wish you the best of luck. After all, you are free to choose what is done to your body. I think you can tell quite plainly where I stand on the issue, and that I think you should choose to keep your sack intact. I could say I make no bones about it, but that would be another awful pun, wouldn't it?

Aside from avoiding bad humor, don't be in too big of a hurry to get your snip, or you may wind up having a major surgery following your "minor" vasectomy. According to Howard (1982), "Almost all men requesting reversal emphasized that vasectomy had been carried out in a time of crisis, when they were convinced that sterilization was the only way out of their difficulties."

Be particularly cautious in approaching a vasectomy if you have any history of hydroceles, hernia, epididymitis, mumps or other testicular maladies. Many of the men I have corresponded with who are suffering chronic post-vasectomy pain had a history of testicular problems and either didn't think to mention it to their doctors or the doctors proceeded anyway, considering it to be no big deal.

In terms of how these men should have been counseled: "Conditions that may increase the risks or difficulties of performing the [vasectomy] operation include previous scrotal trauma, large varicocele or hydrocele, previous surgery for cryptorchidism, inguinal hernia, and certain coagulation disorders.… When any of these conditions are present, the patient should be informed about the possible increased risk" (Schwingl, et. al., 2000). How often do you think this disclosure actually happens? Similarly, "it may be reasonable that men who already have multiple cardiovascular risk factors such as smoking, hypertension, and or hypercholesterolaemia may be more cautious before deciding on a vasectomy" (Frances, et. al., 1983).

For example, one man I corresponded with had experienced a hernia as a child. When the doctor was performing the vasectomy, he spent an hour and a half trying to find the man's vas deferens, causing a great deal of damage in the process. At the point I last heard from him, the man had to have the damaged testicle removed and was still in pain all of the time after already suffering for months and months.

Additional evidence necessitating caution before having a vasectomy is found in research showing that men who have hydrocele cysts in their scrotum will often not know it prior to vasectomy. The hydroceles can be perforated during a vasectomy procedure with "potentially alarming" results (Seidi, et. al., 2000). This would reinforce the case for a thorough physical examination prior to the surgery.

If you are still determined, you may want to consider having the procedure done as a no-scalpel vasectomy, combined with the open-ended vasectomy technique. This may give you the least chance of encountering long-term painful problems. Doctors may resist you on this, insisting that they know the better way, based on their chosen technique. Decide for yourself. Would an open-ended procedure have worked for me if it had been done originally? I'll probably never know because of the damage that was done the first time around and in the months that followed.

Statistically speaking, it appears that you're better off with the open-ended procedure, as far as pain goes, at least. Also, know that there is conflicting evidence as to the benefits of the no-scalpel vasectomy, beyond its marketing potential for urologists. Christensen, et. al., (2002) reported "No significant difference found between the two [bilateral and no-scalpel] methods with regard to effectiveness, time of operation, the patient's pain and discomfort, and per-operative and post-operative complications. Overall, vasectomy was inadequate [failed] in 5%, haematoma was found in 13%, infection in 9%, and scrotal pain or painful ejaculation in 9%", putting another nail in the coffin for the "one-in-a-million" theory.

Having your testosterone level checked by a blood test before a vasectomy is a good way to establish a baseline for potential future hormonal changes that may occur after the procedure. If you wait until afterwards, you may never know what your body's natural balance point was beforehand, and the range of "normal" testosterone doctors will check for is quite wide.

You would be well advised to discuss the method of anesthesia with your doctor. "In one study, men in whom the anesthetic bupivicaine was injected into the vas deferens during the operation had neither acute nor chronic pain afterward" (Simon, et. al., 1998). This was the same anesthetic (bupivacaine) that the pain specialist used during my caudal epidural, and was the most effective of the numerous varieties of anesthesia I received. To quote one study on the issue: "It has now been shown that the incidence of this common [chronic pain] complication can be significantly reduced by the injection of a small volume of local anesthetic into the vas deferens at the time of surgery" (McConaghy, et. al., 1996). I wish someone had told me about that prior to my surgery.

This point was furthered by the same authors in another study: "Previous workers have shown that chronic testicular discomfort may occur in up to 33% of men following this relatively minor procedure, although this may be significantly reduced by the injection of bupivacaine into the lumen of the vas deferens during surgery.... The possible benefit of pre-emptive local anesthesia is thought to be due to inhibition of excitability at the dorsal horn of the spinal cord caused by nociceptive [nerve] impulses from the injured tissue. Increased spinal excitability has been shown to contribute to pain following tissue trauma in animals which may persist for a long time following the tissue injury" (McConaghy, et. al., 1998). Translation: If you stop the nerves at the surgery site from becoming sensitized during surgery, you will stop the central nervous system, i.e. the spinal cord, from becoming sensitized too, which greatly diminishes the perception of pain.

Wilson (2001) advocates the use of a "No-Needle Anesthetic" in conjunction with the no-scalpel vasectomy. In this method, a jet injection device creates a fine stream of anesthetic that disperses quickly into the tissues. Wilson claims that patients liken the sensation to the snap of a rubber band against the scrotum [rubber band or bungie cord?] versus the stick of a needle, not that either are my idea of fun on a Saturday night, but if you gotta choose.... Interestingly, Wilson also claims that this approach to anesthesia lessens the risk of hematoma.

Another study found a supplemental inguinal block (in the groin) to be effective in decreasing pain during the procedure (Rasmussen et. al., 1994). The key to remember here, as many men and doctors have related to me since my own vasectomy, is that the procedure is not supposed to be excruciatingly painful. If it is, something is wrong.

Yet another study (Cooper, 2002) found that use of a topical anesthetic cream (ELMA) prior to the injection of local anesthesia lower pain responses in patients during the surgery. If I had know the possibility, I would have insisted on these types of pain mitigating measures in any of the procedures I had. Unfortunately, they weren't offered. I can't help but believe that some simple, inexpensive precautions like these just mentioned might have made a huge difference.

I have been told of studies being done with a new form of No-Scalpel Vasectomy where the vas is not severed, but a slit is made in it, and a plug inserted (personal correspondence, 2002). A lot of the details of this are unclear, such as what effect the inevitable long-term inflammation we have discussed here will have on the plugs. Also in question is if this can be combined with the open-ended technique to avoid epididymal congestions and rupturing, but the idea is to develop a vasectomy procedure that is much more reversible than what is currently done since so many men are eventually requesting reversals.

Your susceptibility to autoimmune disease can be estimated beforehand with a test for HLA, which can help to determine your genetic predisposition to these types of maladies. It may be difficult to find a doctor who will allow this before vasectomy, but you need to determine if you want to take the risk. If the test is unavailable, look at the rest of your family and see how many have autoimmune diseases such as lupus, rheumatoid arthritis, psoriasis, Graves' disease, Crohn's disease, fibromyalgia, and multiple sclerosis among many others. If there is a propensity for these types of diseases in your family, chances are good that you have an increased chance of developing autoimmune disease of some sort, though not necessarily exactly the same disease as the other members of your family (Rose, undated). You will then need to question whether potentially creating a strong immune system reaction due to a vasectomy is a good idea.

Several months after your vasectomy, have your blood checked for sperm antibodies and do whatever is appropriate to minimize their effect. Since this appears to be one of the greatest areas of potential problems, you would be wise to guard your health in this aspect. The Indirect Immunobead Assay antisperm antibody test performed on blood is reputed to be the most accurate way to determine this (Broderick, et. al., 1989). Also, you would be well advised to continue to do a testicular self-exam (as will be described shortly) on a regular basis, given the incidence of problems after vasectomy.

Antibody tests, hormone level tests, and testicular exams become especially important if you begin to experience the kinds of symptoms that have been discussed. It is important to become familiar with this information and make the connections your doctor is unlikely to make for you. Have any tests done by a competent lab in your area that processes a fresh sample if at all possible. Out of the area labs analyzing frozen samples are notoriously inaccurate in my experience.

If you are a man who has already undergone vasectomy, regardless of the outcome, ask yourself this question: If you had been aware of the information presented here, even if it were presented as being "controversial", would it have influenced your decision to have the surgery? I am sure that for myself and for many others, the unhesitating answer would be "You're damned right it would have made a difference!"

Let's be clear about this: It's OK to look at the vasectomy you opted to have done in ignorance and say it was a bad idea. I have come to surrender my pride in this process enough to do that, and I know it is not easy. Given what I know now, my wife and I would have chosen another way, even if I had not wound up in chronic pain.

Your Honor, I move that the witness be disqualified
on the grounds that he's nuts!

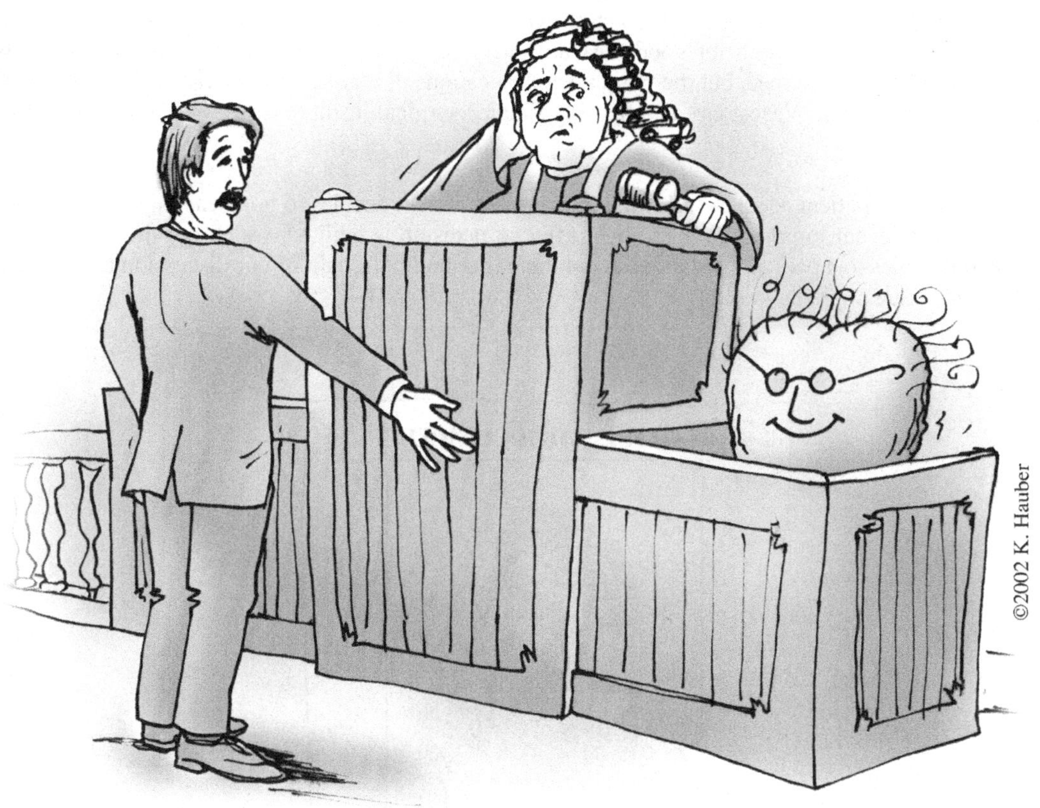

"Consent to perform surgery is a contract, whether it is verbal or written" (Schmidt, 1988). This leads to the issue of informed consent, one of the hottest topics in medicine today. Basically, the idea is that when the doctor knows that something can go wrong, the doctor needs to tell you. In so doing, you, as patient can make an informed decision about whether you want to be cut, medicated, radiated, or whatever is being proposed. The old idea of "I as your doctor know what is best for you and you need not know or question my opinions" has become a thing of the past, legally at least, if not in practice.

"Informed consent is the legal embodiment of the concept that each individual has the right to make decisions affecting his or her well-being. It is generally accepted that individuals should consider- that is, trade -off - the risks and potential benefits flowing from their decisions. To do so, decision-makers must have knowledge of those risks and potential benefits. The law protects the individual's right to give informed consent by requiring the disclosure of information by the party to whom consent is given.... The law places on one party a positive obligation to disclose information regarding risks to the party or parties who are 'at risk,' that is, those who will suffer injury if a chance event arises" (Merz, undated).

Various courts have confirmed this in practice, legal practice, that is. In California, review of Supreme Court literature on the subject yields the following: "The scope of a physician's duty to disclose is measured by the amount of knowledge a patient needs in order to make an informed choice, and the physician should give the patient all information material to that decision. Material information is that which the physician knows or should know would be regarded as significant by a reasonable person in the patient's position when deciding to accept or reject the recommended medical procedure…. Additionally, if the physician knows of a patient's unique concerns or lack of familiarity with medical procedures, the scope of required disclosure may be expanded…. The duty to disclose material information may require the physician to reveal various schools of thought regarding a specific course of treatment" (California Torts, 2000).

It is not just the legal types who express these opinions. Examine this statement by Dr. Malcolm Carruthers (1997) regarding the issue of informed consent: "In order for patients to make an informed decision about whether to take it, a drug has to have in the packaging a formidable list of every complication, however rare, ever recorded in association with the use of that compound, and often for good measure every related compound. The same should apply when an operation such as vasectomy is prescribed, but the possible complications discussed here are rarely mentioned and certainly not covered in the detail deserved. Vasectomy is, after all, a major surgical insult to a very sensitive, delicate and highly tuned organ."

If a doctor gives the patient adequate relevant data and the patient decides to go ahead anyway, understanding the risks, that's OK. But if relevant information that would affect a decision is omitted, watch out. In other words, a doctor can't play God when it comes to a patient's decisions about his or her body. In light of our discussion about vasectomies so far, do you see how this issue might be raised?

Raising the issue is exactly what I did. My research and discussions with other vasectomy patients suggested that most doctors tended to be very reluctant to change their disclosure practices. By all indications, even my original urologist was still failing to disclose the kinds of issues he had seen patients like me experience. Unfortunately, I only found this out after a friend of mine had a vasectomy done by him. Also unfortunately, my friend experienced periodic testicular discomfort after his vasectomy which caused him great concern after he found out about what I had been experiencing.

These and numerous other factors led me to the decision to follow my attorney's advice and file legal action. It was clear that my medical case was not enough to impress my original urologist that there might be a flaw in his approach. But doctors listen to their malpractice insurance companies. They must. That seemed like a likely place to start. So I embarked on a legal attention-getting campaign with the doctor, who would be defended by his malpractice insurance company.

This is not something that I undertook lightly. I cannot think of a more unpleasant subject to sue over. In addition, I did not relish the tremendous amount of time and effort that would no doubt be required in such an exercise. I was right in this regard. Two years after my initial legal filing, I hadn't even seen the mediation table yet, let. al.,one the inside of a courtroom.

The attorney for the doctor's malpractice insurance company continually papered us to death, in many cases in duplicate and triplicate. Since I had kept copious records of conversations, memorandums and expenses, many trees were sacrificed in this process. I also soon became aware of the kind of intimidation tactics that attorneys of this type will use to try to scare you off. What was intended to be a way to force telling of the truth and an attempt to recover some of my medical expenses and lost wages was turning into a parade of egos. The attempt to wear me down was obvious, but then, he didn't know me very well.

They say that 98 percent of attorneys give the rest of the bunch a bad name (OK, I couldn't resist throwing in an attorney joke, but it was just too good of a target). If that's the case then I was blessed with one of the remaining two percent for my own attorney. When you find an attorney to work with who is communicative, human and ethical, you have been truly blessed. Such was the case for me. I can't say the same about the other side. I hold great hope for all humanity and our innate ability to show kindness, empathy and courtesy to each other. Unfortunately, the malpractice insurance attorney chose not to demonstrate those characteristics in my presence, but then again, maybe he thought that was what he was being paid for. Who knows? I hope he made up for it elsewhere.

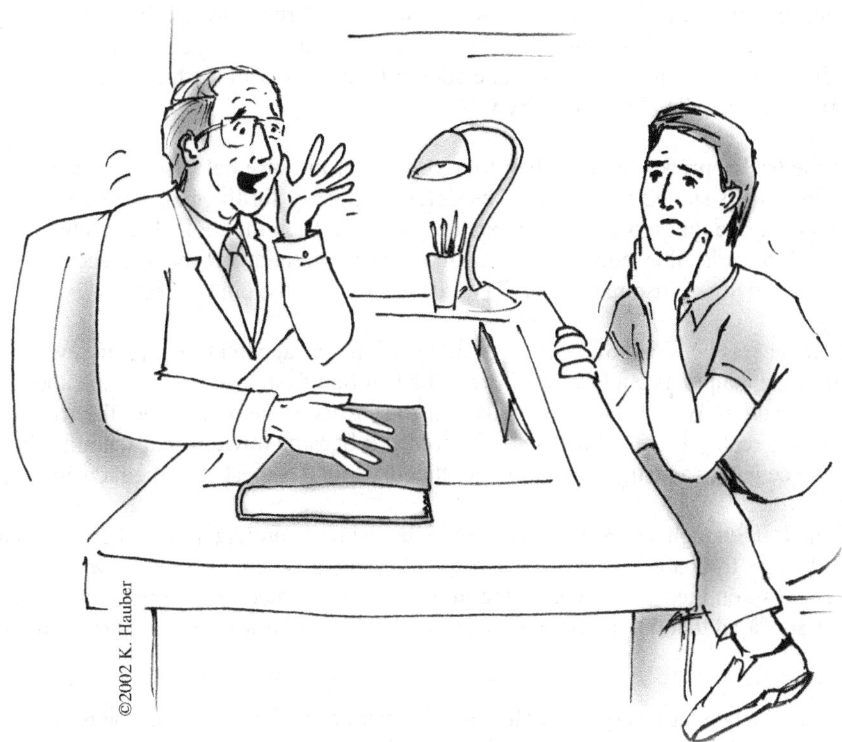

Your injury has been resistant to every form
of treatment so far... I strongly recommend a three-year
course of intensive litigation as your next move.

It was also apparent that vasectomy malpractice suits were hard to win, since most doctors did not disclose potential problems, which set a standard of practice that effectively protected any doctor who chose not to. This sounds a bit twisted, doesn't it? But that is in fact the case; if all the doctors in an area hang together and choose to disclose or not disclose something, even if the ethics are questionable, there is legal precedence that says that it is Okay. Sometimes, at least. Then again, sometimes not.

The other issue that became quite obvious in the process is that, as a rule, doctors will not testify against each other. Whether this is due to the brotherhood closing ranks, or real or perceived pressure from the malpractice insurance companies, or both, is a matter of speculation. This unwillingness to testify against another doctor is particularly true in the field of urology. It is interesting to note that most of the urologists I had seen were all clients of the same malpractice insurance attorney who, incidentally, was also defending my original urologist. It was surprising to note the difference in tone of the remarks the doctors were willing to make before and after the attorney had conversations with them. The circle is truly small.

The doctors who were willing to make the most open commentary were doctors from other specialties, such as pain specialists, who often end up trying to clean up after numerous failed surgeries. One pain doctor I saw told me that the average patient he saw was the recipient of four failed back surgeries and the best that could be hoped for when the patient walked through the pain specialist's door was to find some moderate control for the pain: Not a cure mind you, but some mild relief at best. So much for the idea of back surgery as a course of treatment at any time in the future.

There have been some notable exceptions to this "code of silence" strangle-hold on the legal recourse of vasectomy patients. In 1999, "An upstate [Pennsylvania] jury awarded $4.5 million to a Philadelphia law firm's client who now suffers debilitating pain as a result of a botched vasectomy.... The trial was the second for the medical malpractice case. In 1997, a jury gave the plaintiff $950,000.00, but that award was reversed on appeal. This time around the plaintiff was also awarded nearly $2 million in delay damages [serves them right- sorry, I couldn't resist the editorial comment]....

"The plaintiff was a 33-year-old married father of two when he underwent a vasectomy... Instead of making an incision on the scrotum, the surgeon made the cut on the base of the penis, injuring a nerve that runs from the abdomen to the right leg. The misplaced incision, and the resulting scar tissue caused reflex sympathetic dystrophy [sound familiar?], leaving the plaintiff with chronic pain in his penis, testicles, groin and abdomen. The damages included the wife's loss of consortium [that means she received an award because she couldn't have sex with her husband any more]. Also, $1 million was awarded for lost earning capacity" (TRC Public Newsletter).

As the date for the trial approached more than four years after my original vasectomy and over three years after I filed the lawsuit, interesting things started to happen. The defense attorney for the malpractice insurance company started making motions (13 of them at one time) to attempt to exclude evidence from the trial. These attempts included motions to keep many of my medical records, this book, volumes of medical research on the subject of vasectomy and Post-Vasectomy Pain Syndrome, and my "conspiracy theory" (whatever that means) out of court.

I was amazed! What was he afraid of, as if I didn't know? It was apparent that, as my evidence had become more compelling (and damning), the malpractice attorney's interest had shifted from trying to grill me about the facts to trying to eliminate the evidence altogether. We are taught as kids that the justice system is about "the truth, the whole truth, and nothing but the truth," but the reality is something quite different. It became obvious that winning this case was becoming a contest to see what evidence would actually make it before the jury, not a contest over the facts themselves.

My hope was that if enough cases like this could be won, including mine, then the malpractice insurance companies would force doctors to change their disclosure and treatment practices, since it was obvious to me that most doctors were unwilling to do so on their own, even in the face of evidence such as my case and the numerous others I was repeatedly learning of. It appeared that the inertia within the medical practice was just too strong to allow for change from within.

In the words of researchers at Henry Ford Hospital in Detroit: "Chronic scrotal pain is the most common post-vasectomy complication that may adversely affect quality of life in men undergoing vasectomy." This has more than ethical considerations for doctors. Also noted in the same article: "Vasectomy is the leading cause of urological litigation, the most common reasons for which are failure to provide proper informed consent and a surgical complication.... Regardless of the technique used, the high litigation potential of this procedure warrants thorough counseling of factors that may affect quality of life (Choe, et. al., 1996)." There it was, right in the medical journals!

However, I was prepared for an uphill climb since the truth seemed to matter less than legal maneuvering and tactics. In many states, and in my home state of California in particular, insurance companies have been very successful over the years in getting various initiatives and legislation passed, often under the guise of "reforms," that limit the ability of injured parties to seek damages from their doctors. What I found is that when you sue your doctor because of some gross mistake he has made, you are not just suing the doctor, but you are taking on his insurance company with their battery of resources, and in fact your are taking on the entire insurance industry with its massive legislative and judicial influences.

Dr. Malcolm Carruthers (1997) characterizes the legal situation this way: "There are powerful lobbies both inside and outside the medical profession with vested interests in maintaining the 'safe' image of vasectomy. First, doctors who have been promoting it for many years don't want to change their tune and have to face the possibility of being in the wrong.... The reluctance of the medical profession to discuss vasectomy issues is likely to be even greater when the financial considerations of the vasectomy industry are taken into account."

This broaches another un-discussed and undisclosed aspect of vasectomies. It is commonly known in the medical industry that vasectomies are a moneymaker. Oliver Stone could probably spin a great conspiracy theory here. Actually, it would be more of a training and indoctrination theory. Without going that far, just consider this: At $500 or so per snipping session for a few minutes work times a million or so guys per year. Add an apparent lifetime of follow-up treatment for many, and an inevitable percentage of very expensive reversals, and there is a lot of cash shifting from the coffers of the OB-GYNs and pediatricians to those of the urologists. In his deposition, my urologist claimed to do about 200 vasectomies per year and that his four partners did about the same. Let's see, that's 1,000 vasectomies a year times $500 average each plus follow-ups, which comes out to more than a half a million dollars per year, straight to the bottom line. Was my doctor, or almost any other, likely to sacrifice this easy income source without a fight? I think not.

One study claimed that a doctor using the no-scalpel technique is able to do an average of 57 procedures a day, compared to 33 per day with the standard method (Nirapathpongporn, et. al., 1990)." Do the math; you'll get the idea. It became apparent also that promotion of the "No-Scalpel Vasectomy" technique was as much about economics as it was about being beneficial to the patient. Can you see the economic reasons as to why an industry has built up around this? Nobody ever said change was going to be easy.

What was the final outcome of my lawsuit? During the three-and-a-half years the lawsuit was pending, an appellate court in California handed down a decision tightening the testimony requirements regarding medical malpractice. What it boiled down to was that another "expert witness" urologist with credentials in California would have to testify that it was below the "Standard of Care" to not disclose Post-Vasectomy Pain Syndrome, and that it was below the "Standard of Care" to perform a vasectomy and cause significant nerve damage that led to the formation of traumatic neuromas and a chronic pain syndrome. Seems pretty simple, doesn't it. I mean, anyone can put two and two together and come up with that right?

No one would do it. The malpractice insurance reptile, I mean attorney, had systematically eliminated anyone who hinted at willingness to be an expert witness. Evidently they all had the same insurance, and, hence, the same legal representation. Guess who that was? The wagons were circled and common sense was not admissible in court. So with the prospect of more agony and a trial scheduled to start during the holidays, which was likely to cost me a whole lot more with no favorable outcome, my attorney recommended I drop the case and focus on my health.

This experience was a huge disappointment and demonstrated just how far the legal system was from "The truth, the whole truth, and nothing but the truth", and how bad the ethics were with many of those within the system. No wonder Shakespeare said, "First, we kill all the lawyers." Since that course of action was likely to create more problems, I settled on a few new focuses. Next, I intended to see legislators about this informed consent issue. If the way lawyers were twisting the law was wrong, change the law needed to be changed to keep 'em from doing it. It was also apparent to me that as much outside pressure as possible was needed to affect this type of change since it was unlikely to come from inside either the medical or legal professions.

A little media campaign wouldn't hurt in this regard. Most of the media coverage regarding vasectomy up to this point gave only the positive spin offered by the medical community. A friend of mine advised me, "If you don't like what the media is saying, don't get mad at the media. Become the media!" This sounded like good advice. The experiences outlined in chapter Twenty-Six entitled "Extra, Extra" were the outgrowth of this decision. So my decision was to sacrifice whatever concern I might have remaining for my ego or privacy in this process and tell the truth as often and as widely as possible. My sense was that the media would eat this up.

Doc, It Hurts When I Do This

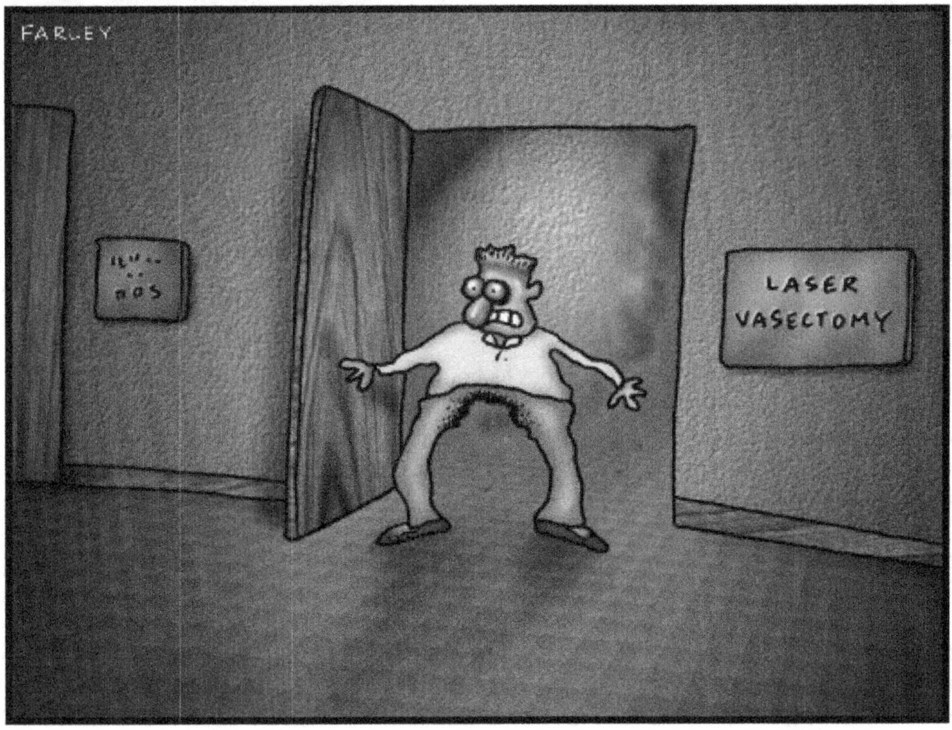

This is one of my father-in-law's long standing, favorite bits of humor:

The patient comes to the doctor and says, "Doc, it hurts when I do this."

The doctor looks for a moment, and the replies, "Hmm, well, don't do that."

This is good advice when it comes to vasectomies to begin with, except you don't end up hurting until afterwards, sometimes years afterwards, when the damage is already done. Turning that situation around can be tough, as you can see by now.

So the best answer is, "Hmm, don't do that to begin with." Available research shows that once a man has scrotal surgery for any reason, especially vasectomy, the trouble begins, and he will pay dearly to stop it.

If you are a man who has already undergone a vasectomy procedure, I sincerely hope that you have not experienced any of the problems discussed in this book. I hope this information comes as a complete surprise to you. Nevertheless, based on the research presented, you would do well to guard your health also.

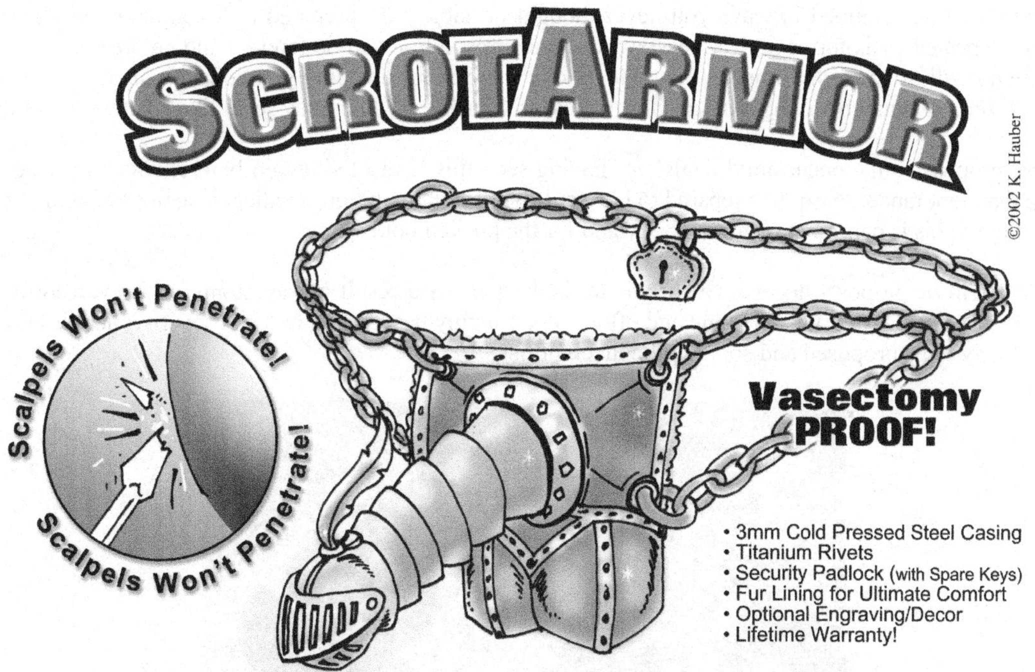

This may involve clean living, exercise, and a good diet as best as you are able. It may also involve medications or supplements to minimize any antibody action your system may be developing. A worthwhile precaution would certainly include regular PSA and other screening tests, as are warranted anyway as we pass age 40 and beyond, especially if you have a family history of prostate cancer.

As previously described, chronic pain resulting from a vasectomy can come in the form of a dull ache in the testicles and/or prostate and/or groin and abdomen that is constant or periodic. It can also come in the form of shooting pains in the groin. It can occur only during sexual arousal, in which case the issue becomes "Doc, it hurts when I do it."

While we're on that subject, Dr. Stanwood Schmidt (1979) has characterized the pain that can result from chronic inflammation after vasectomy in this way: "Localized pain during sexual excitement was common, often severe at ejaculation, so that the patient would avoid sexual intercourse because of fear of pain. The pain could also be experienced with a steady, severe onset during sexual excitement, or as a testicular ache after ejaculation. It could radiate to the flank – in which form it could be most severe: in three such cases the patients required hospitalization." Have you ever had an orgasm that put you in the hospital? Talk about crossing the line between pleasure and pain!

If you are really unlucky, like I have been so far, chronic pain can come in all of the forms I have just mentioned, all the time, with spikes during your attempts at sex. It's kind of like hitting post-vasectomy pain lotto. This can occur days, months, or years after the procedure. It's not just the pain that needs to be mentioned: Hormone imbalances, erectile dysfunction, inflammation, prostatitis, testicular atrophy, and a host of other maladies have been described as post-vasectomy symptoms deserving notice.

If something goes wrong, start taking notes. This might make your doctor nervous, but do it. Get copies of your medical records. I found these to be some of the most useful practices in understanding what was going on and in developing a treatment plan that suited me. Start doing your own independent research as an adjunct to whatever your doctor is offering you in the way of information. Try to make as balanced a decision as you can and be insistent about what you want, or don't want for that matter.

If you do end up with some form of chronic pain or other complications, and choose to have medical assistance in the resolution of it, be prepared for a highly invasive and unpleasant experience. You may be confronted with being medicated and sliced and stabbed in ways you never thought possible. Be prepared to be coming and going in cups on command, on a repeated basis for years if necessary, if in fact a resolution can be found. And be prepared to have medical professionals who will offhandedly propose the removal of parts of your anatomy you consider quite valuable, and others who will say, "Well, you may be living with this for the rest of your life," which may seem like an eternity at that moment.

These proposals may occur amid denials of having seen this kind of situation before, which may be due to legal liability more than ignorance. Also, be prepared to have a difficult time with your medical insurance coverage for what you need to have done. This is painful stuff for the body and for the pocketbook.

What might be proposed to resolve chronic testicular pain as a result of vasectomy? It took a lot of research to learn about this, so let me save you some time and effort. In a roughly descending order of severity, here is at least a partial list of what is likely to be proposed and some of the inherent risks:

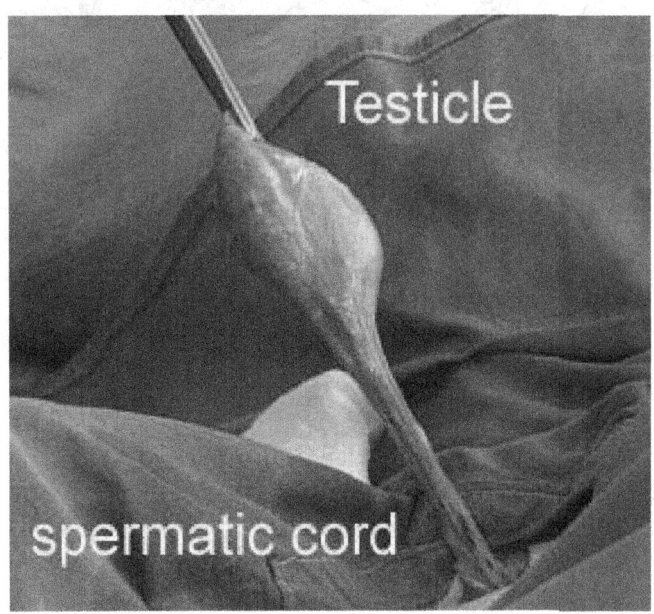

- Inguinal orchiectomy - this is a form of castration where the doctor cuts your groin and pulls out the testicle(s) along with the cords, thereby attempting to alleviate the source of the problem and creating several others in the process. These problems can include unresolved pain for various reasons, lifelong hormonal imbalances and inherent need for medical treatment, and psychological. As with any surgical procedure there is also the possibility of some really yucky infections, causing you to lose a lot more than your testicles, up to and including a "life-ectomy". "Patients often can be insistent about having testes removed for persistent pain but, clearly, they must be counseled that orchiectomy may not provide relief" (Davis, et. al., 1990). This is true even if only one testicle is affected by pain before surgery. Witness the previous discussion regarding sympathetic orchiopathia. Expect doctors to lead off by offering the castration option to get your attention and make the other options sound better.

- Scrotal orchiectomy - this is a similar form of testicular deforestation as above, but the incision is made in the scrotum and the spermatic cord is left in the groin. The risks are similar, save that the risk of unresolved pain is higher, since the source of the pain may be nerve damage along the cord. In fact, studies on the use of orchiectomy to resolve testicular pain show up to an 80% failure rate (Costabile, et. al., 1991). So in the majority of those cases the patient was still in pain and was missing his testicle(s). This is not a very compelling track record. Other doctors make more favorable claims regarding the use of orchiectomy for pain resolution, but the number of men I know who have continuing pain and other complications after losing one or both testicles makes me wonder how much data is being swept under the carpet.

- An epididymectomy may be proposed as a sure-fire method of resolution. It is not sure fire, and studies have been mixed as to the extent of pain relief from this procedure, with many results showing about a 50% success rate. The chief advantage, of course, is that the man remains sterile, which he probably wanted to begin with, and retains his testicles, which he probably also wanted to begin with. Unfortunately, he may only keep his testicles for a short while longer after an epididymectomy since the blood supply to the testicles can be damaged in the procedure, causing testicular atrophy, along with numerous other possible complications.

- Neurectomy, or surgical denervation (nerve-stripping) is another major surgery that can be performed which *may* block the pain if not resolve the problem at the source. This might be okay, if being numb from the groin down through the testicles and possibly into the inner thigh doesn't bother you. I have yet to speak with a man who has had this done successfully and is still able to have a completely normal life, including a normal sex life without any further pain. I know of one man for whom the nerve stripping surgery was a failure. In fact, he was one of the men in one of the studies I have quoted. I know of one other man for whom the nerve stripping surgery brought his pain level down to half of what it was previously, but he wasn't completely cured by any means, and his recovery time was extensive. Several doctors claim good success with this method. Notably, Heidenreich, et. al., (2002) claim a 96% success rate in a series of 35 patients with chronic testicular pain after an "extensive preoperative work-up (urine/semen cultures, transrectal ultrasound, testicular sonography, pain and orthopedic consultation)." Thoroughness of this nature is typically German, as is Heidenreich, but it sure helps to take the guesswork out of the process before removing parts that can't be put back. In examining these claims in the literature versus the stories of the men I have met, I had to question what is considered a "success" in this type of surgery. I have yet to talk directly with anyone who has had a complete cure by this method. This is not to say that it hasn't happened, but just not in my experience. Not yet, at least. Don't get me wrong: Pain reduction is a good thing, mind you, but pain elimination is far better, and not being in pain to begin with is best. On the other hand, several doctors have told me that nerves severed in this way can grow back together, form painful neuromas, or find alternate pathways to transmit signals, and when they do the sensations are "angry." The proficiency of the surgeon at this procedure would seem to be of vital importance. Be forewarned also that even though this surgery is referred to as a neurectomy, more than just the nerves are removed. I found this out by reading the articles on the procedure and asking extensive questions of the doctor/author without climbing onto the operating table and having another one of those "What do you mean you're taking all that out?" experiences. See, you can teach an old dog new tricks. Along with the nerves being "divided", so is the cremaster muscle, resulting in your testicles becoming, essentially, free-floating. Also typically removed or "transected" are some of the lymph glands. This can lead to hydrocele formation resulting in decreased testicular function, i.e. hormone deficiencies, low energy, erectile dysfunction, etc. The veins along the cord are removed, leaving only the testicular artery, and a section of the vas is commonly removed to rule out the possibility of nerve signals along the vas itself. There go the benefits of your reversal if you have had one as I did. Actually, my greatest concern in this regard has been the potential recurrence of ruptures in the epididymis and subsequent autoimmune responses, scar tissue formation, chronic inflammatory responses, etc., ad nauseum (literally) as a result of performing what is effectively another vasectomy plus a lot more, just in a new intimately personal location higher up in the groin. You probably understand some of these implications by now. If you have had any trouble or suspicions about any of these structures as a result of your vasectomy, consider and discuss the subject at length with any surgeon pointing his scalpel at you before getting too close.

- Reversal of the vasectomy may be proposed by vasovasostomy or vasoepididymostomy as necessitated by the degree of congestion you have in your epididymis and vas. This is the closest surgical option to the "just leave me as you found me" approach. However, as you may have gathered by now, this procedure is quite unpleasant and quite expensive. Some men have had good results with reversals to relieve their pain, while others like me have not. If your intent is to ever attempt fathering children again, the chances are reduced substantially from your pre-vasectomy state. In fact, if you have a blood test done before a reversal and the sperm antibody titre is higher than 64, it is quite likely that you will have antibodies in your semen after reversal, which will limit the possibility of impregnation (Linnet et. al., 1981). The flip side of this is that you will need to reinstate some other form of contraception if you are trying to avoid another pregnancy. The medical community in general wants to warn against a panic that would cause a rush to get reversals. The jury's still out on that one as far as I can see, and you have to weigh the potential effects of continuing to retain sperm in your body against the potential effects of fathering additional children. This is not an easy call. If I had it all to do over again, knowing what I now know, I would have had the reversal done, but would have pursued hormone therapy beforehand to reduce the inevitable autoimmune response that the reversal unleashes when everything is opened up. Of course if I knew then what I know now, I wouldn't have had the vasectomy in the first place. I'll discuss the hormone treatment in more detail, or you can refer back to Chapter Fourteen.

- Redoing your vasectomy as an open-ended vasectomy may be an option if the damage from the initial procedure isn't too severe. Such was not the case for me, unfortunately, but then it is hard to tell the extent of internal damage until you get in there. The open-ended vasectomy redo has the advantage of maintaining a sterilized state if that's what you still want, and not increasing the risks of an unexpected pregnancy, if properly done that is. It might be a good idea to ask the surgeon how many open-ended procedures he or she has done. That answer only became clear in my case when I was on the operating table.

- Removal of potentially painful granuloma(s) or other cysts may be proposed. This still carries all the aforementioned surgical risks and may or may not resolve the pain. With this and all of the previously noted surgical procedures, remember the adage "When all you have is a hammer, everything looks like a nail." Surgeons are taught to cut things out of us and then sew us back up to try to resolve problems. If you have already had one or more troublesome surgeries, your body is likely to object quite vehemently to more invasions. Remember, *surgery is not natural and traumatizes the body!* That is why there is always a projected recovery period from any surgery. Be careful what you allow, and be good to yourself in the process.

- A spermatic cord nerve block, an epidural, or even a hypogastric block may be proposed. My experience has been that the farther away from the source of the pain the better when it comes to sticking good-sized needles full of anesthesia into your privates. Some doctors like Heidenreich, et. al., (2002) recommend this type of block be performed with both local anesthesia and steroid injections, an idea which makes some sense. The most successful nerve block I have experienced was a superior hypogastric nerve block, which, while very effective, didn't last very long, and was followed by a lot of those "angry" nerve responses due to sticking needles and caustic substances into sensitized nerve plexuses. A series of nerve blocks may be proposed to try to break the pain cycle. Don't let anyone fool you, these are not pleasant procedures, and they can be dangerous. Pursue this course judiciously if you do. This is what I looked like several weeks after one of the cord blocks I had done hit a vein:

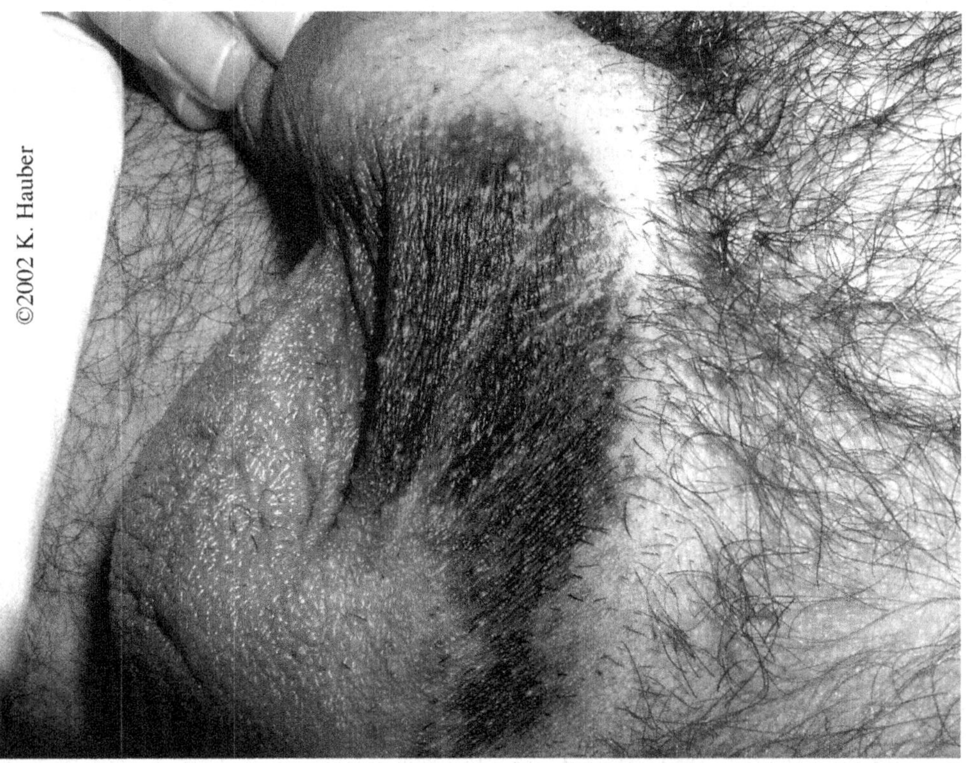

This little beauty mark lasted for over a month. I sent a message to the doctor with this picture attached a little over two weeks after the nerve block asking him to take a Rorschach test and tell me what the blot on the screen made him think of. My interpretation was of a man praying that this shit would end. His response: "Wait it out."

- Conservative measures are likely to be suggested by doctors before any of the invasive procedures noted above are undertaken. This probably means medications aplenty, so be careful of drug interactions and addictive or dependency producing properties. Antidepressants, anti-seizure medications, anti-convulsants, various painkillers, hormone (testosterone) therapy, and anti-inflammatories are all serious medications for which you will need to weigh the potential benefits against the risks. Among the anti-inflammatories, I have found Vioxx to be the most helpful medication, and Quercetin and Wobenzym to be the most helpful herbal formulations. Other guys have reported good luck with Celebrex, which didn't do much for me. Use whatever works best for you. Just remember the warning that my dentist gave me: "Be careful, medications are all selective poisons," which is why you don't eat a lot of them like you would food. Reducing the effects of continued sperm production and the inflammatory responses that occur are an avenue worth considering as conservative measures before any surgery. Use of hormone therapy beginning with an anti-androgen injection such as progesterone followed by testosterone therapy with injections and topically applied Androgel worked well for me and has been shown to be a safe protocol for suppressing sperm production in numerous World Health Organization studies. Some doctors have used moderate doses of corticosteroids to suppress immune system responses (Hargreave, et. al., 1983). See Rosenberg et. al., (1980) for a comparison of the effectiveness of hydrocortisone, methylprednisolone, and dexamethasone for this purpose. Be careful though, since long-term use of steroids can cause "bilateral aseptic necrosis of the femoral heads" (Hendry, 1982). Translated, this is a condition wherein the tops of your femur bones deteriorate and you wind up getting hip(s) replaced. My take on this steroid vs. testosterone therapy argument is that using steroids as an anti-inflammatory may be a good way to treat the symptom, but the hormone therapy is a good way to treat the cause. Again, it really comes down to whatever works best for you, but be careful.

- Acupuncture has been one of the more effective pain relieving methods I experienced, about as effective as most forms of anesthesia with far less dramatic aftereffects. I found an abstract from a Chinese medical journal that addressed this very issue, which my acupuncturist and I adapted to my situation. This form of treatment was quite relieving for me, even if the relief was only temporary. I'll quote the abstract in it's entirety for your information (This gets a little technical): "Cui SY [the author], Treatment of epididymal stasis after vasoligation with audio-frequency therapy applied on the points. *Chinese Journal of Integrated Traditional and Western Medicine*, 6:2, 89, 1986. An audio frequency instrument, model NY-2, with adjustable frequencies 50-500 Hz. & 50x15x1 mm lead plate electrodes, with a 60x20 mm lining, were used. Two electrode protocols were used once per day for a 10-day course. (a) In course one, two electrodes placed symmetrically at bilateral ST30-LV12-LV11 along both sides of the genitals (200 Hz, 20mA). (b) In course two, two electrodes were placed along the course of CV, Chongmal and KI channels at CV01 + CV03-K112 (200Hz, 20-30 mA). Protocols (a) and (b) were alternated between courses, using the principle of combination of related points. The intensity used in the third course depended upon the patients' conditions, but the maximal intensity was kept < 40mA. 10/11 cases were cured." If this nomenclature makes little sense, which is probably the case, take this to a reputable acupuncturist who will use his or her secret decoder ring to help you interpret it. A reference for this type of acupuncture for post-vasectomy pain and other disorders can be found in the bibliography under Rogers. My Chinese-born and trained acupuncturist has told me that there are many other journal articles on the subject of treating post-vasectomy pain with acupuncture, but you need to be able to read Chinese to understand them. I have enough trouble understanding the doctors who are supposedly writing in English!

- Other conservative therapies outside the normal medical realm have actually been the most helpful in my case. These have included, in order of appearance: Warm baths, swimming, yoga, therapeutic massage, hypnotherapy, network chiropractic (or other non-traumatizing methods of chiropractic), diet and nutrition counseling, physical therapy including electric muscle stimulation, TENS units, ultrasound, biofeedback, and myofascial release of the pelvic floor, abdominal, and low back muscles. I found all of these therapies are helpful in unwinding some of the stress that chronic pain puts on the body without putting me at a higher risk of complications. Again, do what you body tells you is right, but be conscious of consistently unwinding that stressful pain spiral, lest you end up in the hospital with bleeding intestines, as I did, or with some other dramatic result of ignoring or covering up your body's signals.

- The other treatment option that deserves mentioning is time. This is a tough one since post-vasectomy pain syndromes can go on for years. "Chronic pain progressively leads to limitation of physical, mental, and social activity with accompanying anger, depression, and family and socioeconomic disruption" (Nader, et. al., 2001). To help you through this, I would suggest that you consider some form of pain and stress management training because you will need it. The program modeled after the University of Massachusetts Medical School program designed by Jon Kabat-Zinn was a tremendous benefit to me. Likewise, forming a relationship with a good counselor can help you through the anger and depression that are inevitable aspects of chronic pain. Learning to recognize and control anger is a key. Have you ever seen a movie where someone kicks a guy in the balls and he's so angry about it that he grabs a gun and shoots the kicker? That's what you will feel like, often, I might add. Recognizing and getting a handle on the anger response will help you hurt less, quite literally. An excellent summary about the psychological aspects of what surgery can cause in the way of trauma to the body is in a book by a therapist named Peter Levine titled <u>Waking the Tiger: Healing Trauma</u>. He states: "Intellectually, we may believe in an operation, but on a primal level, our bodies do not. Where trauma is concerned, the perception of the instinctual nervous system carries more weight- much more." What do you think the primal level of your body feels about the imminent threat of emasculation? Levine continues: "It is difficult enough to deal solely with the symptoms of trauma without the added anxiety of not knowing why we are experiencing them or whether they will ever cease. Anxiety can crop up for a variety of reasons including a deep pain that comes when your spouse, friends and relatives unite in the conviction that it is time for you to get on with your life. They want you to act normally because they believe you should have learned to live with your symptoms by now. There are feelings of hopelessness, futility, and despair that accompany being incorrectly advised that the only way your symptoms can be alleviated is through a lifelong regimen of medication or therapy. Estrangement and fear can arise from the thought of talking to anyone about your symptoms because your symptoms are so bizarre you are certain that no one else could be experiencing the same thing. You also suspect that no one will believe you if you do tell them, and that you are probably going crazy. There is added stress associated with mounting medical bills as you go in for a third and fourth round of tests, procedures, referrals, and finally, exploratory surgery to ascertain the cause of your mysterious pain. You live with the knowledge that the doctors think you are a hypochondriac because no cause for your condition can be found." Does this sound at all familiar? Do you see why I recommend having good, competent, professional help along the way, and developing good stress management skills?

- Finding out if you are having any autoimmune reactions by blood or semen analysis may be appropriate. Be sure the test is looking for antisperm antibodies. Most labs need specific instructions about this, or you may get a false negative result. Ask for an indirect immunobead assay antisperm antibody test to be done on your blood if you have not had a reversal, and a direct immunobead assay antisperm antibody test on your semen if you have had a reversal and are fertile again. The blood test will tell you what the level of antibodies floating around in your bloodstream, while the semen test reveals what level of antibodies exist in the genital tract. Expect to have to explain what you want and why. Look for a test that gives an actual percentage result, not just a positive or negative at a certain threshold. That way you can track any trends. This is experience talking; I drained a lot of blood to figure this out. It also may be worthwhile for you to have your testosterone and other hormone levels checked, since this seems to lead to so many other possible problems following vasectomy. A "Free Androgen Index" test is reputed to be best in this regard. Unfortunately, no one has been able to tell me a good way to eliminate the autoimmune response your body is likely to have after a vasectomy, other than the approaches I have tried along the way. This is probably the most daunting aspect of the procedure, even if you're not experiencing chronic pain as result. Careful use of steroids such as Prednisone or testosterone therapy may be worth exploring in this regard as previously mentioned.

- You would be well advised to start doing a regular testicular self-exam if you don't do so already. Whether or not you do this daily as comedian and testicular cancer survivor Tom Green suggests is up to you, but you are more likely to detect some change, pain, or abnormality than to wait for the doctor to find something with infrequent checks. Besides, the doctor is checking testicles all day long. How do you expect him or her to remember what's normal for yours? Here's a good description of the self-exam as offered by <u>www.discoveryhealth.com</u>:

  "Follow the simple steps listed below once a month, after a bath or shower. The warmth helps loosen and relax the tissues, and moist skin enhances the ability to feel any lumps.

  "1. Examine one testicle at a time.

  "2. Gently grasp the testicle between your thumb and index finger, rolling it between them to feel for any lumps on its surface. Be sure to feel the entire surface, top to bottom.

  "3. Be aware that a small soft structure, the epididymis, is attached to the top and back of the testicle. Soft blood vessels and a firm cord-like structure, the vas deferens, also may be felt behind and above the testicle. Become familiar with the normal shape and feel of your own testicles; in that way changes from the norm will be more apparent to you. If a new lump is found, do not panic. Remember that most lumps are benign, but that all of them merit investigation and evaluation by an experienced doctor. Resist the temptation to repeatedly check the lump, since doing so might make it more swollen or tender and hamper the doctor's evaluation."

Here's an example of what an unusual lump might look like:

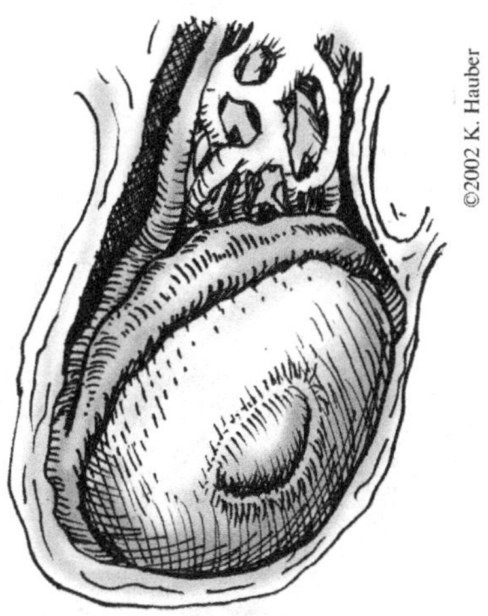

- Testicular massage may be a benefit for men who have had a vasectomy as well as those who have not. In their book <u>The Multi-Orgasmic Man,</u> authors Mantak Chia and Douglas Abrams Arava make several observations and recommendations pertinent to our discussion about vasectomy and sexual health. The reader may not necessarily be interested in cultivating the ability for multiple orgasms (who wouldn't be?), but from a health standpoint it is stated by the authors that "with a vasectomy, the vas deferens is cut just above the testicles and the sperm have nowhere to go…. Many men complain about feeling congested in the testicles and pelvis." That's one way to put it. The authors go on to recommend a form of testicular massage developed by Taoist monks of antiquity. These Taoist monks believed that the production of millions of sperm cells a day takes a tremendous amount of energy, and in this I'm sure they are right. They also believed that regularly ejaculating those millions of sperm cells is a huge drain on the body's energy system. Hence, daily ejaculating may be okay for 15-year-olds, but as we age, conserving energy becomes an issue. So the Taoists developed a non-ejaculatory sexual practice premised on the retention of sperm cells called the Tantra. This goal of not ejaculating had to be balanced by their belief that orgasms were good for the body and soul, and the more, the merrier. This beats the old sin and guilt model all to heck, doesn't it? To mitigate the effects of sperm cells retained in the body (sound familiar?) the Tantrists developed a series of self-massage techniques since it is unlikely that you can get anyone else to do it for you anyway. The intent of these massage techniques is to clear congestion and dead cells from the testicles and improve blood flow. These are worthwhile goals. However, this should be approached cautiously and gently at first, especially if you are experiencing any testicular pain. If all of this sounds too much like self-pleasuring instead of just good self-care, I would offer two observations. First, you probably haven't tried it. These massage techniques can be quite uncomfortable and take you to the edge of what you can stand, especially if you are already having symptoms of congestion and pain. Secondly, dare I point this out, it is far easier on your body than surgery and you might just feel better. Enough said? So put away all of those "the body is a bad thing and shouldn't be touched" concepts from childhood for a little while and give it a try.

Here is the method recommended by Chia and Arava:

"Testicle Massage:

"1. Rub your hands together to warm them up.

"2. Hold one testicle between the thumb and fingers of each hand [see below]. Your testicles should feel like small apricots between your fingers [If they feel like large eggplants you might be in trouble.].

"3. Firmly but gently massage your testicles with your thumbs and fingers for a minute or two. If your testicles ache or are sensitive, rub lighter but longer, until the pain goes away [hopefully]. The pain is caused by blockage, and the massage will help bring blood and sexual energy to the area, which will disperse any blockage.

182

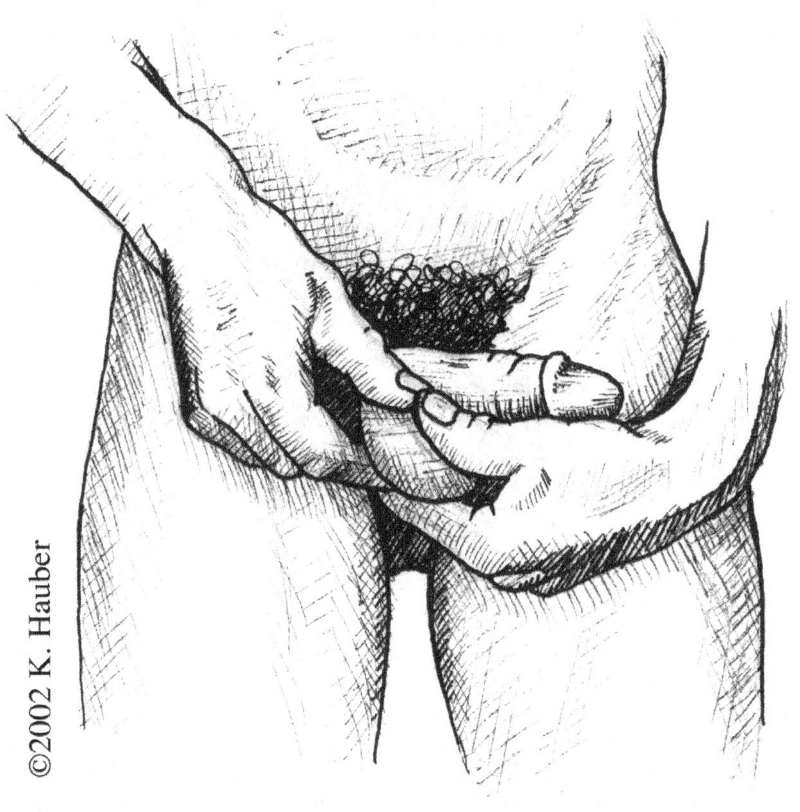

"4. Hold your penis up to expose your testicles and tap with your longest finger for a minute or two [see below and proceed with caution]. This helps invigorate your testes and increase sperm production.

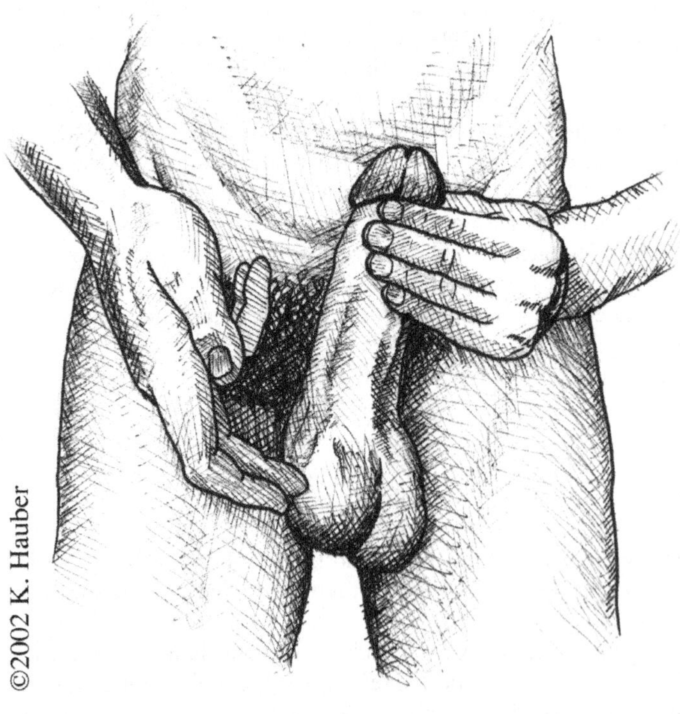

"5. Finally, hold your penis and scrotum with your thumb and forefinger [This is the toughest if you already have testicular pain]. Now lightly pull your penis and scrotum forward with your hand as you pull back with your pelvic muscles. Then repeat, pulling to the right with your hand and to the left with your pelvic muscles. Then pull to the left with your hand and to the right with your pelvic muscles. Finish by pulling your hand down and your pelvic muscles up.

"Do this exercise nine, eighteen, or thirty-six times. It will keep the ducts that carry your sperm healthy."

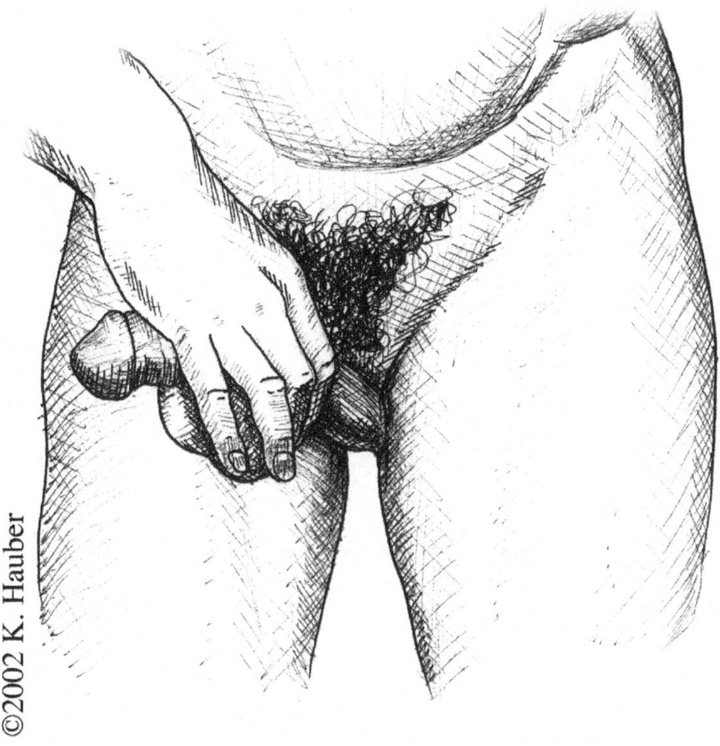

- If you are concerned about the prostate cancer risk aspect of vasectomy, or just about the general risk of prostate cancer even if you haven't had a vasectomy, there are a number of simple preventative measures you can take. Chan, et. al., (1998) states "nutritional factors, especially meat, fat, and dairy intake, have been linked to greater risk of disease. Higher consumption of selenium and Vitamin E, fructose/fruits, and tomatoes all have been associated with reduced occurrence of prostate cancer...." So it appears that eating in a more healthy fashion is good for you in ways you might not have expected. The article goes on to call out risk factors for prostate cancer including smoking and exposure to cadmium, and low levels of physical activity and exercise. Oh, by the way, vasectomy is also mentioned as a risk factor for prostate cancer in the article. Surprise, surprise!

You might find many of these forms of treatment quite unsavory to consider, particularly the more invasive medical ones. They are. Let your doctor know of any distress this causes you and insist as politely as possible that his or her disclosure practices change in the future. Let your doctor know that you expect to have his or her support in monitoring your health for any potential problems. Consistent checks for prostate cancer and other common maladies would be advisable. This constitutes a minimum of active steps for a prudent man to take, in my opinion of course.

In case there is any dispute over the availability of information about post-vasectomy pain syndrome and the need to disclose the possibility, check out the short treasury of relevant quotations at the end of the book that you may want to have on hand. Speaking of quotations, here is a good summary offered by Dr. Malcolm Carruthers in his article "Vasectomy – The Unkindest Cut of All": "Personally, I would strongly advise against vasectomy, which is a major trauma to the testis, a delicate and complex organ producing a variety of external secretions and hormones, including testosterone. Any oral contraceptive, used either with men or women, with an equivalent range of short and long-term complications, would surely have been taken off the market by now and the manufacturers heavily sued. Why not apply the same stringent conditions to vasectomy?"

I like Dr. Carruthers' (1997) historical summary also: "The first recorded vasectomy was done by a British surgeon, Sir Astley Cooper, who in 1823 vasectomized his dog. My clinical experience over the past 15 years has made me firmly of the opinion that it shouldn't even happen to a dog. If you or a friend are thinking of having the knot of vasectomy tied, my earnest advice to you would be: Don't!"

Thank you, Dr. Carruthers for being willing to go against the herd and speak out!

Chapter Thirty

Let There Be Light

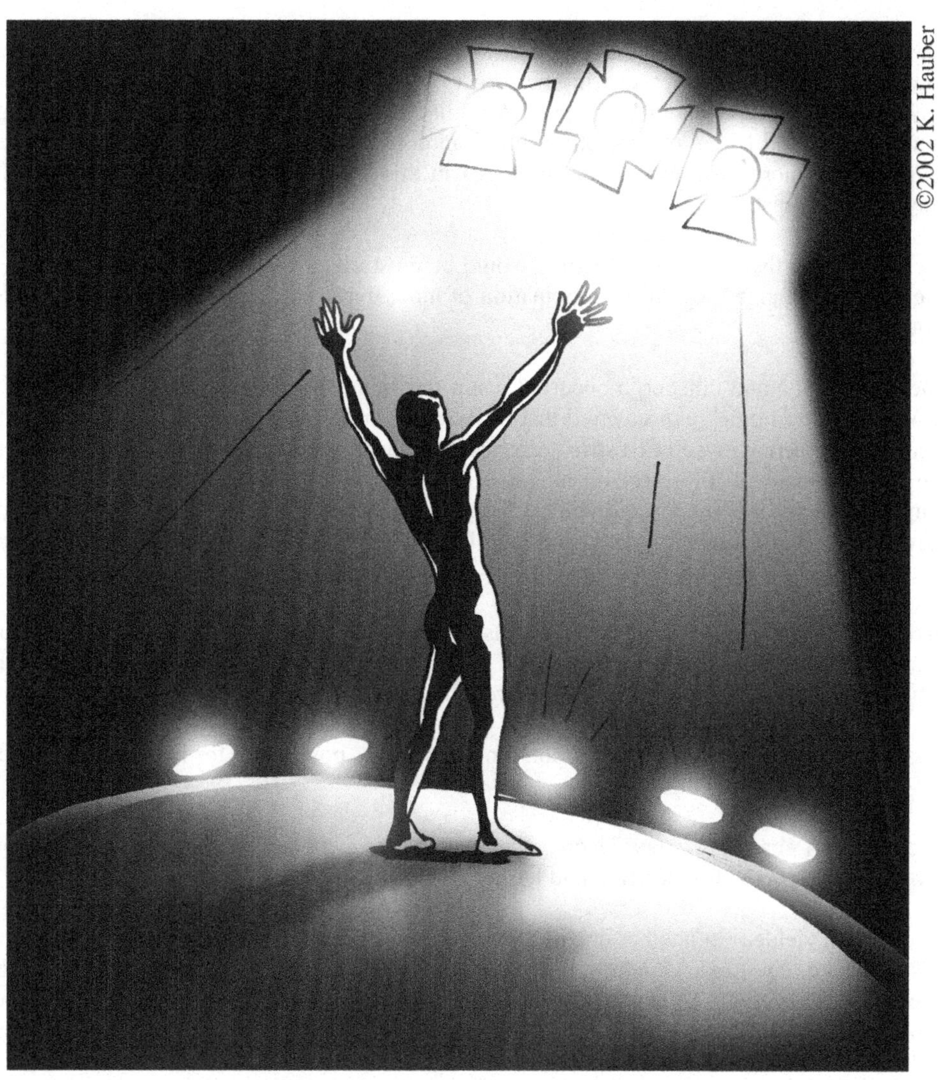

About two and a half years into my post-vasectomy experience, my internist, Dr. Stephen Hilty, made what I considered an unconventional but interesting suggestion. He had another patient who had experienced significant reflex sympathetic dystrophy (RSD) chronic pain symptoms following an auto accident. Like me, she had tried just about everything to cure her pain. Dr. Hilty came across a new approach to the treatment of chronic pain called "Photon Therapy". Evidently, this therapy had been used for some time in veterinary medicine, but had only recently won FDA approval for use on humans.

The concept is to use a wand that emits infrared light at specific frequencies to stimulate the regeneration of damaged nerve tissues. Evidently the research behind this technique showed that cell growth is very responsive to certain bands of light, namely the infrared bands used in the "Photon Therapy". The information I received from Dr. Hilty was that a Dr. Connie Haber (no relation to me) in Pittsburgh had been instrumental in developing this technique and had a great track record of positive results.

The literature I subsequently received from Dr. Haber told of a little girl who had been struck by lightning, causing severe nerve damage and RSD symptoms throughout one entire side of her body. One week of Photon Therapy had cured her. Other testimonials were equally dramatic. I discussed this possibility with Dr. Hilty and we both reached the same conclusion: This type of therapy had little or no downside risk, save having to go to Pittsburgh, and the potential for healing in a non-invasive manner was substantial. So I scheduled myself for a trip to Pittsburgh in December hoping that the infrared light would be enough to keep my thin California blood from freezing. Well, at least my balls might stay warm. Or not.

As if this wasn't enough, I took an "as long as I'm going that way anyway" approach and scheduled to see the doctor in Chicago who specialized in the nerve-stripping surgery while on my way to Pittsburgh. He planned to do another cord block, his way this time, while I was in Chicago to determine if the nerve stripping was a viable long-term option for me. I know, why on earth would I want to subject myself to another cord block after my first experience? I was holding out hope that this guy knew more than my original urologist in this regard, and could make it a slightly less agonizing event. That was my prayer at least.

Dr. Haber advised me that the photon therapy would be most effective if I were to shave down, so once again, I found myself perfecting this strange life skill in anticipation of more treatment. At least it wasn't in anticipation of more surgery, at least not yet.

My journey to Chicago and Pittsburgh occurred just a few months after the September 11, 2001, terrorist attacks on New York and Washington. I quickly discovered that traveling by air in the age of terrorists is not what it used to be. It felt like I was practically subjecting myself to a strip search just for mentioning the fact that I intended to travel by plane. I must have had the entire contents of my carry on luggage rifled through at every terminal. When one inspector started looking through my medical records binder and another foraged through my wallet I felt this form of protectionism had gone too far. It gave me a taste of just how much people will surrender their rights and their privacy to feel "safe." It also motivated me to opt for trips by car or train until some of this madness subsided.

Upon arriving in Chicago, I made my way to Rush Hospital and then to the offices of Dr. Laurence Levine. I found him to be as personable in the flesh as he had been on the phone, with a reassuring candor and empathy about the post-vasectomy pain condition his other patients (30 or more of them) and I had experienced.

"With what you've been through, I think I could make you my poster-boy for how bad this type of situation can get," he quipped as he reviewed my records.

"Please feel free to share my story in any way that would get the information out," I implored, "with my blessings." Self-consciousness about the situation had left me long before this.

The physical exam yielded yet another one of those "My, you *are* tender," exclamations, and fortunately he didn't push too far or mash too hard. Dr. Levine couldn't help noticing my shaved down state, and asked, "Is pubic shaving some kind of fashion trend in California?" Evidently, he had seen another patient from California recently who was a body builder and had shaved his whole body save a mustache-like strip above his penis. Put a pair of glasses on the guy's scrotum, and I bet he'd look like Groucho Marx.

I had a momentary urge to spin a great story about the shaving parties and hot tubs we all have in California, but I resisted that impulse. Now, I know that people in the Midwest think everyone from California is more than a little crazy, but I thought that contributing to that myth (or reality, depending on how you look at it) wasn't in my best interest at that point. Besides, urologists are quick to refer patients for psychological counseling when they are experiencing post-vasectomy pain syndrome anyway, and I had no desire to spend more time on any couch other than my own at home. I assured him that it wasn't about fashion for me, but more in anticipation of being bombarded by photons. We reached an agreement that if you don't need to remove all the covering that Mother Nature gives you for some legitimate medical reason, why bother.

After discussing various aspects, symptoms, and options, we decided that pursuing a spermatic cord nerve block would be a productive thing to do that day, and he loaded up his needles. If my original urologist had loaded for bear when he did my first cord block, then Dr. Levine was loading for elephants. Fortunately, my efforts to reduce inflammation seemed to have yielded some benefit, since administering the block was still mighty unpleasant, but didn't feel like he was driving a spike through my groin as had been the case nearly two years prior.

The block actually took effect within a few minutes and worked well to reduce the aching and tearing sensations emanating from my testicles, allowing me to feel closer to normal than I had in quite a while. I know, it's debatable as to whether I have ever been normal or not, but let's not enter that discussion here.

"How are you doing," asked Dr. Levine when he reentered the room after a brief hiatus.

"So far, so good," I responded. "I think you know how to make these blocks work."

"It's all a matter of knowing how much to put in and where to put it," he summarized.

Despite the locker room-like sound of that statement, I had to agree with him. We decided that I would let him know how long the block was effective, and if anything unusual occurred. Then we could assess what to do about any future nerve-stripping surgery. This was lining up to be a good fall back position, depending on how the photon therapy came out, and depending on what happened after I ceased the testosterone therapy and became fertile again, hopefully without the recurrence of any autoimmune symptoms. I had no desire to be fighting two wars at once, i.e. a significant autoimmune response with all of the associated swelling, scar tissue formation, etc. and the need to recover from a surgery in the region at the same time. If anything in this process, I was learning to be patient and methodical.

When I arrived in Dr. Haber's office the next day, I found her singing as she pushed a cart of holiday goodies to the front of her office. In our discussions, she consistently referred to herself as a "little old lady" despite the fact that she darted around her office like a kitten with its tail on fire. Little old lady, my foot! Nuclear power plants should hope to have that much energy.

First, she gave me instructions on all of the supplements and good organic food I was to ingest during the week she was treating me, including some liquid supplements that were "a real ass-kicker." "We're gonna teach these nerves some respect and get you your life back," she belted out. I liked her already.

Then she became serious for a moment. "Now, I'm going to have to start off by being mean to you," she stated. Uh oh.

"What do you mean by 'mean'," I wondered out loud.

"Well, I need you to stand naked in front of a fan for 20 minutes to cool you off so I can get good thermal images as part of the photon therapy," she replied.

This was a new brand of weird. How anyone could think I needed cooling off with as little action as I had been getting I'll never know.

"You're going to have to work a lot harder at being mean if you want to beat what I've had done to me so far." I hoped she wouldn't take the challenge.

So I got an opportunity to flap in the breeze for a while, quite literally, in an attempt to create an ideal skin condition for thermal imaging. The imaging process itself was fascinating. I could stand in front of the camera and see the different gradients of heat emanating from my body displayed on the screen, with noticeable "hot spots" showing in the most tender areas and other "cold spots" showing a lack of circulation due to vascular constriction (I'll leave the exact locations to your imagination). After taking an initial set of images, Dr. Haber pulled out her magic photon wand and began bombarding these various hot and cold spots, some of which were larger than just spots. Within minutes, the treated areas would begin to equalize temperature with the surrounding tissues and become less tender, which I could see on the monitor and feel by touch.

"You're going to get the patient of the day award," exclaimed Connie. We were on a first name basis by this point, which tends to be the case for me when someone gets as close to the tender spots as she was.

The thermal imaging and photon therapy were the most amazing use of medical technology I had seen yet and one of the easiest to administer, despite the shaving and flapping in the breeze that preceded it. The visible difference in balance and symmetry that resulted was remarkable. The entire treatment process took about three hours the first day.

"I'm not done with you yet," Dr. Haber ordered as I readied to leave. "Go back to your room and rest now for at least an hour. No exercise, no TV, just rest."

"Yes ma'am."

Who am I to argue with someone telling me to take a nap? The one-hour nap turned into three, which I must have needed, followed by several hours of significantly reduced pain. I was keeping my fingers crossed that I was onto something.

The next day brought four more hours of the same kind of treatment in some really fascinating positions with camera angles that I never considered to be my best side. But if this worked, I was going to have the images framed and then made into a billboard. That day's efforts included the use of the photon therapy to clear my lymphatic system. What a concept! Again, a substantial reduction in pain followed the treatments for a number of hours.

"Do you think you can stretch this relief interval out a bit," I asked, "like for the rest of my life?"

"That's what I'm aiming for sweetheart," Dr. Haber replied in her typical manner.

During my third day at her clinic, Dr. Haber called me into one of her exam rooms and introduced me to another one of her patients.

"He's having testicular pain after multiple hernia repair surgeries," she told me, "and his doctors are recommending nerve-stripping surgery now. I think you two have something to talk about." I think I had just joined the photon therapy sales team.

Evidently, no one had talked with him yet about some of the potential risks of this type of surgery, so I mentioned the possibility of infertility, testicular atrophy, infection and increased pain. I offered to copy some medical journal references on the subject of this type of neuropathy and send them to him. He was quite thankful to be able to talk to someone else who was having a similar experience of pain and could offer an alternate perspective and some resources for him. He seemed content with the idea of using photon therapy to try to melt away the nerve entrapments that were causing his pain before allowing himself to be cut on again; a good choice in my book.

So each day Dr. Haber would use her magic photon wand to make my hot spots cooler and my cool spots hotter in a never-ending attempt to bring me back into balance and get my nervous system to talk nicely to itself instead of all of the rude messages it had been giving for the last several years. Each day she would add to this regimen something new; an energy measuring device here, a laser there, you get the idea.

About mid way through the week, she said, "OK, now we're going to magnetize you."

She took me to a room containing a large machine with two long arms with plates at the ends. She picked up a light bulb with a wire wrapped around it and waved it over the plates. The light bulb lit up spontaneously.

"Very strong electromagnets, "she commented, "You might want to take off anything metallic."

She then maneuvered the arms so that one plate was in front of my groin and the other was on my lower back.

"We're going to make a testicle sandwich out of you here for about 10 minutes," she said.

"Hold the mayo, if you will," I quipped.

It was yet another unusual and fortunately painless treatment modality. I think it was a good thing that I didn't have any metal implants anywhere in the region from prior surgeries, despite the "balls of steel' reputation I was getting by that time.

And so it went. Each day I would assume positions that usually get reserved for dancers in really seedy bars. And each day streams of photons would assault the sorest parts of me. The funny thing was, it actually seemed like the intensity of the pain was beginning to diminish. I had several days in a row when I didn't need to resort to painkillers by the time evening rolled around. That was truly exciting. It's not like I stopped hurting all at once, but it sure seemed like I was making progress in the right direction. By now I was keeping my fingers and toes, and everything else that would cross, crossed.

As I left Pittsburgh at the end of my week's treatment, I saw a new moon rising in the winter sky as my plane climbed into the heavens. It seemed such an appropriate symbol for the sense of new opportunity this therapy had offered me, even if it had not been a complete cure as yet. Being patient and methodical appeared to be paying dividends. Even in the following days when normal activity would bring on a familiar pain cycle, the intensity of it was at least somewhat diminished from what it had been before. My intuition said to keep with this approach somehow. How that would unfold, only time would tell.

I close this chapter with a thought from Albert Schweitzer (who was an M.D., by the way): "Each patient carries his own doctor inside him. We are at our best when we give the doctor who resides within each patient a chance to work."

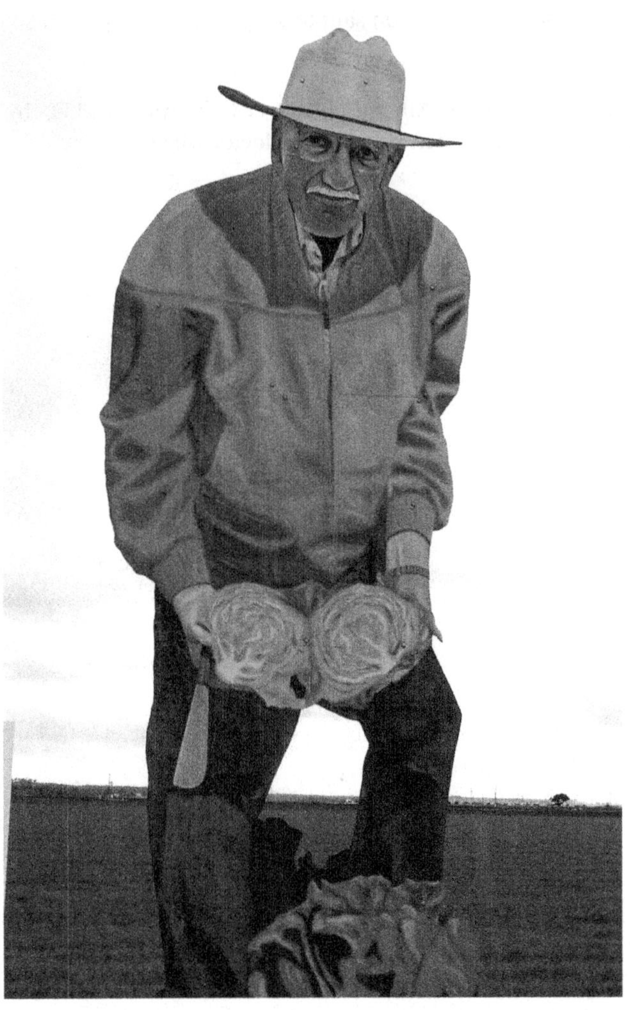

And you think you have problems?

"He is the best physician who is the most ingenious inspirer of hope." – Samuel Taylor Coleridge

"Valid social ends do not justify invalid, unscientific means…. The desirability of zero population growth cannot excuse the routine resort to irreversible, controversial procedures, be they drug or surgical" (Soderdahl, 1982).

People have an amazing ability to bury their heads in the sand about important issues, even when those issues affect their health. Doctors aren't immune from this tendency. As an example, consider the following:

One of my doctors was at a medical conference and happened to attend a seminar on urology. There was a question and answer session at the end, and one of the General Practitioners in attendance asked about chronic pain following vasectomy. The panelist doctor waved off the question saying that he must be talking about post-vasectomy pain syndrome and he didn't want to discuss it. Why the heck not? That was exactly the kind of forum in which the subject needs to be discussed.

Another variation on this theme of not wanting to acknowledge a problem is found in a research article by Dias (1983). The purpose of this article was to study whether vasectomy had any effect on the volume of the testis. The article stated that there were no complications experienced by the 15 patients in the study. Then the article went on to note "except for patient #13, who had a scrotal oedema [sic] when examined on the fifth day. The wounds all healed well and the patients had no complaints except for occasional pain in the scrotal and inguinal region" for the duration of the one-year study. Do you see the same red flag here that I do? How can it be said that no complications resulted, and in the next breath state that oedema and pain resulted. Supposedly, complete informed consent was obtained from each man before surgery. Do you think that the discussion included the possibility of chronic pain? This doesn't seem very likely if the doctors don't consider it a problem. But, then again, it's not the doctors who are in pain, is it?

In addition to the doctors I chose to see, another doctor was consulted about my case on request of an insurance company. When asked about disclosing the possibility of chronic pain and other serious complications of vasectomy to patients, he replied that these issues were routinely not discussed because it would frighten and traumatize patients. No kidding! I should send the doctor a copy of this book so he can know what being scared and traumatized about this issue really feels like.

As another example, Dr. Lars Linnet (1983) advocates that men be tested for sperm antibody levels before having a vasectomy reversal and informed about the impact on their ability to father children that high antibody titers will likely have. Amazingly enough, other doctors have objected to this practice of informing the patient. So let's see, these other doctors are advocating that a man allow his testicles to be cut open (again) in what can be a significantly painful operation, spend thousands of dollars on the procedure, which is commonly not reimbursable by medical insurance, all in the anticipation of making babies that are not likely to be conceived. What is wrong with this picture? In Dr. Linnet's words, "it would seem correct to inform a man with a high titer that he might encounter additional problems." This seems like common courtesy, in addition to good medical ethics.

"For men considering vasectomy, it's the pain they're worried about, not the permanence..." (ABC News, 3/12/01). For many doctors, however, the opposite is true. My original urologist once stated to me in a prideful manner, "I don't have vasectomy failures." Period. End of story: like it was a huge deal. I told him to knock on wood. He couldn't state with such vehemence, though, that he had never seen one of his patients writhing in pain because of his surgical expertise. So, whose feelings matter more in this situation, the surgeon who is proud of his record, or the patient in endless agony?

It has been noted that "men, like women who seek sterilization, are often dissatisfied with their previous form or forms of contraception" (Sandlow, et. al., 2001). This can be a very stressful subject for the patient, especially if a "whoops" baby or two has occurred. But an automatic response of offering surgical sterilization in any form when patients are under duress is a dangerous proposition, as has been shown repeatedly throughout this text.

As you might be able to tell by now, the complications I continue to experience haven't stopped yet. This situation has given me a unique and continuing motivation to be an advocate for change in this area of medicine. From that perspective, I wish to issue the following challenge:

Medical science, you've created this monster. Now it's time to help us find a way to tame it. There are many men who are likely to suffer needlessly if current vasectomy practices are not changed. Advocate the change instead of resisting it.

Data that doesn't endorse current practices is just simply that, opposing data. This doesn't automatically make it wrong. This game of life we all play has so many unquantifiable aspects that putting blinders on is dangerous. Put the scalpel down for a moment, give complete information, stand back, and let your patient decide.

Take a stand for health which says that the negative long-term health consequences due to any form of contraceptive use by men or women are not acceptable. Let your peers and the public know how you feel.

We all need safe, effective means of birth control in our modern society. We also need that means of contraception in a way that doesn't cause more harm than good. It is my opinion that a majority of the medical community, the media, and the general public are asleep about risks related to vasectomy. When people are in a deep sleep, often they need to be shaken a little to wake up when needed. I hope this book provides an earthquake!

Chronic genital pain and lifelong autoimmune responses with significant implications for numerous diseases are not an acceptable outcome of an elective surgical procedure. This is especially true when there is no disclosure of these facts beforehand and no effective treatment for these conditions afterward.

There is another more basic motivation for medical professionals to be better informed about post-vasectomy pain and other problems: personal safety. What do I mean by that? Consider this: when Miller, et. al., (1991) surveyed several hundred post-vasectomy couples about any regret they had about the procedure, an interesting, unexpected result occurred. The researchers found that a "vocal group of men in our sample expressed considerable dismay and anger over the occurrence of lasting soreness and pain in the genital area following the surgery." I understand these sentiments, and note the word "anger." Numerous men with whom I have spoken have been extremely angry at the doctor who performed their vasectomy which left them in chronic pain, only to be abandoned by that doctor afterward. Many of these men have admitted contemplating violence to "give that S.O.B a taste of what this is like." A large portion of our population owns weapons. My prediction is that sooner or later, someone is going to get hurt or killed because of this, if in fact, it hasn't happened already. I hope it doesn't take something like that to get the medical community's attention.

It is my greater hope that in waking up and looking at this issue, the research which is needed will be done and not continually swept under the carpet, and we will come up with better individual and collective options for the problems we face. This is not an issue that can be solved by men and women passing the contraceptive hot potato back and forth. It is a mutual issue for men and women, with significant health consequences for both genders.

I'll close this chapter, and this challenge, with a quote from Nobel Peace Prize winner Dr. Alexis Carrell: "The hope of humanity lies in the prevention of degenerative and mental diseases, not in the care of their symptoms." With any luck, the mindset of the medical community in regard to the negative effects of vasectomy will shift in this direction.

Chapter Thirty-Two

How Does This All Add Up?

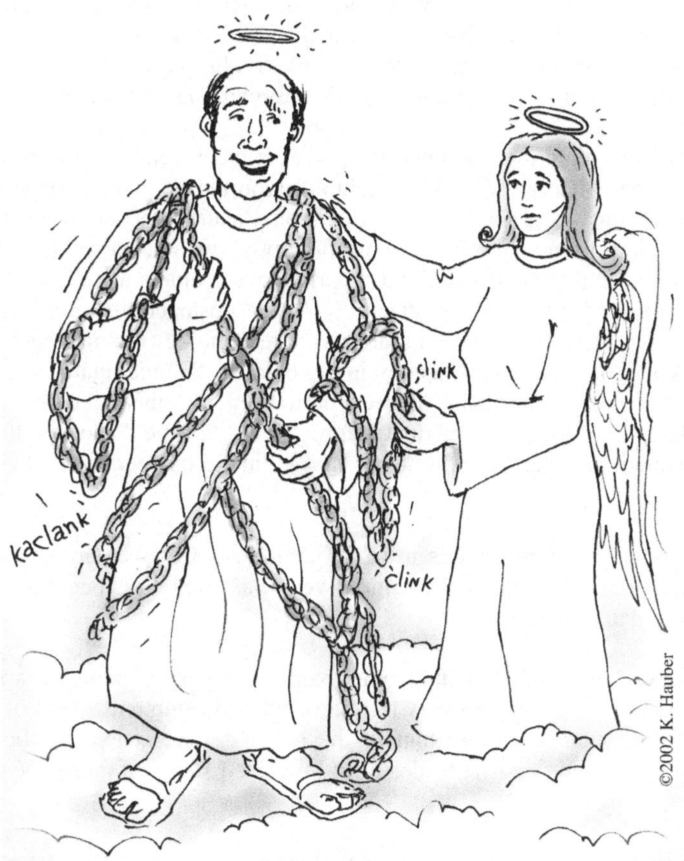

Oh, the chains?... well, tonight I'm going back to haunt the doctor who did that "simple procedure".

"All truth goes through steps:

First it is ridiculed,

Second it is violently opposed,

Finally it is accepted as self-evident."

-Arthur Schopenbauer, German Philosopher

"Follow-up studies of vasectomy series seem as often as not conducted rather to show how good the operation is than to uncover its effects" (Wolfers, 1973).

So how extensive are the problems created by vasectomies? You may have asked yourself that question by now. This book has cited many studies and individual examples of the problems that can result from the procedure. But how extensive is this, really?

Well, if you take the 75% estimate of men developing autoimmune reactions from the studies on the subject and use the recent estimate of 100 million men having had the procedure (that number is at least several years old, by the way) you come up with 75 million men who are now experiencing an immune system reaction because of their vasectomies. That seems like a lot of people to be putting at risk, doesn't it?

Let's look at the numbers another way. We've already discussed the reluctance men have to reveal or do anything about genital problems. The embarrassment, shame, and fear that accompanies such conditions keeps many men away from doctors altogether. But what about the available studies and individual cases of those willing to disclose the problems and seek treatment? How do those add up? Here is some of this information presented chronologically (more or less):

The earliest recordation of a significant number of men experiencing chronic post vasectomy pain that I have been able to find was way back in 1966 when Dr. Stanwood Schmidt reported on a series of vasectomies in which "delayed postoperative, diagnosed as not due to granuloma or other complication, occurred in 4 men," while another man experienced pain that prevented him from "returning to work promptly" without saying how long this pain lingered. Still another man complained of postoperative impotence, and "spermatic granuloma arising from the cut end of the proximal vas occurred in 21 patients, who had a total of 28 attacks." Also, "postoperative epididymitis, not of bacterial origin [hmmm], occurred in 21 patients." Despite the lack of more recent terminology that had been applied to these situations, it is quite easy to see what was going on. Quite significantly in my opinion, Schmidt makes mention of "2 cases of gangrene of the testis after vasectomy" in operations that had been performed by other "junior doctors," and another case of "gangrene of the testis after ligation of the entire spermatic cord." Couldn't the doctor tell the difference between the vas and the entire cord? That's enough to make me refuse to be first in line to be operated on by someone just recently out of medical school.

Esho, et. al., (1973) reported complications in 62 (15.5%) of 400 vasectomy cases reviewed, with some cases experiencing multiple complications. Eleven of these men were classified as experiencing "testicular and epididymal congestion," i.e. post-vasectomy pain syndrome.

Schmidt (1979) reported a series of 83 symptomatic [painful] spermatic granulomas forming in patients following vasectomy. Sixty-three of these cases required surgery to relieve painful symptoms. One of the patients was a physician who encountered pain significant enough to send him to the hospital. He stated that he had "experienced the most agonizing pain in my life," and "the pain finally subsided after I received 15mg. of morphine on five occasions in less than two hours."

Shapiro (1979) reported on nine patients who experienced "chronic and persistent post-vasectomy orchialgia [testicular pain]." These men underwent vasectomy reversal to attempt to relieve their symptoms.

Silber (1980) reported on the results of 10 men who were referred to him for "persistent discomfort many years after vasectomy." Eight of those 10 men chose to undergo surgical reversal of their vasectomies even though they did not wish to become fertile again.

The deaths of seven men resulted from scrotal infections following their vasectomies as reported by Grimes, et. al., (1982).

In 1982, the *British Medical Journal* carried several articles describing men who were experiencing chronic pain when ejaculating following their vasectomies. I. S. Edwards reported on seven men who had experienced painful ejaculation symptoms and had undergone a second, open-ended vasectomy to seek relief (Edwards, 1982).

Schned, et. al., (1984) reported 14 men who underwent epididymectomy in hopes of relief from their "severe, unremitting scrotal pain" following their vasectomies. This report served as the basis for several future reports.

Eighteen patients who had experienced chronic post-vasectomy pain for five to seven years underwent epididymectomy, as reported by Selikowitz, et. al., (1985). One man required castration because of complications that became apparent during his epididymectomy. There was no comment on the long-term consequences for the other patients.

Cui (1986) reported treating 11 men with a form of radio-frequency acupuncture for chronic pain following their vasectomies. Ten of the 11 men were reported to have experienced resolution of their pain by this treatment.

Schned, et. al., (1986) reported on four men who had experienced long-term post-vasectomy pain and underwent epididymectomies in an attempt to resolve the pain. This was a continuation of Schned, et. al.,'s 1984 report, but several new findings were noted in this new article. When the epididymides were examined following surgery in each case, a chronic inflammatory phenomenon the authors termed "epididymitis nodosa" was found in each case. The authors concluded that this inflammatory reaction is likely very common, and "recognition is important to prevent misdiagnosis as a neoplasm [cancerous tumor]."

Alderman (1991) found complications in 124 vasectomy cases which represented 10.6% of the study population. This included 23 instances of "congestive epididymitis," i.e. post vasectomy pain syndrome with varying times of onset from the date of surgery up to two years afterwards in several cases. Orchitis was diagnosed in another two men who had swollen testicles Another 12 patients who experienced no inflammation of the epididymis or testicles as the others had, but had "intrascrotal pain." Methods of classification are interesting and varied, aren't they?

Chen, et. al., (1991) reported on ten patients with chronic post-vasectomy pain who underwent subsequent epididymectomy. Half of these patients experienced relief. There was no mention of how many patients required subsequent castration following their epididymectomies due to testicular atrophy or other complications.

Fifty-six of 172 patients (33%) experienced chronic testicular pain following their vasectomies in the study by McMahon, et. al., (1992).

Moss (1992) reported congestive epididymitis following closed ended vasectomy in 6% (185) of 3081 cases. Open-ended vasectomy resulted in 2% (63) cases of the same complication. Other complications were not discussed.

H. J. Roberts, M. D. (1993) reported on 74 cases of significant post-vasectomy diseases that he had treated or reviewed as a doctor.

Buchholz, et. al., (1994) found 18 men out of a group of 180 vasectomized men that attributed their erectile dysfunction to vasectomy.

Choe, et. al., (1996) reported post-vasectomy scrotal pain in 34 (18.7%) of 182 patients. This was noted as a "late" complication of vasectomy. Early complications were reported in 23 (12.6%) men.

Levine, et. al., (1996) reported on the results of microsurgical nerve-stripping for four patients with post-vasectomy pain that had continued for up to 20 years. Three patients had relief after the nerve-stripping procedure. One patient eventually had a testicle removed to seek relief.

Ahmed, et. al., (1997) found a group of 108 men who experienced chronic post-vasectomy testicular pain. This represented 27.2% of the study population. The pain was severe enough to motivate 17 of these patients to have the nerves surgically stripped from their spermatic cords to seek relief, and numerous others needed to use pain medication for extended periods of time.

Brunning (1997) reported nerve-stripping of the spermatic cords to have been successful in alleviating chronic post-vasectomy pain in two other patients. There was no mention of how many other procedures did not succeed, but it was noted that this was a way to try to avoid eventual castration. Not a bad motivation to my way of thinking.

Myers, et. al., (1997) reported on 32 men who underwent vasectomy reversal for treatment of their post-vasectomy pain syndrome. Several of these patients underwent subsequent epididymectomy and eventual castration.

Ninety-four of 1223 men experienced complications following their vasectomies in the Labreque, et. al., (1998) study. That's an overall rate of 7.6%.

Five men posted messages on the Prostatitis Website – Vasectomy Page in 1998 discussing their experience with vasectomy and the chronic prostatitis they developed following the procedure. Their conditions had persisted for up to nine years.

Sweeney, et. al., (1998) reported on eight men who suffered with "post-vasectomy epididymal engorgement." These patients underwent epididymectomy in an attempt to relieve their symptoms.

Fervenza, et. al., (1999) outlined three cases of Staph infections of the heart valves in men following vasectomy. Major courses of intravenous antibiotics and subsequent surgical reconstruction of the heart were described.

Nangia, et. al., (2000) reports on the results of 13 men who underwent vasectomy reversal one or more times in an attempt to resolve their post-vasectomy pain syndrome. Only nine of the 13 became pain free.

Levine, et. al., (2001) reported the results of denervation surgery on the spermatic cords of an additional three vasectomy patients following his 1996 report. The report actually included the results of this surgery for a total of 27 men, seven of whose pain was due to vasectomy as previously mentioned, with others seeking relief after hernia surgery, trauma to the testis and other causes. Overall, 76% of the men achieved complete relief by denervation, but the specific percentage of vasectomy patients achieving complete relief was not mentioned.

Speaking of nerve-stripping, Heidenreich, et. al., (2002) reported on a series of 35 patients who underwent the procedure, 34 of whom had "durable" relief without significant complications. Six of those men had experienced chronic testicular pain due to vasectomy. Interestingly, in five others their pain was due to inguinal hernia repair which affects the same nerves.

That's a total of well over 1,000 cases of significant complications in just a handful of reports. Then there are the individual cases. I am personally familiar with some of these cases.

The longest lasting case I'm aware of is the friend of a friend who had his vasectomy done about thirty years ago. After his vasectomy failed the first time and he fathered another child, he had it done a second time and ended up with chronic pain during sexual activity and occasionally at other times. He says he still gets a burst of pain from time to time.

Another man I met and talked with had his vasectomy about 25 years ago. He had pain afterward that lasted several years.

A retired doctor I met had his vasectomy done 22 years before. The doctor doing the surgery goofed and tied off his testicular artery instead of the vas on one side. As you might guess by now, testicles and other organs don't do well without a blood supply. This man ended up losing a testicle because of the other doctor's error and has suffered chronic pain ever since.

The *British Medical Journal* (1982) reported the following: "A 38-year-old man says that for two years, starting two years after a vasectomy, he has often experienced sudden severe pain in the right testicle, groin, and lower abdomen at the moment of ejaculation…. There is no abnormality on examination of the genitals, spermatic cord, or prostate, and he is mentally and sexually normal." Dr. G. Barry Carruthers responded to this that "the history of vasectomy is probably coincidental," suggesting that the patient was probably experiencing prostatitis. We'll give the doctor the benefit of the doubt that he was not hiding something since information about post-vasectomy pain syndrome was not readily available at that time.

"In 1983, a 57-year-old man presented to the Elliot-Smith Clinic, Oxford, for a vasectomy. Two semen tests at 16 and 18 weeks after vasectomy were negative for spermatozoa. Eighteen months later his wife became pregnant; he subsequently had two further negative semen tests. As it was thought that he could not be the father, his wife had an abortion. Over the intervening years, he had intermittent right testicular discomfort. His wife again became pregnant in 1995 and was 14 weeks pregnant by the time the pregnancy was confirmed. Subsequent semen analysis performed in October 1995 [12 years after the vasectomy] showed a sperm count of 14 million per ml. (Khan, et. al., 1997). There was no comment about the couple's feelings about having aborted a baby that was probably theirs after all, but the authors did conclude that the man was intermittently fertile all along due to partial recanalization.

In one of the Internet forums, a woman wrote of her husband who had a testicle removed during his vasectomy 15 years before. She was concerned because he was now facing further surgery recommended by his doctor because of testicular pain he had been experiencing in the prior year.

Balogh, et. al., (1985) reported the case in which a "29-year-old man noticed painful swelling of the scrotal skin after vasectomy." One has to wonder who could help but notice. This led to another surgery for the man, and when the lesion was examined it was found that he had developed vasitis nodosa and spermatic granuloma of the scrotal skin.

Also reported in 1985 by Auman was the case of a man who's doctor evidently pierced both an artery and a vein with a suture when sewing the man up during his vasectomy. The patient developed a large hematoma in his right scrotum following the surgery which took three weeks to resolve. Over the next 10 years a large scrotal mass formed. Understandably, the patient declined further surgery until the mass became so painful that he needed to proceed with an exploration. Surgery revealed what was termed a "large, symptomatic spermatic cord arteriovenous fistula" at the site where the suture had penetrated the artery and a vein.

Then there is "Harry" whose quote from Dr. Malcolm Carruthers' (1997) book outlines his pain experience and the resulting life dramas in the 10 years since his vasectomy. That book also recounts the story of "James" which you saw previously, with all of the medical drama that was involved in his post-vasectomy experience.

Charlie had his vasectomy in 1990 and has been in pain ever since despite numerous surgical attempts to remedy the situation, including eventual removal of both of his testicles. I'm sure his quote in the Relevant Quotations chapter will give you some idea of what that has been like.

Steve is a friend of a friend who experienced chronic pain that would periodically bring him to his knees without warning in the years following his vasectomy in 1990. He eventually had a reversal done and the pain has gone away for him. Lucky guy

One of the most dramatic cases was a man who died from gangrene which occurred after his vasectomy. This was reported by Viddeleer (1992). The man's pain experience was relatively brief since he only lived for a few days after much of his anatomy had to be removed once the gangrene set in, but the complications obviously had long-lasting effects.

Richard Barcham had his vasectomy done in 1995, and at the time of his Australian radio news article in 1997, was still experiencing pain following his vasectomy.

Joe A. is another man who has been experiencing pain that significantly affects his life. His saga has been going on since 1995.

Mike is another man I've gotten to know. He had his vasectomy done at age 23 in 1995 and has been in pain ever since.

Cardiac arrest during a vasectomy procedure was reported for one patient by Lamberg, et. al., (1996). I think we can safely call this a complication.

"Paul" posted a message to the Urology Forum describing the pain he had been experiencing since his vasectomy in 1997. His doctor was recommending an epididymectomy at the time of his message two years later.

"Lori" wrote to one Internet forum and described her husband's experience of epididymitis since his vasectomy in December, 1997.

Then there is the case of the friend of mine who had to have one of his testicles removed because of a chronic infection that set in after his vasectomy. He's still seeing doctors to try to get his system back in balance.

"Scotty" is another man who has described his post-vasectomy pain experience since his procedure in February, 1998. He has lived with a "roller coaster" of pain emanating from his right testicle.

My college friend has been experiencing pain since his vasectomy in 1998. He's taking a "Looks dangerous, you go first" approach in my discussions with him about seeing more doctors.

"Dave" described his post-vasectomy pain experience since his procedure in late 1998 in a message posted to the Urology Forum. As of March, 2000 when he posted his message he had been to see doctors 72 times in search of a cure.

Don't forget the guy who wanted the scrotal mole removed and got a vasectomy instead. He was still hurting last I heard, even after his reversal.

"Joe Brown" is a man I came in contact with through several Internet forums. He has been experiencing chronic pain since his vasectomy in early 1999.

My own painful experience has continued since my vasectomy on August 12, 1999. I'd love to tell you that this ordeal is over for me, but it isn't. I continue to pray; a lot!

Ken is another man I have come to know who has also been experiencing post-vasectomy pain since 1999.

Another Aussie, "Peter," described his post-vasectomy pain experience on the Urology Forum. His procedure was done in December, 1999, and he had been in pain up to the time of his posting the message in April, 2000.

Martin is a man I met who lives near me. When I met him in the fall of 2000, he had been experiencing debilitating post-vasectomy pain for nine months, and was scheduled to have his testicle removed. I warned him against this, but his urologist insisted that this was the best possible cure, without discussing the irreversible aspect of castration. After he had his testicle removed, he was still in pain and developed a severe infection that nearly killed him.

De Diego Rodriruez, et. al., (2000) reported a man who developed Fournier's gangrene following his vasectomy and subsequently underwent numerous radical surgeries.

These are just a few of the many individual cases I have found in addition to my own. In all, I have found more than 1,200 cases in the literature thus far. Dozens of other men have written to the www.dontfixit.org web site describing their fear, pain and complications following vasectomies. My instinct tells me that where there is smoke, there's fire on this one.

Keep in mind that the cases from the medical literature are primarily reports from individual doctors or clinics. Many other doctors are reluctant to publicize complications from vasectomy for a variety of reasons. Please note that these results do not include the reports of associations between vasectomy and prostate cancer. These are only the cases where vasectomy was directly linked to pain or other significant complications. Also, these figures do not include vasectomy failures and the pregnancies that have resulted.

Chapter Thirty-Three

On a Personal Note

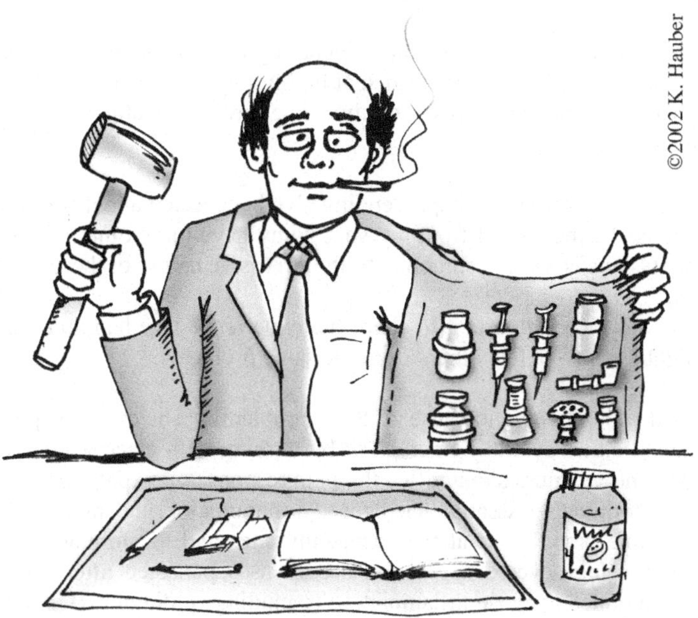

"We can't make your pain go away, but we can do some procedures and create enough other pain that you wont notice the pain you have now nearly as much, And we can give you enough drugs so that you just dont care."

"Any day is a good day when you're not in a urologist's office!"
(Garrison Keillor, Prairie Home Companion, 2002)

"Life consists not in holding good cards, but in playing well those you do hold." (Josh Billings)

What advice might I be able to give about this issue, having learned what I have through my experience? First, obviously, I would implore you not to have a vasectomy performed for the numerous reasons that have been discussed. Consider altering your sexual habits slightly before you consider altering your body surgically. There is a great deal of strong evidence to support this opinion regarding both men and women.

Second, if contraception is an issue for you, as it is for most of us, pick a method that works for you and become proficient at it, whether that is the use of condoms, a diaphragm, foams, or whatever method or combination of methods you and your partner choose and feel comfortable with. There is a great story I have to tell about this: A young couple was about to engage in love making for the first time. As their passions heightened and their clothes came off, they fell into bed together.

The woman said, "Wait just a minute. I want you to wear a condom."

"But I don't know how to wear one," the man replied, "I've never used one before."

"It's simple," she said, holding out two fingers and unrolling the condom onto them to demonstrate, "just put it on like this."

He agreed quickly, they turned out the light and proceeded. After a minute or two, she turned the light back on.

"This doesn't feel right," she said, "are you sure you're wearing that condom?"

"Absolutely," he replied, "just like you told me," as he held out two of his fingers with the condom on them.

The point is that to become proficient at anything, including contraception, you need to be able to communicate completely and practice. This may not be best accomplished at highly impassioned moments. Take your time and have fun with the process. Whether it's glow-in-the-dark, ribbed, or chocolate flavoring features that give you pleasure, go for it and enjoy yourself. Just learn how to be good at it.

As for myself, I'd love to be writing that happy ending I've been asked about by so many people. Unfortunately, the pain and autoimmune response I experienced from my vasectomy have turned into a long-term situation. Obviously, I am not alone in this predicament. This is a real testimonial to the pervasive nature of these kinds of problems.

However, I felt that it was more important to share the experience I've had and the information I found sooner, rather than later. Doing so might just save a few others from the same problems.

So what actually happened in my case to cause all these problems? The evidence points to nerve damage that was caused by the original vasectomy, either by cutting nerves or by burning with electrocautery. When the testicular tissues began to congest and rupture, the nerve injuries magnified the pain response. As sperm cells escaped into my bloodstream, my immune system mounted a formidable assault that caused inflammation and more pain. These factors led to the formation of scar tissue and sizable granulomas at the vasectomy sites and the formation of traumatic neuromas as the nerves attempted to rejoin after being severed. The nerve responses persisted after my reversal surgery, as did the autoimmune responses, which continued to cause inflammation (including epididymitis) and the formation of spermatocele cysts. It took months of hormone therapy and lymphatic massage along with numerous other therapeutic approaches to begin to unravel just the autoimmune response portion of what I was experiencing, which was minor compared to the pain from the nerve damage. That's the best summary I can give based on everything I've seen, read, and experienced so far.

My original vasectomy was performed in August, 1999. What has the time since then been like? Often it has been an unimaginable hell, and at other times an unimaginable forced learning experience. Life changing is a minimal description.

To this point, I have undergone more than a dozen invasive procedures of various types plus various trigger-point injection therapies and some subsequent cutting on my scrotum to alleviate the infections that followed my reconstruction surgery. I have been cut apart and sewn back together in ways that I had never previously imagined. Even when I have had procedures performed that have been purported to be "minor" and "simple," disaster has continued to result.

The pain that resulted over the past few years has been amazing to me, even when I try to look at it from a detached perspective. In regard to the pain, I have been advised by numerous doctors that my only remaining medical option is to start cutting out various parts of my privates. None of these surgeries, even removing the testicles altogether, can guarantee a cure. In fact, the doctors I give the greatest credibility tell me the chances of more surgery of any type reducing my pain are 50/50 at best. And then, it could get worse too. This is not an exciting prospect.

It is also quite possible that any of these proposed procedures would result in a lifelong need for medical treatment along with the possible loss of various functions. This not very exciting either. As a result, I have decided to declare my body a scalpel-free zone and avoid further surgeries for some time to come, since surgeries only seem to aggravate what has already been injured. I have not seen enough evidence yet to convince me that there are any surefire surgical cures to this type of surgically-induced problem. In fact, most of the conversations I've had with other men and several doctors who have encountered similar circumstances bolster this opinion.

Most of the men with whom I have spoken who have confronted similar circumstances say that it has often taken years for their symptoms to subside. Many have chosen to not seek any further medical intervention, which is an understandable choice in my book and one that I am inclined to pursue myself barring any miracle cures developing. This has become an exercise in developing a patient and gentle approach to a painful and complex problem. Needless to say, patience in this situation is not easy.

I have sought assistance from more than 50 different providers of varying specialties in the past several years for innumerable therapies (many of which I swore I would never do) in an effort to resolve the pain and other complications. Let me remind you, I started out as a person who didn't see doctors or take medications. Speaking of medications, as of this writing I am on substance number 192 in this process, and have become exceedingly judicious about what I will allow to be put into my body as a result.

The medical costs and lost earnings I've encountered in this process thus far have exceeded $500,000 and continue to mount without compensation. I have considered changing the title of this book to <u>The Six Million Dollar Manhood</u> since it seems that is where I'm headed. It has been a continuous jousting match to get insurance coverage for any of these costs, even after leaving my HMO. My income was roughly half of what it was prior to the first vasectomy for more than a year afterwards due to lost focus and time away from work. Even after learning how to compensate for and mitigate pain as best as possible, medical costs and lost time at work continue to be an issue for me. The bottom line: it has been painful physically, emotionally, and financially.

The strain on family and personal relationships has been tremendous, but I am glad to say that I have been lovingly supported all along. I feel quite blessed in this regard, since I know this is not universally the case, and many marriages have broken up because of such problems. I have had to limit my formerly active athletic interests, civic and social pursuits. I have no choice but to focus on the basics of providing for my family and maintaining and improving my health as much as possible. This has been quite frustrating.

Pain is still my constant companion, but I have been fortunate enough to derive a way to mitigate the autoimmune response I was experiencing, at least temporarily. Now I need to determine how to keep the autoimmune responses under control permanently while working on healing the nerve damage that amplifies the pain responses that haunt me.

What I have learned in this regard is that medical science has only minimal success in treating this type of injury. So this is the position I get to spend hours of my day in, often several times on any given day:

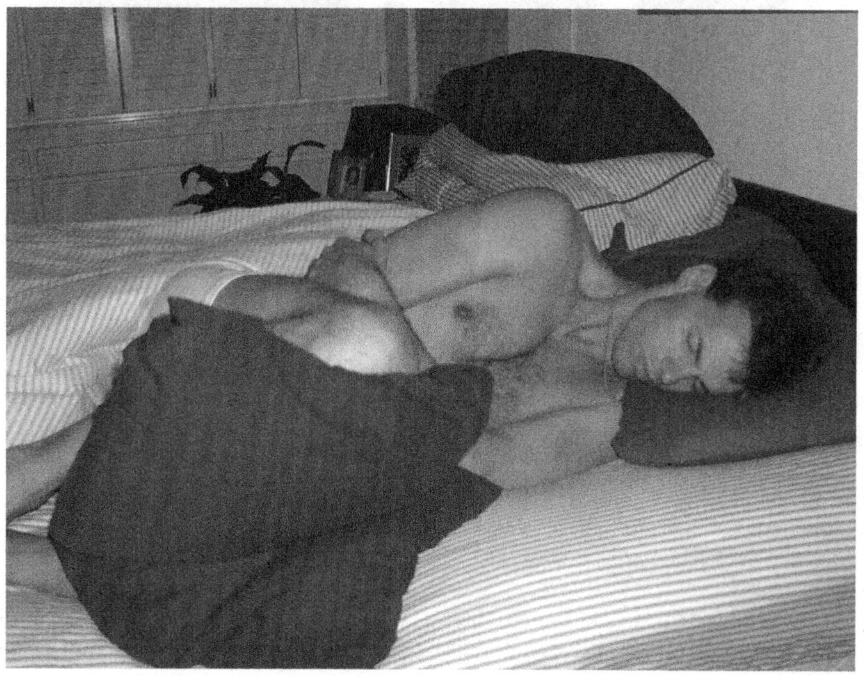

A recent issue of the *New England Journal of Medicine* characterizes the prospects this way: "Treatment of painful sensory neuropathy presents enormous challenges and is currently inadequate.... Patients must understand that complete relief of pain is unlikely to be achieved with our current armamentarium of agents [medications]" (Mendall, et. al., 2003). This is an accurate reflection of my experience thus far. Now, it would appear to be time to hang out and wait for the science to improve.

To give you a more visual clue of the internal reasons for my continued pain, here is an image from a neurography imaging study done three years after my vasectomy showing chronic "Neurogenic Inflammation" from my testicles up to the inguinal ligaments near the hips on both sides. The white areas are the ones that hurt. I share this since it was the visual evidence that finally gave many of the doctors I worked with a better idea of what was going on. You may benefit from doing the same type of neurography study, if needed, although it is a very expensive test.

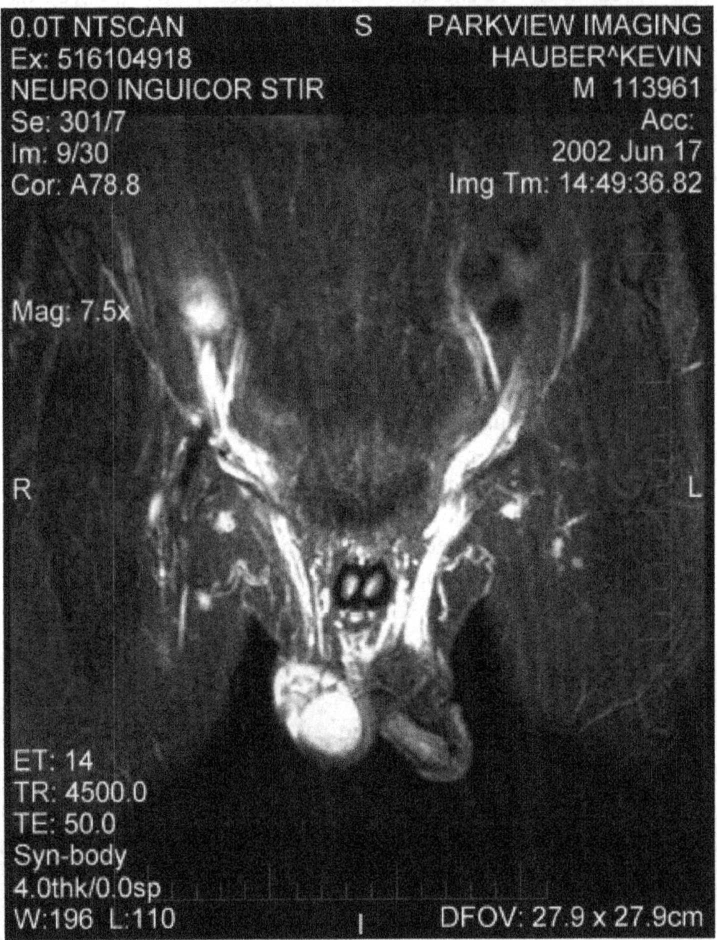

I share this summation not as a "poor me" effort to evoke sympathy, but as a simple statement of the huge impact this type of medical situation can have on one's life. Obviously, if I had known beforehand what I know now, I would have made a different choice. I hope this information has helped you in making informed choices for yourself.

What specific advice can I give to those who are experiencing post-vasectomy pain and other problems based on what I've learned? Let me tell you a story first, as it was told to me by my endocrinologist, who could probably do stand-up comedy if he ever decided to change careers.

A man starts getting splitting headaches every day. He goes to see numerous doctors, including many specialists, but to no avail. His headaches continue viciously, and finally, he is so desperate that he contemplates suicide.

A friend knows of his plight and tells him, "Hey, I have a great doctor I go to. Go see him. I'll bet he can help you."

So the man goes, and after a through examination, the doctor says, "I think I can help you, but it's pretty radical therapy."

"Anything, Doc, just help me to stop these headaches," the man pleads.

"Well," the doctor explains, " it will require cutting off your testicles."

"I'll have to consider that for a while. Let me get back to you," the man states.

Several days later, the man comes back to the doctor and says, "I just can't take it anymore, Doc, go ahead and do the procedure."

Immediately after the operation, the man gets dressed and notices that his headache is completely gone. He hugs the doctor jubilantly and exclaims, "I feel like a new man. I'm going to go out and celebrate. And I think I'll buy myself an entire new wardrobe."

So the man finds a skilled tailor and asks him to measure him for the new suit he wants.

The tailor looks at the man and quickly says, "Looks like your jacket will be a 38 regular, and your pants will be a 36 inch waist with a 31 inch inseam."

"Wow, that's amazing," exclaims the man, "I'm surprised you can tell all of that by just looking at me. The only thing you got wrong was the inseam; I wear a 30 inch inseam."

"Oh no," said the tailor, "if you wore a 30 inch inseam it would put pressure on your testicles and give you terrible headaches."

So, what's the point? Don't be too quick to accept the most radical treatment proposed to you, despite how desperate you may be. There may very well be a much simpler solution that is not so dramatic.

All of that being said, here are "Kevin's Post-Vasectomy Survival Suggestions" (remember, this is just between us guys since I'm not a doctor):

First, hunker down and prepare yourself for what could be a really long haul. It is terrifically difficult to be patient in the face of pain and other post-vasectomy complications. Form whatever support team you need to make it through and don't be afraid to ask for help whether it is from family, friends, counselors, doctors, or whoever suits you best. You will need to surrender a good deal of pride and any modesty in the process. The payoff is that you can be less angry and hurt less as a result.

Second, become conversant with your pain and other conditions that plague you. This means doing some medical research. Beyond that, learn to quiet the swirl of thoughts, reactions, and feelings swimming around in your mind. Notice the characteristics of what you're experiencing. What circumstances or activities aggravate the symptoms? Conversely, what improves them? Is there a daily or periodic pattern? Can you notice a center of the pain, or notice how the pain spreads as it increases? Are there different types of pain that you experience?

For example, I've noticed that the nerve damage pain I experience was with me from the time of my initial vasectomy, and worsens with activity such as anything more than brief periods of standing, walking or sitting. Simply put, this nerve pain gives the sensation of my testicles and spermatic cords being squeezed and torn off. I agree with Dr. Levine (1996, 2001) in his several articles that discuss the Reflex Sympathetic Dystrophy-like characteristics that this type of nerve injury causes. I also agree with McConaghy, et. al., (1996) that this type of chronic pain response in the nervous system causes a sensitization of the nerve roots in the spinal cord, wherein even simple movement like walking aggravates and exaggerates pain.

In addition to the nerve pain, I noted the onset of a cyclical aching in my testicles beginning several days after my vasectomy that would increase and decrease in intensity every few days. My reversal surgery and subsequent hormone therapy have helped to alleviate much of the intensity of this particular pattern of pain. This is the type of late-onset congestive pain that has been noted by many post-vasectomy pain sufferers and gives the sensation that one's testicles are exploding (which, effectively, they are).

These close observations of your own condition will help you in your discussions with medical and other health care providers in choosing an appropriate path of treatment that suits your particular case. The bottom line is listen to what your body is telling you, and become responsive to its messages.

Third, determine that you will find a way to do what is in your own best interest regardless of any nay-saying from your insurance company or pessimistic doctors. In all likelihood, you will hit a lot of resistance in this regard, so expect it and don't let it faze you. Choose doctors to work with who will be truly supportive of you and your health, even if you have to go some distance to see them. Let those providers who don't seem to have your best interest at heart fall by the wayside. Be prepared to pay for good help and advice.

Fourth, pick your drugs and other therapies judiciously. Remember that many of the medications prescribed in these types of circumstances can have substantial side effects and addictive, dependence, or tolerance properties while offering at best only a cover for symptoms, not a cure. You don't want to end up with more problems than you already have. Utilize conservative therapies that help you open and unwind the spiral of pain in you body, and when it comes to trying different medications, remember that, "Therapy is imperfect because understanding [by medical science] is incomplete" (Turek, 1999).

Likewise, pick any invasive or surgical procedures judiciously. My experience tells me that traumatized bodies don't like to be re-traumatized. I was very impatient to end my pain saga in the first year, and incurred a lot of additional stress and pain as a result. But as time went on, I learned how to be kinder to my body. I have already hurt a lot, and have learned to avoid more as best I can.

Do the best you can to take care of the rest of your body. When you hurt all of the time, it is easy to rationalize not exercising or eating poorly. Many guys have told me they gain a lot of weight due to sitting around in pain constantly with low energy. Work with a nutritionist if possible to create the best fuel and balance possible for yourself, including any supplements needed. Doctors have recommended Zinc supplements to me for general genital tract health in men.

Also several studies have found L-Carnitine to be a helpful supplement in improving the natural function of the epididymis which is commonly affected by vasectomy (Lewin, et. al., 1981 and Menchini-Fabris, et. al., 1984). It is interesting to note that the aforementioned studies discussed the positive effects L-Carnitine had on sperm motility, sperm count in men with fertility problems. I tried adding this supplement to my diet on the recommendation of another post-vasectomy pain patient who had good results himself, and I can tell you that the apparent positive effects on my energy level were noticeable.

Finally, find a way to stop the war going on inside yourself to allow for complete healing. There is a physical battlefront as has been discussed at length in this book, and there is also the internal war that this situation brings out at the spiritual and emotional levels. These parts of your being need as much care and compassion as your body does.

That's enough advice for now. Here's the way another guy put it (I agree with him wholeheartedly, by the way): "I've learned a lot along my path to pain-free living. If there is one main thing I would recommend to any man experiencing pain following a vasectomy it is to exhaust all non-surgical therapies before allowing an urologist to perform any further surgeries. The more surgeries a guy receives in the groin area, the more problems can arise. This may require going through numerous physicians/urologists until you find the right one who wants to help without cutting on your privates. This may require being persistent with your HMO to get approval to see the right physician. Having to find the right doctor may be exhausting, but I highly encourage a guy to run from the doctor who quickly mentions surgery.

"I would also recommend a guy who is experiencing PVPS to speak with another guy who understands. For me, I was very depressed when this pain controlled my life. I felt like I had made the worst mistake in my life and would often end up in the fetal position on my bed to 'sleep away' my pain....thanks in part to my large collection of strong pain medication I had been prescribed. I felt no one understood and it was not the easiest subject to talk about with family and friends. I felt very good after talking with other guys who were experiencing the same thing I was" (Mike, from Ohio, in a personal correspondence to the author). This is precisely why this book and the Internet site associated with it are so important.

Some would say that I have been too explicit in writing of this book. Sorry, I tried to warn you. But as you can see, it is a pretty explicit experience with some big implications that someone should tell you about if you're in the market for surgical contraception.

By the way, I tried to focus on the parts of the story that included some bit of humor to make it more palatable. There were a lot of other very unpleasant aspects I left out. And please note, I refrained from writing the chapter entitled "Honey, I Shrunk the Testicles!"

Others would contend that this information is poorly founded or controversial. My experience tells me this information is quite well founded as I have lived with exactly what a lot of the research talks about, and I'm more than a little miffed that it wasn't presented to me in advance. As for controversial, I suppose anything that runs counter to a commonly promoted perception can be termed controversial, but look at the evidence, both anecdotal and factual. Get copies of the research articles and read for yourself. Or read the excerpts in the "Relevant Quotations" chapter from patients who have encountered a similar experience.

If you will notice, I'm not quoting the *National Enquirer* as a source for this book. Most of the research material came directly from doctors and the medical journals they write and use for reference. Hopefully, this information mixed with my personal experience and the experiences of numerous others has made some kind of lasting impression.

I think we can safely dispense with the "one-in-a-million" argument also. Claiming the supposed rarity of the types of complications that have been described in this book is either blindly ignoring the facts or a vain attempt to have men hide in embarrassment and not bring this issue to the fore.

Finally, I suppose there are those who would say that this book is just angry and reactionary. Me, angry? Actually, I was spittin' mad over this for months before I began writing this book, and the book turned into an excellent tool for processing that anger. The anger turned out to be quite a motivator.

In a strange way, I guess I owe a debt of thanks to my original urologist who started the ball rolling, so to speak. But at this point, I would rather fix the problem than fix the blame. That goes for me and everyone else. The first step in this process of fixing the problem is to tell the truth, which, so far, has been a missing piece in some important circles.

As for reactionary, it appears that this book is nowhere near as strong a reaction as what starts happening inside a man's body after a vasectomy. I'm just willing to talk about it in very human terms. This is an amazingly human experience, not just a statistic contained within a study. Ask anyone who's had a similar condition.

My personal prediction is that in 50 years we will look back on the practice of performing vasectomies with the same regard most people now have for the idea of castrating young choirboys so their voices won't change. Future generations will see both procedures as equally vain and with incredulous disdain: "Men used to have what done to themselves, Grandpa?" There will be better birth control methods developed, and vasectomy will be seen for what it is: a quick fix for a complex issue, and a fix that has many problems associated with it.

During the course of the last few years, several people have asked my wife why she didn't just go get her tubes tied instead of me getting a vasectomy. To this she has responded, "After what Kevin has gone through with his 'simple' procedure? Forget it!" I might add that this was before we found out about the high incidence of hysterectomy after tubal ligation in women. One reactionary author in the family is enough.

At this point, I don't know if the answer to the medical problems I've been experiencing will be found in yet another medication, or another surgery, or in a prayer, or simply in the passing of time. That is, if there is a solution at all. For this answer, I have to trust in God's great plan, which I'm sure is grander than any of us can imagine. In the meantime, my practice remains to learn to find a joyful life in the midst of pain. I now know that I am not alone or unguided in that experience. My guidance tells me it is time to speak out about this issue, just like it was time for women to speak out about problems with the pill, the IUD, or breast implants. It can affect your life too much for you to not be told.

As for the rest of the story, with the happy ending, I guess we'll all have to wait for the second edition. In the meantime, I'd like to hear your feedback about the information I've shared here. Sign onto the web site at www.dontfixit.org and post a message to the vasectomy forum, or email me directly at sadsacks@dontfixit.org. Sign up on the mailing list on the web site for periodic updates and late breaking news.

Or, if you see me in person, tell me. It will be easy to pick me out; I'm the one walking slowly and slightly bow-legged, carrying the package of frozen peas. I hope loose pants stay in style for a while. And if the testosterone therapy needs to keep up for very long, you may recognize me as the guy with the nicely developed breasts.

Good health to your, and try to keep you sack intact!

Chapter Thirty-Four

As If That Wasn't Enough

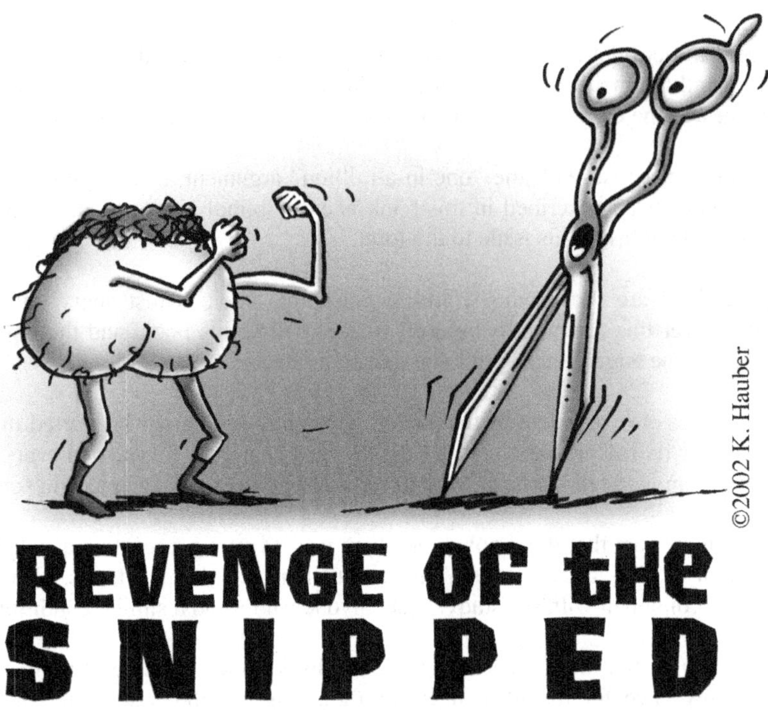

There are two things I found out while living through my vasectomy disaster and talking with others about it. First, almost every guy who has had a vasectomy has a great funny story about it, some of which the guy is willing to tell, some of which only his wife is willing to tell. Second, there is a lot of research on the subject out there that we just plainly don't get told about, lest it would confuse our pea-size little brains and make us not want to do the procedure.

So this section is dedicated to the stories, outtakes if you will - "Adventures of the Vasectomites." Following this section is a summary of relevant quotes regarding disclosure of the possibility of chronic pain and other complications due to vasectomy, should you ever find yourself in need of such references. I will also follow with a list of references on vasectomies and related subjects that you may find of interest if you want to do some more reading on your own.

Here are the stories first, of course, since they are typically more fun:

One guy I know had his vasectomy done many years ago by a doctor who was quite aged at the time. The doctor's hand shook like a wet dog as he approached the man's scrotum, with the scalpel glistening alternately in the operating light like a disco ball. This made the patient quite anxious, as he contemplated how severe of an injury he might receive if he bolted from the table. Just as the scalpel made contact with the skin, the doctor's hand stopped shaking and he cut a nice straight incision. The patient resumed his normal breathing.

A friend of mine was a nurse in a family doctor's office. While she assisted in a vasectomy procedure one day, the doctor was getting ready to make the incision, and she tapped him on the shoulder. He wheeled around angrily.

"What!" he demanded.

"Uh, doctor," she said calmly, "don't you want to give the patient the local anesthetic before cutting?"

"Oh" the doctor replied sheepishly.

207

Another acquaintance of mine told me that his vasectomy procedure was a rough one, too. Why, I inquired? Well, it seems that the doctor at his medical clinic was a he-man ex-military type. Being so predisposed, the doctor didn't see any need to use local anesthetic to numb out any of the pain from the cutting, pulling, and snipping on a patient's genitals during a vasectomy. Just gut it out soldier, you'll get to enjoy yourself later! The man said he'd never been in so much agony in his life.

Speaking of anesthesia, when another friend had his snip, the doctor didn't let the local take effect long enough. The doc started cutting, my friend's reflex actions took over, and he kicked the doctor in the head. I wonder if the doctor now shows up to do vasectomies dressed like an ice hockey goalie.

Another friend had his vasectomy done a number of years ago. The doctor attempted a "new" technique at the time making the incision in the groin instead of the scrotum, snipping the vas and tying it off there. Only problem was, as the doctor was working on the first side and prepared to seal off the upper end of the vas, zip, oops, the vas slipped back into my friend's body and disappeared. The doctor fished around extensively trying to find the errant vas, only to finally give up and seal off the remaining end as best he could.

The doc then decided that maybe this new technique wasn't all it was cracked up to be, and proceeded to do the other side by the "old" method, making the incision through the scrotum. Time was wearing on and the anesthetic was wearing off. My friend was really sweating by this point. Understandably, he was quite sore for some time afterwards, both high and low.

Then there's the story of the guy who had his vasectomy done and then continued to father children afterward. Not all that unusual, you say, given what you've read in this book? Turns out that when he went back to the doctor, it was determined that he had three testicles and the doctor had only disconnected two of them. Why the doctor, and more importantly the man, never noticed triplets instead of twins to begin with remains a mystery.

I heard another vasectomy war story from a fellow post-vasectomy pain sufferer. A friend of his had a vasectomy done and then went home. He was hurting quite a bit, so he called his buddy and asked what to do.

"Put some ice on it and keep the swelling down," his friend advised.

That was fine except that the guy put the ice directly on his scrotum and then drifted off to sleep. You can imagine what happened next. The ice stuck to his scrotum and wouldn't come off. In his panic he called the paramedics, who wound up blasting him with a blow dryer to dislodge the frozen mass from the man's scrotum. How would you like to be the fireman who had to write up that report?

See what great stuff you hear when you're willing to share? Got any good stories of your own?

Here's a good one that's been around for a while: A man goes into the hospital for a vasectomy.

Shortly after awakening from his anesthetic, the surgeon comes in and tells him: "Well, I have good news and bad news for you."

"Give me the bad news first," says the patient.

"I'm afraid that we accidentally cut your balls off during the surgery, son" said the doctor.

"Oh my God!" cried the patient, breaking into tears.

"But the good news," the doctor adds, "is that we had a biopsy done on your testicles and we are relieved to know that they weren't malignant."

Not had enough yet? Here's another: After having their 11th child, a backwoods couple decided that was enough (they could not afford a larger double-wide). So, the husband went to his doctor (who also treated mules) and told him that he and his wife/cousin didn't want to have any more children. The doctor told him that there was a procedure called a vasectomy that could fix the problem. The doctor instructed him to go home, get a cherry bomb (fireworks are legal in the backwoods), light it, put it in a beer can, then hold the can up to his ear and count to 10.

The man said to the doctor, "I may not be the smartest man, but I don't see how putting a cherry bomb in a beer can next to my ear is going to help me."

So, the couple drove to the next county to get a second opinion. The next physician was just about to tell them about the procedure for a vasectomy when he noticed that they were from the backwoods of the neighboring county. This doctor instead told the man to go home and get a cherry bomb, light it, place it in a beer can, hold it to his ear and count to 10. Figuring that both learned physicians couldn't be wrong, the man went home, lit a cherry bomb and put it in a beer can.

He held the can up to his ear and began to count. "1, 2, 3, 4, 5 . . . . ," at which point he paused, placed the beer can between his legs and resumed counting on his other hand.

Here's one man's story, as it was relayed to me that is a least somewhat related to the sensations we've been talking about: "Calling in sick to work makes me uncomfortable. No matter how legitimate my illness, I always sense my boss thinks I am lying. On one occasion, I had a valid reason, but lied anyway because the truth was too humiliating. I simply mentioned that I had sustained a head injury and I hoped I would feel up to coming in the next day. By then, I could think up a doozy to explain the bandage on my crown.

"The accident occurred mainly because I conceded to my wife's wishes to adopt a cute little kitty. Initially the new acquisition was no problem, but one morning I was taking my shower after breakfast when I heard my wife, Deb, call out to me from the kitchen. 'Ed! The garbage disposal is dead. Come reset it.'

"'You know where the button is.' I protested through the shower pitter-patter. 'Reset it yourself!'

"'I'm scared!' She pleaded. 'What if it starts going and sucks me in? (Pause) C'mon, it'll only take a second.'

"So out I came, dripping wet and buck naked, hoping to make a statement about how her cowardly behavior was not without consequence. I crouched down and stuck my head under the sink to find the button. This is the last action I remember performing.

"It struck without warning, without respect to my circumstances. Nay, it wasn't a hexed disposal drawing me into its gnashing metal teeth. It was our new kitty, clawing playfully at the dangling objects she spied between my legs. She had been poised around the corner and stalked me as I took the bait under the sink. At precisely the second I was most vulnerable, she leapt at the toys I unwittingly offered and snagged them with her needle-like claws.

"I lost all rational thought to control orderly bodily movements, while rising upwardly at a violent rate of speed, with the full weight of a kitten hanging from my masculine region. Wild animals are sometimes faced with a 'fight or flight' syndrome. Men, in this predicament, choose only the 'flight' option. Fleeing straight up, the sink and cabinet bluntly impeded my ascent; the impact knocked me out cold.

"When I awoke, my wife and the paramedics stood over me. Having been fully briefed by my wife, the paramedics snorted as they tried to conduct their work while suppressing hysterical laughter. At the office, colleagues tried to coax an explanation out of me. I kept silent, claiming it was too painful to talk about.

"'What's the matter, cat got your tongue?' they asked. If they had only known."

(Author anonymous for good reasons.)

I guess we should all consider ourselves lucky, though. I heard once that, in prior centuries, Chinese eunuchs used to pickle their penises after being cut off and carry them around in a jar as their resume for prospective employers. Talk about your restrictive job market.

The Chinese must have a penchant for extreme measures when it comes to their genitalia. A Taoist philosopher named Chan Tze-tan has become renown for his power lifting ability of up to 350 pounds. This in itself is not that big of a deal, except that he does so with the weights tied to his scrotal sac. I knew that meditative practice was helpful in getting through pain, but isn't he putting himself in harm's way more than he needs to? Upon witnessing this thick-skinned feat one commentator noted "The audience applauded after a long silence."

I know those last few stories weren't about vasectomies, but I couldn't resist including them. Here's another story that I can't resist telling. A man who looked to be in his sixties or seventies at the time I met him had grown up in Germany. When a much younger man, he had referred to an old German medical textbook to find information on a particular condition. While scanning for the information he was looking for he noted that the textbook claimed that masturbation was highly detrimental to health and, in fact, caused insanity. It was also noted, however, that for medical students who had no time for female companionship, masturbation was an acceptable temporary practice.

Aside from the obvious double standard and the assumption that all medical students would be male, I am led to this question: Knowing what you now do about vasectomies, who's crazier, the doctors who perform them, or those of us who allow them to be performed? It's your call.

Chapter Thirty-Five

Getting a Firm Grasp on the Obvious:

Relevant Quotations Regarding Post-Vasectomy Pain and Other Side Effects of Vasectomy

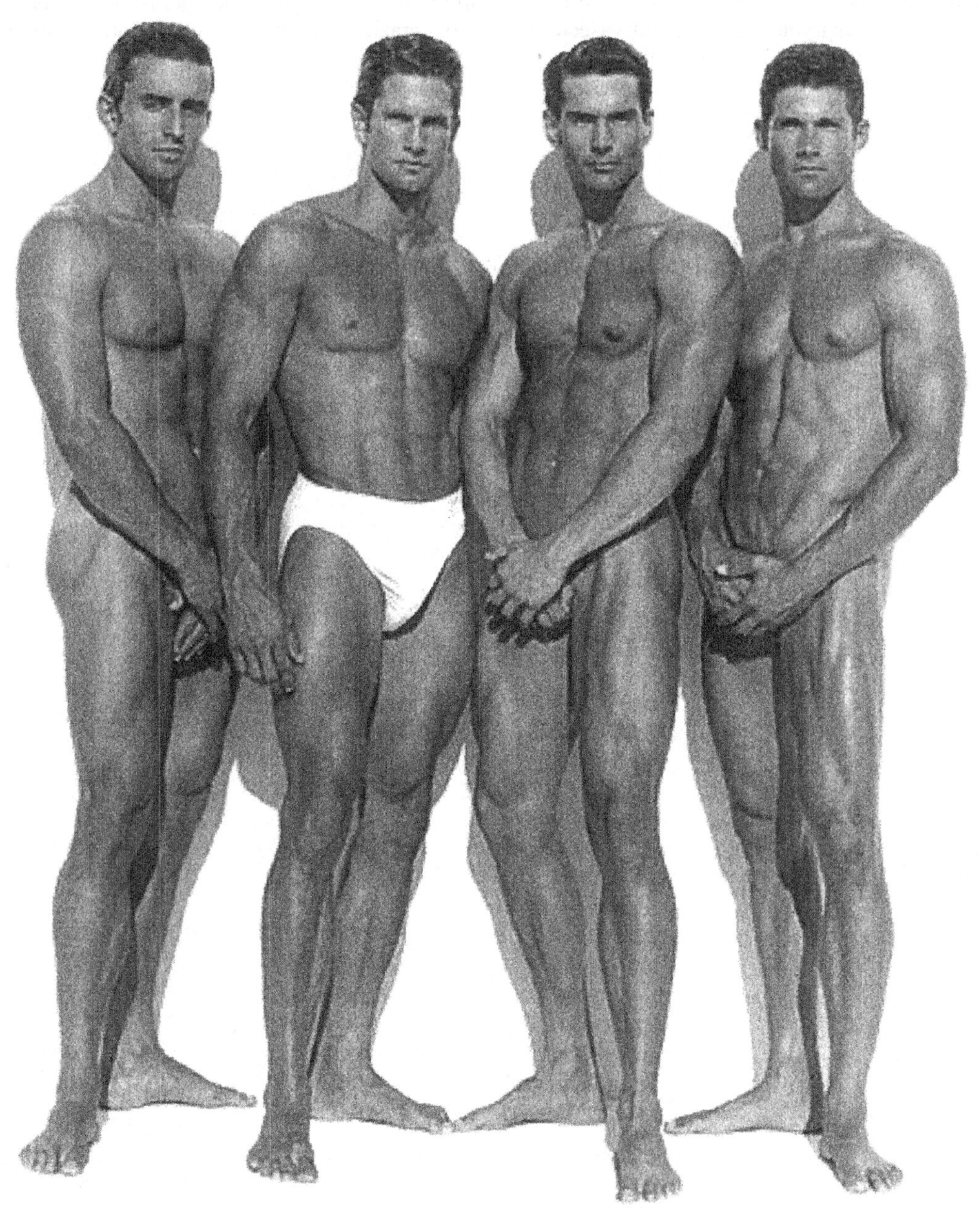

This picture is to remind you that three men out of four will develop an immune system reaction to vasectomy that can leave them "holding the bag" with problems for years to come. These guys don't look very happy about that, do they?

Do you think there are only a few of us who are left holding the bag like this? In case you might doubt that this vasectomy stuff we've been discussing is a loaded gun with a hair trigger, just keep reading a little longer. In this chapter you will find statements from doctors and researchers on the subject. What's more, you'll find the statements and stories of some of those who have paid the price: the patients themselves.

1. "Pathological findings revealed features of long-standing obstruction and insterstitial and perineural fibrosis [scarring and nerve entrapment] which may have accounted for the pain. It is important to recognize this late complication of vasectomy" (Chen, et. al., *British Journal of Urology*, 1991).

2. "Family physicians should be aware of the potential effects and complications of vasectomy so they can appropriately counsel patients seeking sterilization. Vasectomy produces anatomic hormonal and immunologic changes and…has been reputed to be associated with atherosclerosis [hardening of the arteries], prostate cancer, testicular cancer, and urolithiasis [kidney stones]. Complications of vasectomy include overt failure, occasional sperm in the ejaculate, hematoma [bruising], bleeding, infection, sperm granuloma, congestive epididymitis [a synonym for post-vasectomy pain syndrome], antisperm antibody formation, and psychogenic impotence" (Raspa, R. F., *American Family Physician*, Nov. 15, 1993).

3. "We have carried out a survey by postal questionnaire and telephone interview of 172 patients four years after vasectomy…Chronic testicular discomfort was present in 56 patients (33%)…. Prior to vasectomy, all patients should be counseled with regard to the risk of chronic testicular pain" (Mc Mahon, et. al., British Journal of *Urology*, February, 1992).

4. "Future studies should include evaluations of the long-term effectiveness of vasectomy, evaluating criteria for post-vasectomy discontinuation of alternative contraception for use in settings where semen analysis is not practical, and characterizing complications including chronic epididymal pain syndrome"(Schwingl P. J., et. al., *Fertility and Sterility*, May, 2000).

5. "There is a small but significant incidence of CPTP [chronic post-vasectomy testicular pain] and patients should be warned of this possibility when counseled before operation" (Ahmed I., et. al., *British Journal of Urology*, February, 1997).

6. "In our study chronic scrotal pain was the most frequently reported complication of vasectomy with an incidence of 18.7%. Pain adversely affected quality of life in 2.2% of our study population. A review of the literature would suggest that techniques in which the epididymal vas is not ligated can reduce the incidence of post-vasectomy scrotal pain. Regardless of the technique used, the high litigation potential of this procedure warrants thorough counseling of the factors that may affect quality of life" (Choe, J. M., et. al., *Journal of Urology*, April, 1996).

7. "Problems mentioned concerned sexual performance, long lasting pain, and wanting children in new relationships" (Ehn, B. E., et. al., *Scandinavian Journal of Urology and Nephrology*, December, 1995).

8. "Because of the frequency of chronic pain syndromes following vasectomy, concern regarding the long-term complications of this procedure has revived…. The disorders that are now being linked with autoimmune reaction after vasectomy include unexplained thrombophlebitis, prolonged fever, generalized lymph node enlargement, recurrent infection, skin eruption, multiple sclerosis, liver dysfunction, and rheumatoid arthritis. In addition to these health problems, several studies have revealed a statistically significant association between the risk of prostate cancer and a history of vasectomy. The risk of prostate cancer in men who have had a vasectomy is more than three times that of those who were not vasectomized" (Dr. Anthony H. Horan, [Online]).

9. "Congestive epididymitis [a synonym for post-vasectomy pain syndrome] was diagnosed in 6% of [6220] cases utilizing closed-end vasectomy and 2% of cases where the open-end vasectomy was performed. Open-end vasectomy is recommended because the incidence of congestive epididymitis is reduced" (Moss, W. M., et. al., *Contraception*, December, 1992).

10. "Chronic epididymal pain following vasectomy is a well recognized clinical entity…. The post-vasectomy pain syndrome is a well recognized complication of vasectomy…. Reports of pain involving the testis and epididymis after vasectomy range from 3 to 8%…. Most urologists will encounter a significant number of patients with the post-vasectomy pain syndrome during their career…. The post-vasectomy pain syndrome is a rare but serious complication of vasectomy" (Stanley A. Myers, et. al., *Journal of Urology*, February, 1997).

11. "Although vasectomy reversal is often successful, it cannot be guaranteed even in the best of circumstances, and when the vasectomy has caused epididymal obstruction, reversal is often unsuccessful" (Peterson, H. B., et. al., *Obstetrics and Gynecology*, September, 1990).

12. "Spermatic granulomas are specialized abscesses which frequently occur at the site of vasectomy. Although some are often silent, others can be agonizingly painful. A series of 154 granulomas is presented. Of these, 83 were symptomatic and 63 required surgery for relief of pain" (Schmidt, S. S., *Fertility and Sterility*, February, 1979).

13. "A group...with a previously unappreciated syndrome of unremitting epididymal pain and induration five to seven years after vasectomy was collected.... Recognition of this late post-vasectomy syndrome, which represents a major complication of vasectomy, might be expected to increase as cohorts of vasectomized individuals age.... Patient discomfort usually was constant, often disabling, exacerbated by sexual activity and, occasionally, radiating along the spermatic cord structures.... because the vasectomy procedure is so prone to medico-legal complications, we believe that the late post-vasectomy syndrome should be included in the informed consent form for vasectomy" (Stuart M. Selikowitz, et. al., *Journal of Urology*, September, 1985).

14. "Several studies report on the incidence of post-vasectomy scrotal pain and different names for these pain complaints were mentioned.... Dependent on the way of documentation and patient population, recurrence rates vary from 0.9% in a cohort of 10,590 men studied by Massey, et. al., (1984) within one year after vasectomy up to 54% in a group of patients with post-vasectomy scrotal granuloma.... Since the major reason for dissatisfaction after vasectomy was reported to be chronic pain, pre-vasectomy counseling of the patient on this problem should take place" (Van Der Poel, H. G., et. al., [Online], June 17, 1999).

15. "In more than 50% of men, vasectomy leads to auto-immune pathology. The auto-immune response to sperms following vasectomy is triggered by the phagocytosis of sperm in the epididymis. In the humoral immune response, sperm agglutinating, sperm immobilizing, and antibodies to sperm nuclear protamines occur, as early as 3-4 days after vasectomy. The incidence reaches 60-70% within 1 year and remains almost the same even after 20 years" (Shahani, S. K., et. al., *Archives of Andrology*, September, 1981).

16. "Any technique of vasectomy carries a very small risk of orchialgia [chronic testicular pain], whether due to the presence of a sperm granuloma at the vasectomy site or to increased epididymal pressure" (Shapiro, E. I., & Silber S. J., *Fertility and Sterility*, November 1979).

17. "Post vasectomy pain syndrome... can turn a previously fit man into a chronic invalid. Even if the operation was painless, and not accompanied by the bruising and immediate post-operative discomfort which is quite common, weeks, months or years after the operation, nagging pain begins at the site. Sometimes tender cysts, or lumps called granulomas, can arise around the cut ends of the vas, and even if further surgery is performed to cut them out, the pain persists. This can be one of the most difficult problems in andrology to treat, especially as the precise cause is usually unknown. More research is urgently needed to prevent and treat the condition" (Dr. Malcolm Carruthers, [Online]).

18. "The vasectomy is not free. It can cause frightening and frustrating long-term effects which are about as permanent as the sterility that it was intended to produce. The numbers of dissatisfied vasectomized men are increasing, primarily with the affliction of post-vasectomy pain, (about 20%, but that number is adjusted upward every year). Once one finds out that there are others like him, he is more likely to drop stoic pretenses and admit that his balls hurt.... A vasectomy is almost always referred to in terms of 'harmless,' no 'secondary long-term effects.' It's a good sell, but it is not the whole truth. Little or nothing is said about life after except for the benefits of sterility.... In more true to life terms, a vasectomy is having your vas deferens cut in two, the ends are cauterized or sutured, interrupting the flow of sperm from the testis, sterility is achieved. Unfortunately the testis aren't informed and continue to function normally, producing sperm cells.... With the holes on the tubes bunged up and the testis of a normal healthy man still dedicated to the production of sperm, something has to give... and it does. The sperm backs up and eventually forms a toothpaste-like sludge. As the sperm backs up so does the pressure and blowouts begin to occur along the epididymis. Because the body is not ordinarily exposed to sperm (with leakage after the blowouts) antibodies to the sperm are produced and the problems begin. The sperm cells are actually quite irritating and resistant, they have to be to withstand the hostile environment of someone else's body in a reproductive role. They were never meant to be out in the blood stream.... Reports of secondary long-term effects are rising to the surface. I have collected a few assorted references to this 'politically incorrect' malady. They are fairly hard to find.... Surgery has always meant the 'remedy' for a pathological condition. The

truth is that a vasectomy is an attempt to use surgery to correct a social problem. Further, plugging up a healthy organ system and expecting 'no side effects' is just plain idiocy. Medically speaking, symptoms from an injury provoked on a healthy organ system could take years to manifest, and that manifestation could be almost anything.... On the same tangent... Why would public health or other medical 'authorities' not raise questions about the procedure? We can't expect a cohesive group of professionals to be self-incriminating. Repercussions from iatrogenic illness (produced by the physician's activity) are always very damming and damaging. Medical authorities (public and private institutions responsible for public health) always provide a very quick response to negative news... and the answer is always the same...' it's safe, don't worry'.... Many vasectomized men find it hard to admit that they have problems. Most mention the 'it's all in your head' response they get from the same M. D.'s that did the procedure. There's a lot of frustration and anger and there is no place to take it to.... Being responsible (in a reproductive sense) does not mean you have to sacrifice your health. Remember that the vasectomy is not the treatment of a pathological condition, it is the cutting into a healthy organ system with the deliberate intention of plugging it up.... The vasectomy creates some real problems, post-vasectomy pain is too common and should be a sign to halt present policies. But we will see no restraint or real informed consent until the medical establishment is held accountable by legal action" (Hall, Michael, [Online]).

19. "Urolithiasis [kidney stones] causes substantial morbidity among otherwise healthy, middle-aged men who account for two-thirds to three-quarters of cases. This is precisely the population that is most likely to undergo vasectomy. Nonetheless, we were surprised to find a previously unreported, statistical relationship between vasectomy and urolithiasis in an epidemiological study.... Even though the association between vasectomy and urolithiasis is unexplained, it is important. Confirmation of the finding that vasectomy substantially enhanced the risk for urolithiasis suggests that patients be informed about this risk before vasectomy.... The increased risk for urolithiasis associated with vasectomy may indicate a need to reevaluate the risk-benefit ratio of vasectomy compared with other methods for contraception" (Kronmal, et. al., *American Journal of Kidney Diseases*, February, 1997).

20. "Chronic intrascrotal pain may occur in up to a third of patients after vasectomy and in approximately half the pain is considered troublesome" (Padmore, et. al., *The Journal of Urology*, July 1996).

21. "Vasectomy is a common operation and even if short-term complications only occur in a small proportion of people, or it has just a slight influence on the long-term chances of developing a serious illness such as prostate cancer, this makes it important that we learn much more about it, and that people who have it done, or are considering it, are better informed.... There is, however, one consideration which might give American doctors in particular cause for thought before they continue to recommend and perform vasectomies. If convincing evidence were produced that serious damage might result from either the antibody formation or hormonal changes which many studies have already shown to occur after the operation, it would open the floodgates for a torrent of highly emotive litigation cases. Even now, drug companies are having to defend some very large-scale group actions for everything from breast implants to drugs such as Thalidomide and Norplant" (Dr. Malcolm Carruthers, 1997).

22. "When a patient elects to have a vasectomy, he must understand that pressure build-up proximal to the vasectomy site, congestion of the epididymis, and, indeed, epididymal blowouts are inevitable consequences of this surgical procedure. In more than 800 vasovasostomy patients whom we have seen, there is always some degree of epididymal engorgement and congestion. Indeed, after one explores these post-vasectomy patients micro-surgically, it becomes difficult to understand why the vast majority of such patients have no pain or discomfort" (Shapiro, E. I., and Silber, S. J., *Fertility and Sterility*, November, 1979).

23. "The greatest anatomic effects of vasectomy occur in the rete testis, epididymis and vas deferens. The rete testis and epididymis frequently sustain damage induced by back-up pressure. Blow-outs and secondary sperm extravasation commonly occur at the body and tail of the epididymis. Vasectomy usually causes loss of tone and luminal dilation of the testicular end of the cut vas deferens.... Antisperm antibodies can be measured in the serum of up to 70 percent of men after vasectomy" (Raspa, Robert F., *Journal of the American Family Physician*, 1993).

24. "Men with antisperm antibodies may be at risk for the development of immunologically mediated diseases. Furthermore, immune complex orchitis, glomerulonephritis, and exacerbated atherosclerosis have been demonstrated in vasectomized animals.... It was reasoned that such antibodies, or possibly immune complexes containing such antibodies and sperm antigens, might cause disease, either locally in the testis or epididymis, or in

the organs remote from the operative site…. As expected there was a notable excess of epididymitis-orchitis in the vasectomized men" (Massey, et. al., *JAMA*, August, 1984).

25. "Chronic testicular pain can be a more troublesome long-term complication [of vasectomy]…. If the patient is not seen after the procedure he is assumed to have had no problems: this potentially underestimates complications…. Orchialgia [testicular pain] is thus the most common complication after vasectomy. Because it is potentially chronic, this risk must be mentioned…. Very few patients require further surgery for orchialgia and the outcomes after intervention are not uniformly successful…. The issue of prostate malignancy is yet to be resolved, with conflicting evidence and methodological deficiencies in some studies…. Preoperative counseling, consent, postoperative support and follow-up are key issues in avoiding medicolegal problems with vasectomy…. The man should understand the complications of haematoma, infection, and orchialgia" (Preston, J. M., *BJU International*, 2000).

26. "Vasectomy may have some long-term sequelae, for the majority of vasectomized men develop antisperm antibodies that persist for many years…. Genitourinary disease… is much more common in the post-vasectomy period than at any time in the population at large. Men who have recently undergone vasectomy are more likely to come to medical attention for various chronic genitourinary disorders, such as benign prostatic hypertrophy or phimosis…. Hospitalizations for arthritis, rheumatism, and connective tissue disorders became more common in vasectomized men with the passage of time" (Walker, et. al., *JAMA*, June 12, 1981).

27. "Three main reasons have been offered for the well-known discrepancy between continuity of the vas and low fertility rates after vasovasostomy: (1) microsurgical techniques are essential; (2) the appearance of autoantibodies after vasectomy causes the low fertility rate; and (3) during vasectomy the innervation of the epididymal portion of the vas is destroyed, leading to reduced sperm transport during ejaculation…. Large numbers of nerves are resected by routine vasectomy in man. That would be compatible with the idea that the nerves of the vas deferens play an essential role in the outcome of vasovasostomy" (Esk, et. al., *Fertility and Sterility*, March, 1981).

28. "Chronic testicular pain may have numerous etiologies, the majority of which are secondary to nerve trauma to the spermatic cord. Chronic scrotal pain after vasectomy has been reported in 1% to 33% of patients, with occasional discomfort noted in as many as 70%. There is an increased incidence of pain in patients with a spermatic granuloma (54% or less) with the likely cause being disruption of the autonomic fibers surrounding the vasa deferentia" (Levine, et. al., *Journal of Urology*, June 2001).

29. "Hematoma is the most common [early] complication of vasectomy with an average incidence of two per cent but a range of 0.09 to 29 per cent. Infection is surprisingly common with an average rate of 3.4 per cent, but several series report rates from one to 38 per cent…. Long-term effects of vasectomy include vasitis nodosa, chronic testicular pain, testicular function alterations, and epididymal obstruction, and the postulated effect of vasectomy on the cardiovascular system…. Vasitis nodosa has been reported in up to 66 per cent of vasectomy specimens in men undergoing vasectomy reversals…. The brunt of pressure-induced damage after vasectomy falls on the epididymis and efferent ductules. These structures become markedly distended and then adapt to reabsorb large volumes of testicular fluid and sperm products. It is likely that, in time, all vasectomized men will develop 'blowouts' in either the epididymis or efferent ducts. Sperm granulomas may form at the site of rupture, and secondary epididymal or efferent duct obstruction may result…. Vasectomy results in violation of the blood-testis barrier producing detectable levels of serum antisperm antibodies in 60 to 80 per cent of men" (<u>Campbell's Urology</u>, sixth edition, 1992).

30. "Thirty-two per cent of men undergoing ligature vasectomy develop granulomas, and as many as 10% have symptoms" [i.e. pain]…. Vasocutaneous fistulas appeared [after vasectomy] as either recurrent, painful 'pimples' that would spontaneously break and drain, closing and appearing later in an adjacent area of skin, or as a constantly moist spot in the scrotal scar" (Schmidt, S. S., *Fertility and Sterility*, 1979).

31. "The post-vasectomy [pain] syndrome or chronic testicular pain following the procedure is a recognized complication of this procedure in addition to some acute pain" (Paxton, et. al., *British Journal of Anesthesiology*, 1995).

32. "Short-term complications [after vasectomy] are well-established. The most frequent ones are not serious (scrotal swelling, ecchymosis, and local pain). One or more of these may occur after up to 50% of vasectomies" (Kaufman, et. al., 1996).

33. "Vasectomy performed with the traditional technique changes testicular structure. At first, the injuries are slight and restricted, but gradually, and in a time-dependent manner, become more severe and extensive…. We propose that the increase of intraluminal pressure [after vasectomy] is the essential factor that provokes testicular atrophy" (Whyte, et. al., *International Surgery*, 2000).

34. "The major source of anxiety for men before vasectomy was fear of pain. There was also a significant percentage of men who were anxious about the potential side effects. Almost half were unaware of the reversibility of vasectomy. This study demonstrates the need for adequate pre-vasectomy counseling, particularly in the area of postoperative expectations as well as reversibility" (Sandlow, et. al., 2001).

35. "Following vasectomy, spermatogenesis continues, the human epididymis and ductus [vas] deferens may distend and leak, and extravasated spermatozoa stimulate formation of a sperm granuloma. Granulomas may occur at 60% of vasectomy sites…. About 3-5% of patients experience pain [in this location].… Distension of the epididymis is common after vasectomy and may lead to granuloma formation there. Up to 6% of patients have [painful] symptoms…. " (McDonald, *Clinical Anatomy*, 1996).

36. "Chronic testicular pain (CTP) is defined as uni- or bilateral, intermittent or continuous testicular discomfort of at least three months duration that interferes with the patient's daily activities and prompts him to seek medical advice is a rather common urological manifestation of chronic pain syndrome. Diagnosis and treatment of CTP has been a difficult and often unrewarding clinical situation. Success rates of conservative and surgical measures including epididymectomy and orchiectomy rarely exceed 55-73% and 10-40%, respectively…. CTP as many other chronic pain syndromes may have significant social impact since it results in significant health care costs and loss of work time and productivity. Driven by their chronic pain most patients consult many urologists and physicians, undergo multiple diagnostic and interventional procedures in an attempt to ascertain the definite etiology [cause] of pain and to cure symptoms.… In many cases, radical surgical procedures such as inguinal or scrotal orchiectomy and epididymectomy have been favored to manage CTP with failure rates as high as 57%" (Heidenreich, et. al., 2002).

37. "There is a well-recognized condition that can occur after a vasectomy among a small number of men, known as a post-vasectomy pain syndrome. This syndrome can begin immediately after the vasectomy or many months or even years after the vasectomy has been completed. The frequency of post vasectomy syndrome varies amongst given practitioners. Some studies report as high as one-third of men after vasectomy have some type of lingering discomfort. Other studies report that the frequency of post vasectomy pain is one case in thousands.

   a. "Causes: A non-meticulous "rough" surgery where significant amounts of tissue and nerves have been disrupted and/ or tied that have caused lingering irritation of the nerves. While this may be one of the more frequent causes of post vasectomy pain syndrome of post vasectomy pain syndrome one can imagine that it would be less common in the patients of experienced vasectomists.

   b. "A sperm granuloma could develop post vasectomy that becomes inflamed and aggravates the surrounding nerve endings. The sperm granuloma is a build up of extravasated sperm at the end of the cut vas tube end. The reason why a sperm granuloma may develop is not well understood.

   c. "A congestive state in the epididymis from back pressure to the epididymis and testes from performing a closed-ended vasectomy. Some authors believe that by blocking both the upper and lower cut ends of the vas tube the normal passage of sperm from the penis and away from the epididymis and testes causes a build up of pressure and ensuing pain. Studies have shown that this situation can be prevented to a large degree by performing an open-ended vasectomy. This is one in which the lower end or testicular end of the cut vas is left open thereby allowing the sperm to drain out of the tube preventing a build up of pressure.

   d. "A vasectomy carried out too close to the epididymis can cause chronic pain and inflammation at the epididymis.

   e. "Some speculate that post vasectomy pain could be mediated by an immune reaction. It is known that antibodies to sperm are produce by the body after vasectomy. It is possible that these antibodies can react with testicular epididymal and or scrotal tissue to cause an inflammatory reaction.

f.	"Certainly shorter term causes of post vasectomy pain include infection and post operative inflammation which should resolve easily with the appropriate medications and not linger long enough to fall into the category of becoming a syndrome.

"Treatments:

1.	"In regards to a rough surgery, this would likely be the most difficult to treat and to identify as a cause of pain. Possible treatments could include exploration of the area to remove scarred or inflamed tissue, manual manipulation or stimulation of the painful area, or just allowing time to heal.

2.	"In the case of a sperm granuloma, injecting it with steroids or actually cutting out the inflamed granuloma has been found effective in the past. Surgery should always be viewed as a last resort in this case.

3.	"In regards to pain resulting from a congestive state from a closed ended vasectomy, converting that vasectomy to an open ended vasectomy or considering a vasectomy reversal have been identified as being effective in the past.

4.	"Surgery carried out too close to the epididymis causing chronic epididymitis may respond to medications or require an epididymectomy.

5.	"Some advocate the use of a steroidal anti-inflammatory like Prednizone for 1-2 weeks. This treatment may be particularly helpful in treating an antibody/immune mediated cause of the pain.

6.	"Regarding treatment of shorter post-vasectomy pain like post operative inflammation or infection, the use of anti-inflammatories for inflammation and appropriate antibiotics for infection have been shown to be effective in dealing with this type of pain.

7.	"Getting a second or third opinion from different practitioners with an expertise in treating post vasectomy pain is always advisable.

8.	"Time, sometimes 1-2 years, without doing anything at all, may heal the problem.

"Some investigations that may help sort out the cause of post vasectomy pain include:

a) "a careful physical examination of the scrotal contents by a qualified physician.

b) "scrotal ultrasound

c) "semen culture and sensitivity and gram stain

d) "anti-sperm antibodies

e) "scrotal exploration

f) "probing of the testicular end of the vas."

(Vasectomymedical.com, No-scalpel vasectomy; post-vasectomy pain. [online] http://www.vasectomymedical.com/no-scalpel-vasectomy-pain.html, updated 8/15/02.

38.	"Chronic testicular discomfort remains one of the commonest post-vasectomy complications....Pain following this procedure may in part be caused by sensitization developing at the dorsal horn neurons receiving neural input from the site of surgical trauma during the intra-operative period" (McConaghy, et. al., 1998).

39.	"Vasectomy is perceived by all men, on some level, in some way, as a castration. We believe this attitude is supported by our data on reactions of friends and relatives told about the operation, reasons given by the

217

respondents for not telling, worries before the operation, and heightened defensiveness shown by the respondents when being questioned about the meaning of the operation.... We consider mastering the psychodynamic factors of 'I will be sterile, castrated, no good,' as one of the tasks a man must go through during the adjustment to vasectomy" (Ferber, et. al., 1967).

40. "Vasectomy...is associated with a high incidence of chronic pain symptoms.... Chronic post-vasectomy pain... in our experience can be a disabling condition refractory [unresponsive] to treatment" (Baylis, et. al., 1998).

41. "Medical mistakes kill between 44,000 and 98,000 hospitalized Americans each year. And according to the federal Agency for Healthcare Research and Quality, these numbers are probably on the low side" (*American Medical News*, 42: 48).

42. *"Vasectomized patients have 'congestive' epididymitis.... Sperm granuloma is an inevitable consequence of vasectomy... it would be inappropriate for us to suppose that one can perform vasectomies without the risk of some scrotal discomfort... a certain tiny percentage of vasectomized men are going to experience some pain no matter what technique is used..."* [emphasis added] (Silber, 1980).

From the patients:

1. "I had my vasectomy 10 years ago now and I haven't had a happy, pain-free day since. It's been a nightmare from the beginning to the end and it's not over yet.... After seven years on the pill, my wife was advised to stop taking it and so I decided I'd have a vasectomy. On the day of the operation at our local hospital I had no second thoughts at all because I had heard that the procedure was quite straightforward. I was surprised therefore to wake from the general anesthetic with a tremendous pain in my stomach.... for the next few weeks I was only comfortable when I was lying down. Walking or lifting things was impossible and there was no question of being able to work. I was getting increasingly anxious as I had never really been ill before, but since both the hospital and my doctor were adamant there was nothing to worry about, I was prepared to give it time.... Then two months after the operation I found two small painful lumps in each testicle...and they, together with the continuing ache in my stomach region, were causing me such discomfort that it was interfering with my whole life.... The new consultant [doctor] performed an operation to remove the lumps. Afterwards he told me he believed too much of the vas had been cut away during the vasectomy, which explained the painful pulling sensation in my stomach, and I felt very angry. The lumps kept recurring and this was complicated by bouts of urinary infection that caused a painful inflammation in both testicles. To help this, the surgeon finally had to remove the inflamed outer casing of the left testicle, the epididymis. Even this went wrong.... Five months later, the testis on that side began to shrink, and I had to have it removed and a plastic prosthesis put in.... Last year I had to have the same series of operations on my right testicle, with removal of granuloma, and then the epididymis, and now the testicle gets inflamed and is shrinking, so I may have to have even that removed.... It's been such a terrible time since the first operation. My job as a fork-lift truck driver, which I'd had for 18 years before the vasectomy, is gone, and my wife left me because it all got too much and we weren't having any fun or any sex. There have been times over the last few years when the pain and worry have made me think of ending it all, but things are slightly better now.... All this has been a result of a vasectomy gone wrong, probably because it was performed in a hurry by someone inexperienced, though I'm told it sometimes happens in the best of hands. This surgery sentenced me to 10 years' pain and misery" ("Harry" as quoted from "<u>Maximizing Manhood: Beating the Male Menopause</u>" by Dr. Malcolm Carruthers, 1997).

2. I received the following letter from a college friend of mine. At the time of his writing this, it had been two-and-a-half years since his vasectomy and he was still in pain consistently. He had experienced a real peak pain sensation during his procedure, and then "...the day after my vasectomy I was following my doctor's instructions which were not to do anything different. The process was "so simple" that it wouldn't have ANY impact on my life, even the day after surgery. So the next day I was out working in the garden when all of a sudden I almost passed out from what felt like a horse kicking me in the groin. I went into the house, told my wife to get me ice (and quickly) as I crawled to get to the couch. After pumping down three or four Advils and securely placing several pounds of ice on my sack I began to feel somewhat human... at least the spinning feeling and the nausea were subsiding. However, I still had "discomfort." Much to my chagrin, I did the proverbial sack check and "the boys" were completely black and the bruise continued up the shaft of the mother ship, if you know what I mean. Basically, the next two to three days I sat on my butt with ice as my newest best friend. I went to the doctor on Monday or Tuesday and after telling me he had never seen such a thing (actually he told me that I was one in a

thousand; sound familiar?), He prescribed massive pain medication and antibiotics. Eventually the black and blueness (mostly black) went away. The pain, however, did not. Let me describe it. It could be anything from a dull and minor pain/discomfort throbbing sensation to an incredible sensation of a very sharp, intense and hot (yes, hot) shooting pain – somewhat similar to an ice pick in the nuts – that would start at the bottom area or side area of BOTH testicles and go all the way to my stomach. I would learn later that there was this wonderful nerve that "somehow" got impacted during the surgery that goes up through the stomach area. My doctor advised me to wear tight whites [briefs] to keep the boys snug at all times and gave me more prescriptions of a HIGHER dose of pain medication and more STRONGER antibiotics. Of course, it is very important to note here that neither medications even dented the pain at all. This went on for months (10+) and the good doctor all along couldn't fathom that this could ever occur... one in a thousand? Eventually, I asked my doctor the question: "If I was to have a vasectomy reversal, wouldn't it stop all the pain and problems since we would simply be taking my gear back to its original condition?" His response was interesting. Something along the lines that "No, once you have a vasectomy, we have found that the reversal process never helps to alleviate pain and problems, it is a waste of time." What I heard, of course, was nope, I was screwed at this point and that maybe I wasn't one in a thousand since this question had obviously been asked before!!! At this point I internally decided that I had to go this on my own. By then it had been more than one year of various types of pain and frustrations.... I need to tell you that I am not completely pain-free more than two years after this "simple procedure." In fact, today I have pain and discomfort in both testicles that although not overwhelming, it is distressing..... In closing, would I have had a vasectomy if I knew what the true percentages were of complications and/or problems? Not a chance in hell! I suppose I can't complain, however, because the pain and discomfort I experience has become manageable and I can live with it. Begrudgingly, but I can live with it. Should I try a reversal? I don't think I will as I am afraid that the cycle of pain will begin anew or become worse than it ever was.... This seems to me to be information that MUST be put into circulation so that more men don't go through the horrors that other men and ourselves have gone through. Thank you for all of your hard work and especially during what must be an extremely difficult period of your life. Good luck to you and your family. I pray that you soon have all of these troubles behind you" (Name withheld by request).

3. "I had my vasectomy 18 months ago. 'A simple plumbing job' the surgeon said. I have had pain in both testicles every day since. The first two months were the worst; after that the aching has been 'cycling'... a day or two of pain followed by two to 14 days of mild aching. I have been to 72 doctors' appointments since this merry-go-round ride started and there has been no improvement.... Some days are so bad that I have seriously thought about having both of my testicles removed.... Guys, DON'T mess with Mother Nature" ("Dave" as quoted from the Urology Forum [Online], posted March 7, 2000).

4. "...I thought it was time to have a vasectomy. There was a little counseling beforehand, but no medical checks, as I looked and felt completely fit, and was only 34.... "The operation went fine and within a week I was back to my old sexy self, or even better.... Ten months later, though, I didn't feel nearly so good.... I started getting really bad cramps in first my right calf and then my left.... I told my GP about this and he said these symptoms sounded like not enough blood was getting to the leg muscles, but he had never seen this in anyone so young before.... I went back in the hospital having a whole series of complicated plumbing operations, trying to bypass the blockages with plastic tubes. None of these operations lasted more than a month or two.... It got to the point of getting cramps in my right leg at night in bed and the surgeons started talking about amputation.... I was desperate and would rather have committed suicide than live life as a legless cripple. Still, I'm a philosophical sort of man who meditates and I still believed something would happen to save my legs.... A few days after I started on the twice weekly [testosterone] injections, my legs seemed to come alive again.... It's now six years since I started the testosterone treatment and I work out in a gym for an hour most days, swim twice a week, enjoy a great sex life and, having given up the stressful job of being a milkman, I am much happier teaching Tai Chi.... The funny thing is, though, none of the surgeons I used to consult seemed interested in why things went wrong so soon after the vasectomy or why I'm not in a wheelchair now, six years after they said that amputation was the only option left" ("James", as quoted from <u>Maximizing Manhood: Beating the Male Menopause</u> by Dr. Malcolm Carruthers, 1997).

5. "I had a vasectomy about three years ago. Afterwards, I had constant pain in my right testicle. After seeing a urologist for about a year and trying different options, he performed an epididymectomy on the right testicle. The pain has been worse than before. The testicle frequently gets swollen and then returns to its normal size, which is about three times as large as before the epididymectomy. Sometimes the pain is just there as pain, you can feel it but you're used to it. And sometimes the pain is very intense. This type of pain occurs at least twice a month and lasts for three to four days. I started keeping a daily journal so I can show it to my urologist and hopefully get

some more help. But I would definitely not recommend an epididymectomy" ("Paul" as quoted from the Urology Forum [Online], posted on March 19, 2000).

6. "I've been suffering with pain and a 'non-bacterial' prostatitis diagnosis for five years now, following a painful vasectomy" (Posted anonymously on the Prostatitis Website/Vasectomy Page, January 3, 1998).

7. "You guys know as well or better than I that the complications of a vasectomy are understated. I had my vasectomy more than four years ago…definitely not enough anesthesia (certainly a more effective form of torture than pulling out fingernails). Chronic pain, and the urologists telling me to see a psychiatrist…psychiatrists telling me to find a better urologist. I began to feel like people with our problem are just 'collateral damage' like the people in a residential neighborhood in Iraq killed by an errant bomb.... I underwent a vasovasostomy in February, 2000, to put things back together. I figured out that HMO's do not like to do this procedure for pain relief. They don't get paid the $4500 'elective surgery' payment from someone that wants to have children again. My surgeon believed that I was a good candidate for this procedure to help me, after measuring the size of my testicles with a set of templates. Although there were no baseline measurements taken prior to my vasectomy, he believed that my size 10 and size 12 testicles were the result of being swollen and distended. He believes that the surgery will help me, based upon what he saw, but the jury is still out. He told me he has done several hundred of these operations to restore fertility, and a half dozen for pain relief with no complaints.... I'm still waiting for the pain and swelling from the surgery to quit. I should know if it helped me in a couple more weeks. Friends, there is still hope for your pain problems. I pray the Lord helps you find peace and relief from all of your pain" ("Joe A.", as quoted from the Urology Forum [Online], posted March 23, 2000).

8. "I, too, have experienced the pain of epididymitis. A funny way to build character. It all started three months after my vasectomy in 1995. From that time till July 1998, I saw numerous doctors who treated me with every form of meds you can think of. Nothing worked. I convinced the doc to do a vasovasostomy (reversal) in July of 1998 and thank God, the pain has not been back since then. The problem was found that they had used clamps during my vasectomy and clamped too close to my testicle causing enormous amounts of pain.... I recently experienced a case of epididymitis, (the first in nearly two years!) but seems to be curing up with meds (I guess, once you have it, you're prone to get it again). Hope you guys recover from your pain" ("Mike", as quoted from the Urology Forum, [Online], posted April 12, 2000).

9. "I'm in my late 20's, and had a vasectomy a few years ago (had two children and that's it!). A few months after the vasectomy, I began to have pain in my left sack, if you know what I mean. I went to the urologist who did the vasectomy, and he told me I had an enlarged prostate.... He did the usual exams and thought that I should take a medicine also given for blood pressure – Cardura. Well, I've been on that for a while now, and I thought that maybe things should be better, right? They were until I tried to lower the dosage (with his approval). Now I'm getting pain again. Sometimes very sharp. But it is only on the left side. I want to get off of this Cardura, but I can't stand the pain either" (Posted anonymously on the Prostatitis Website/Vasectomy Page, on July 14, 1998).

10. "I had a vasectomy done in Dec., '99. I had right side pain from day one (when I could distinguish from post vas pain). My doctor under-did the local injections and I suffered excruciating pain during the surgery. I thought this was normal until some time after the operation. The pain shot up through my groin to my tummy while the doctor cut and prodded. I thought I had nerve damage.... I have since seen specialists who have diagnosed 'epididymitis post vas' i.e. a likely blockage – the doctor who operated, uses an open-ended cut to reduce the incidence of this but it didn't seem to help me.... I am amazed at how many people told me that there are no complications (the literature indicates two percent).... Suddenly I have encountered all of the two percent and I think there is more than two percent. I have been told to give it another four weeks [May, 2000]. My options (while not guaranteed) are reversal, removal of the epididymis, removal of the testicle, respectively. After all this I am advised that I may still experience phantom pain.... The other victim, my wife, feels guilty, but it's not her fault" ("Peter" as quoted from the Urology Forum, [Online], posted April 23, 2000).

11. "I am a 47 year old male who had a vasectomy in 1980. About seven years ago started to have prostatitis symptoms. These included nocturia, pain in the right testicle during ejaculation, and stiffness of the right testicle" (Posted by "Dave" on the Prostatitis Website on February 26, 1998).

12. "My husband had a vasectomy 15 years ago. There was a problem and they had to remove a testicle. In the last year he has been experiencing pain and his doctor has recommended another surgery to take out a tube (cannot remember name)" (Posted on MEDWEB by Thomas Stellato, M.D.).

13. "I am an active duty officer in the USAF and currently in training. I have finally convinced my docs here to take me out of training so I can deal with my pain…. Tomorrow I go to see a pain management Doc and I am hoping that he will be able to assist me in some way…. I had my vasectomy at 23 (!) and believe me, if I had known even ½ of what I know now, I may have not gone for the surgery. A condom works! If my story can help others decide against a vasectomy, I am all for that…. Doing this alone really takes a toll on you psychologically. How do you explain to other guys that your balls hurt so bad and have them understand? You can't do it. All you get is 'you have to learn how to live with the pain.' I am 28 and this is not how I want to live my life" (Sent to the author personally by another vasectomy patient-name withheld).

14. "This is a BIG problem and if I knew about any of this before the vasectomy I would have never, never had it. Things only seem to get worse instead of better. Having constant unrelenting phantom testicular, vas deferens, prostate, seminal vesicle, pain down the legs, etc. plus being disabled from it having to close my private practice physical therapy office and then getting CASTRATED on top of all of it. Then all of the pain clinic stuff (which is still going on). All of this is something the next unsuspecting man needs to hear about before he has a vasectomy. Also the whole attitude of the medical profession and their lack of investigative fervor and analytic sense and their fear of medico-legal issues all cause the problems to worsen and last longer and longer. They are too busy protecting themselves or too unwilling to say they don't know to aggressively address the problem early on. I have been told 10 times by various docs 'We don't do surgery for pain.' Yet all the articles from the journals around the world advise to do revisions as soon as possible. Let's band together and get this information out there in the hands of men and their wives to help prevent them from going through what we have. I'm researching journals and getting information from patients (you) to put together an expose on this horrible problem…. –Still hopping mad after nine years" ("Charlie" as quoted from the Urology Forum, [Online] posted May 16, 2000).

15. "As a former college athlete and someone who has always been extremely active, my vasectomy surgery has changed my life. I no longer have an active lifestyle. I have two young kids that I cannot play ball with. I can no longer work out or play golf. My wife has been very supportive as she is doing all the housework and mowing the lawn. It has been three and a half years since my vasectomy surgery. At this point, I have made some minimal improvements. I'm no longer in acute pain, but the chronic pain still persists. In all of my research, no doctor or anyone else can specifically diagnose my problem. I have spent countless hours and dollars trying to get well. I cannot believe the medical people are allowed to perform the vasectomy procedure. I understand that thing happen to people, but this was supposed to be such a simple procedure. At this point, I'm just trying to help other people not make the same mistake I did. I'm not ashamed of my problem. When people ask me about my experience, I refer them to the www. Dontfixit.org web site. It is the best resource I know. For all of you who have not had the procedure, all I can say is three simple words: 'Don't do it!' Look at other options that do not require surgery, because, 'You never know'" (Tim, from a personal correspondence, January, 2003).

16. "Being a victim of a bad vasectomy (I should say half a vasectomy, I stopped the doctor after he finished the right side because of the extreme pain I experienced) and in constant pain for the last nine months, I am extremely grateful to Kevin for writing this book. This book does not only chronicle his agonizing story, but helps guys like me know that there are many others out there suffering also. This condition is more common than some would have you believe. I think Kevin's experience and opinions have kept me from making some terrible decisions (such as additional surgery) on my hopeful road to recovery. The crime in all this is not being told before having a vasectomy that a percentage of men develop chronic, disabling pain that can last years (and maybe forever.) I pop Ibuprofen like M & Ms and have to use Vicodin several times a week when I get the "shooting" pains (and I know that I am not as bad as many). I used to be a A+ tennis player, now I'm lucky to be able to go for a casual walk without pain. My greatest hope is that time will heal me in the next couple of years, but I don't know. The information from this book is a must read before undertaking a vasectomy and might be your only chance to see that there could be a less happy side to vasectomy. Unfortunate vasectomy victims should read this book just to find alternatives ways to dealing with the chronic pain; as well as the risks associated with those alternatives. Thanks Kevin, the information you have compiled in this book and on your web site has given me some perspective on this nightmare that I don't believe I could have gotten anywhere else" (Greg, from a personal correspondence, January, 2003).

17. "What I would tell men considering vasectomy is that, in having the procedure, you are taking a chance with their health and happiness. If you are among the percentage of men who will have trouble, you could be looking at years of pain and thousands of dollars spent trying to undue the damage you paid to have done to you. If you have recently had a vasectomy, know that there is a statute of limitations in most states for lawsuits, so you should get

this info and go to an attorney, armed with the statistics in this book, ASAP. The statistics are publicized in enough professional journals that no urologist could credibly claim that they haven't read about the dangers of the procedure. Also, I would encourage men who have chronic pain resulting from their vasectomies to be as vocal as possible to raise awareness and to bring shame to the medical community, which is supposed to help, not hurt, its patients" (Doug, from a personal correspondence, January, 2003).

18. "I was 23 when I underwent a vasectomy. I was not given much information on the procedure, nor briefed in-depth on possible complications. In fact, I remember asking the physician what would happen to all the sperm I would continue to produce. He explained that my body would absorb the sperm. He did not say at what rate…a big issue for a young 23-year-old male producing high amounts. Within four months, I began to experience uncomfortable pressure in my testicles. I was treated with a series of antibiotics and pain meds. This treatment managed my discomfort pretty well until two years later. At that time, I was experiencing serious pain. My doctors recommended surgeries and pain management to help my situation out. By doing research, I found that a vasectomy reversal had proven to be beneficial in helping with post vasectomy pain. I underwent the reversal in July of 1998 and noticed an improvement in my pain within three months. It was found that the surgical clamps used during my vasectomy were extremely close to my epididymis and was probably the cause of my congestion and pain. I thought my experience with post vasectomy pain was through.

"In 2000, I went to an altitude chamber ride due to a new flying job I was entering. By the following day I noticed the pain had returned. I had moved from my original location and was in an area where medical specialists were few. My physician prescribed medications to help and referred me to a Urologist. At my initial visit with the Urologist, he recommended me undergoing an epididymectomy. It was at this time I began to correspond with Kevin Hauberer and learned more about PVPS treatment options. After being treated with many medications and seeing another urologist, I decided to pursue the Testosterone therapy.

"I contacted Dr Larry Lipshultz of Houston's Baylor Medical Clinic for Men's Reproductive Health. The idea of this therapy is with excessive testosterone in your system, your pituitary gland would receive the signal that you had produced enough sperm and would stop your system from producing more. With your system in the 'off' mode you would have the opportunity to heal from any congestion. I began the treatment in May of 2001 and began to have less discomfort within a couple of months. During this time, I also was seeing an Osteopath who worked on aligning my pelvic bone which he found to be seriously out of alignment (which can cause pressure on the numerous nerves going through your pelvic region to your testicles). I stopped the treatment in January of 2002. Following the testosterone therapy, I experienced a significant decline in my pain and a return to a more productive life.

"It has been over a year now since I've completed my testosterone therapy. During this time, I've had occasional testicular pain, but fortunately this is not the norm. I still take pain meds, but the medication is not needed as much as it once was. I have been able to workout and am no longer 'controlled' by the pain.

"I've learned a lot along my path to pain-free living. If there is one main thing I would recommend to any man experiencing pain following a vasectomy is to exhaust all non-surgical therapies before allowing an urologist to perform any further surgeries. The more surgeries a guy receives in this area, the more problems can arise. This may require going through numerous physicians/urologists until you find the right one who wants to help without cutting on your privates. This may require being persistent with your HMO to get approval to see the right physician. Having to find the right doctor may be exhausting, but I highly encourage a guy to run from the doctor who quickly mentions surgery.

"I would also recommend a guy who is experiencing PVPS to speak with another guy who understands. For me, I was very depressed when this pain controlled my life. I felt like I had made the worst mistake in my life and would often end up in the fetal position on my bed to 'sleep away' my pain.…thanks in part to my large collection of strong pain medication I had been prescribed. I felt no one understood and it was not the easiest subject to talk about with family and friends. I felt very good after talking with other guys who were experiencing the same thing I was.

"Who would ever guess that one of the easiest surgeries to be performed on man could cause so many problems? Obviously not the surgeon who created the vasectomy procedure" (Mike, from a personal correspondence with the author, February, 2003).

Bibliography

- ABC News, Few Worries About Vasectomy: Pain, Not Finality, is Most Common Concern, Study Finds., [online] http://more.abcnews.go.com/sections/living/dailynews/vasectomy010312.html, March 12, 2001.

- Abdelmassih, V.; Balmaceda, J. P.; Tesarik, J.; Abdelmassih, R.; Nagy, Z. P., Relationship between time period after vasectomy and reproductive capacity of sperm obtained by epididymal aspiration., *Human Reproduction*, 17: 3, 736-740, March, 2002.

- Ahmed, I.; Rasheed, S.; White, C.; Shaikh, N. A., The incidence of post-vasectomy chronic testicular pain and the role of nerve stripping (denervation) of the spermatic cord in its management., *British Journal of Urology*, 79: 2, 269-70, February, 1997.

- Aitken, H.; Kumarakuru, S.; Orr, R.; Reid, O.; Bennett, N. K.; McDonald, S. W., Effects of long-term vasectomy on seminiferous tubules in the guinea pig., *Clinical Anatomy*, 12, 250-263, 1999.

- Alder, Elizabeth; Cook, Ann; Gray, Jennifer; Tryer, Gillian; Warner, Pamela; Bancroft, John; Loudon, Nancy B.; Loudon, John, The effect of sterilization: A comparison of sterilized women with the wives of vasectomized men., *Contraception*, 23: 1, 45-54, January, 1981.

- Alderman, P. M., The lurking sperm: A review of failures in 8879 vasectomies performed by one physician., *JAMA*, 259: 21, 3142-3144, June 3, 1988.

- Alderman, P. M., The lurking sperm: vasectomy failures., *JAMA*, 260: 23, 3433-3434, December 16, 1988.

- Alderman, P. M., Complications in a series of 1224 vasectomies., *Journal of Family Practice*, 33: 6, 579-84, December, 1991.

- Alexander, N. J., Vasectomy and vasovasostomy in rhesus monkeys: the effect of circulating antisperm antibodies on fertility., *Fertility and Sterility*, 28: 5, 562-569, May, 1977.

- Alexander, N. J., Possible mechanisms of vasectomy-exacerbated atherosclerosis., *Australian Journal of Biological Sciences*, 35: 5, 469-79, 1982.

- Alexander, Nancy J., Similarities between immunopathologic changes after vasectomy and experimental immune complex disease., <u>Reproductive Immunology</u>, edited by T. J. Gill III and Wegman, Oxford University Press, New York, 1983.

- Alexander, N. J.; Free, M. J.; Paulsen, C. Alvin; Buschbom, R.; Fulgham, D. L., A comparison of blood chemistry, reproductive hormones, and the development of antisperm antibodies after vasectomy in men. *Journal of Andrology*, 1: 1, 40-50, 1980.

- Alexander, N. J.; Schmidt, S. S.; Free, M. J.; Danilchik, M. V.; Hil,l W. T., Sperm antibodies after vasectomy with fulguration., *Journal of Urology*, 115: 1, 77-8, January, 1976.

- Alexander, N. J.; Tung, K. S., Immunological and morphological effects of vasectomy in the rabbit., *Anatomical Record*, 188:3, 339-350, July, 1977.

- Alexander, N. J.; Senner, J. W.; Hoch, E. J., Evaluation of blood pressure in vasectomized and nonvasectomized men., *International Journal of Epidemiology*, 10:3, 217-222, April, 1981.

- American Autoimmune Related Diseases Association, Inc., What do these diseases have in common?, East Detroit, MI, http://www.aarda.org .

- Amir, L. H.; Donath, S. M., Rate of vasectomy rises with increasing income., *Australian and New Zealand Journal of Obstetrics and Gynaecology*, 40: 1, 92, February, 2000.

- Anderson, D. J.; Alexander, N. J.; Fulgham, D. L.; Palotay, J. L.; Spontaneous tumors in long-term vasectomized mice., *American Journal of Pathology*, 111:2, 129-139, May, 1983.

- Anderson, D. J.; Alexander, N. J.; Fulgham, D. L.; Vandenbark, A. A.; Burger, D. R., Immunity to tumor-associated antigens in vasectomized men., *Journal of the National Cancer Institute*, 69: 3, 551-555, September, 1982.

- Anderson, Deborah J.; Tarter, Thomas H., Immunosuppressive effects of mouse seminal plasma components in vivo and in vitro., *Journal of Immunology*, 128:2, 535-539, February, 1982.

- Anderson, R. A.; Sharpe, R. M., Regulation of inhibin production in the human male and its clinical applications., *International Journal of Andrology*, 23: 3, 136-44, June, 2000.

- Anderson, R. A.; Wu, F. C.; Comparison between testosterone enanthate-induced azoospermia and oligozoospermia in a male contraceptive study. II. Phamacokinetics and pharmacodynamics of once weekly administration of testosterone enanthate., *Journal of Clinical Endocrinology and Metabolism*, 81: 3, 896-901, March, 1996.

- Armstrong, Lance, <u>It's Not About the Bike</u>., GP Putnam's Sons Publishers, New York, 2000.

- Auman, James R., Spermatic cord arteriovenous fistula: an unusual complication of vasectomy., *Journal of Urology*, 134, 768, October, 1985.

- Banks, Ian, Men's health in Europe: A no man's land? *The Economist*, 46, November 24, 2001.

- Barrett-Connor, E.L., Testosterone and risk factors for cardiovascular disease in men. *Diabete Et Metabolism*, 21: 3, 156-161, June, 1995.

- Bass, C. M.; Rees, D., Homosexual behaviour after vasectomy. *British Medical Journal*, 281, 1460, November 29, 1980.

- Baum, N., Defidio, L., Chronic testicular pain: A workup and treatment guide for the primary care physician. *Postgraduate Medicine*, 98:4, 151-158, October, 1995.

- Baylis, R. J.; Hazelgrove, J., Pain after vasectomy. *Anaesthesia*, 53: 6, 613, June, 1998.

- Bebb, R. A.; Anawalt, B. D.; Christensen, R. B.; Paulsen, C. A.; Bremner, W. J.; Matsumoto, A. M.; Combined administration of levonorgestrel and testosterone induces more rapid and effective suppression of spermatogenesis that testosterone alone: a promising male contraceptive approach., *Journal of Clinincal Endocrinology and Metabolism*, 81: 2, 757-762, February, 1996.

- Belker, A. M.; Konnak, J. W.; Sharlip, I. D.; Thomas, A. J.; Intraoperative observations during vasovasostomy in 334 patients., *Journal of Urology*, 129, 524-527, March, 1983.

- Benet, A. E.; Melman, A., The epidemiology of erectile dysfunction. *Urologic Clinics of North America*, 22:4, 699-706, November, 1995.

- Benger, J. R.; Swami, S. K.; Gingell, J. C., Persistent spermatozoa after vasectomy: a survey of British urologists., *British Journal of Urology*, 76: 3, 376-9, Sep., 1995.

- Bernal-Delgado, E.; Latour-Perez, J.; Pradas-Arnal, F.; Gomez-Lopez, L. I., The association between vasectomy and prostate cancer: a systematic review of the literature., *Fertility and Sterility*, 70: 2, 191-200, August, 1998.

- Bhasin, Shalender, The dose-dependent effects of testosterone on sexual function and on muscle mass and function., *Mayo Clinic Proceedings*, 75(supplement), S70-S76, 2000.

- Bigazzi, P. E.; Kosuda, L. L.; Hsu, K. C.; Andres, G. A., Immune complex orchitis in vasectomized rabbits., *Journal of Experimental Medicine*, 143: 2, 382-404, February 1, 1976.

- Binnette, J. P.; Ohishi, H.; Burgi, W.; Kimura, A.; Suyemitsu, T.; Seno, N.; Schmid, K., The content and distribution of glycosaminoglycans in the ejaculates of normal and vasectomized men., *Andrologia*, 28: 3, 145-149, May-June, 1996.

- Blaustein, D.; Ablin, R. J.; Barthkus, J. M., Immunolgical consequences of vasectomy and consideration of some of their implications. *Allergologia Et Immunopathologia*, 14: 2, 95-99, Mach-April, 1986.

- Bloom, l. J.; Houston, B. K., The psychological effects of vasectomy for American men. *Journal of Genetic Psychology*, 128: 2nd half, 173-182, June, 1976.

- Bohring, C.; Krause, W., Differences in the antigen pattern recognized by antisperm antibodies in patients with infertility and vasectomy. *Journal of Urology*, 166: 3, 1178-1180, September, 2001.

- Bonduelle, M.; Aytoz, A.; Van Assche, E.; Devroey, P.; Liebaers, I.; Van Steirteghem, A, Incidence of chromosomal abberations in children born after assisted reproduction through intracytoplasmic sperm injection., *Human Reproduction*, 13: 4, 781-782, 1998.

- Bonduelle, M.; Joris, H.; Hofmans, K.; Liebaers, I.; Van Steirteghem, Mental development of 201 ICSI children at 2 years of age., *The Lancet*, 351, 1553, May 23,1998.

- Bonsteel, Alan, M.D., Doctor-Patient Relations Threatened., *Plus*, 43-4, April, 2000.

- Boughton, R. Scott; Spencer, Steven K., Electrosurgical fundamentals., *Journal of the American Academy of Dermatology*, 16: 4, 862-867, April, 1987.

- Bower, Keith, Vasectomy: some Questions and Answers., [Online] Available at http://www.ccli.org/vasectomy, 1995.

- Brandell, Roy A.; Goldstein, Marc, Varicocele and its role in male infertility., *Infertility and Reproductive Medicine Clinics of North America*, 10: 3, 471-481, July 1999.

- Brickel, David; Bolduan, Jeffrey; Farah, Riad, The effect of vasectomy-vasovasostomy on the normal physiologic function of the vas deferens., *Fertility and Sterility*, 37: 6, 807-810, June 1982.

- Broderick, G. A.; Tom, R.; McClure, R. D., Immunological status of patients before and after vasovasostomy as determined by the immunobead antisperm antibody test., *Journal of Urology*, 142, 752-755, September, 1989.

- Bruning, Carl O., Re: Vasectomy Reversal for Treatment of the Post-Vasectomy Pain Syndrome (letter)., *Journal of Urology*, 158: 4, 1528, October, 1997.

- Buchholz, N. P.; Weuste, R.; Mattarelli, G.; Woessmer, B.; Langewitz, W., Post-vasectomy erectile dysfunction., *Journal of Psychosomatic Research*, 38: 7, 759-62, October, 1994.

- Burnell, G. M.; Norfleet, M. A., Psychosocial factors influencing American men and women in their decision for sterilization. *Journal of Psychology*, 120: 2, 113-119, March, 1986.

- Caldamone, Anthony A.; Cockett, Abraham T. K., Recent advances in male infertility research., *Urology Clinics of North America*, 8: 1, 63-77, February, 1981.

- Caldwell, J. C.; McGadey, J.; Kerr, R.; Bennett, N. K.; McDonald, S. W., Cell recruitment to the sperm granuloma which follows vasectomy in the rat., *Clinical Anatomy*, 9:5, 302-308, 1996.

- Cale, A. R.; Farouk, M.; Prescott, R. J.; Wallace, I. W., Does vasectomy accelerate testicular tumor? Importance of testicular examinations before and after vasectomy. *British Medical Journal*, 300: 6721, 370, February 10, 1990.

- Campbell's Urology, 6th edition, edited by Walsh, P. C.; Retik, A. B.; Stamey, T. A.; Vaughn, E. D. Jr., Philadelphia, W. B. Saunders Co., 1992.

- Carbone, D. J. Jr.; Shah, A.; Thomas, A. J. Jr.; Agarwal, A., Partial obstruction, not antisperm antibodies, causing infertility after vasovasostomy., *Journal of Urology*, 159: 3, 827-30, March 1998.

- Carruthers, G. B., Painful ejaculation. *British Medical Journal*, 408, February 6, 1982.

- Carruthers, Malcolm, M.D., Maximising Manhood: Beating the Male Menopause., Harper Collins Publishers, London, 1997.

- Carruthers, Malcolm, M.D., Vasectomy – The Unkindest Cut of All, [Online], http://www.goldcrossmedical.com/androscreen/vasectomy.htm, downloaded August 5, 2000.

- Cao, J.; Yuan, J.; Jin, W.;,Clinical Trial of an anti-fertility method with testosterone enanthate in normal men., *Chinese Medical Journal*, 76: 5, 335-337, May, 1996.

- Casella, R.; Luscher, U.; Gasser, T. C.; de Roche, R.; Leibundgut, B., Results of microsurgical reconstruction after vasectomy., *Schweizerische Rundschau Fur Medizin Praxis*, 86: 22, 933-6, May28, 1997.

- Chambers, W. A., Peripheral Nerve Damage and regional anaesthesia. *British Journal of Anaesthesia*, 69:5, 429-430, November, 1992.

- Chan, J. M.; Stampfer, M. J.; Giovannucci, E. L., What causes prostate cancer? A brief summary of the epidemiology., *Seminars in Cancer Biology*, 8: 4, 263-73, August, 1998.

- Chatterjee, S.; Purohit, S. B.; Laloraya, M.; Kumar, P., Vasectomy-induced superoxide dismutase inactivation in the male reproductive tract of rat: A prerequisite for spermatic granuloma formation. *Urologia Internationalis*, 59:1, 23-25, 1997.

- Chen, T. F.; Ball, R. Y., Epididymectomy for post-vasectomy pain: histological review., *British Journal of Urology*, 68: 4, 407-13, Oct., 1991.

- Chi, I. C.; Ko, U. R.; Wilkens, L. R.; Chang, H. K.; Nam, J. J., Vasectomy and non-fatal acute myocardial infarction: a hospital-based case-control study in Seoul, South Korea., *International Journal of Epidemiology*, 19:1 32-41, March, 1990.

- Chia, Mantak; Arava, Douglas Abrams, The Multi-Orgasmic Man., Harper, San Francisco, 1996.

- Choa, R. G.; Swami, K. S., Testicular denervation. A new surgical procedure for intractable testicular pain., *British Journal of Urology*, 70: 4, 417-9, October, 1992.

- Choe, J. M.; Kirkemo, A. K., Questionnaire-based outcomes study of nononcological post-vasectomy complications., *Journal of Urology*, 155, 1284–86, April, 1996.

- Christensen, P.; al-Aqidi, O. A.; Jensen, F. S.; Dorflinger, T., Vasectomy. A prospective, randomized trial with bilateral incision versus the Li vasectomy., *Ugeskr Laeger*, 164: 18, 2390-2394, April 29, 2002.

- Clore, E. R., A guide for the testicular self-examination., *Journal of Pediatric Health Care*, 7: 6, 264-8, November-December, 1993.

- CNN, New male contraceptive found 99 percent effective., April 2, 1996.

- Coghill, R. C.; McHaffie, J. G.; Yen, Y. F., Neural correlates of interindividual differences in the subjective experience of pain. *Proceedings of the National Academy of Sciences*, 100: 14, 8538-8542, July 8, 2003 (abstract).

- Cooper, T. P., Use of EMLA cream with vasectomy. *Urology*, 60:1, 135-137, July, 2002.

- Costabile, R. A.; Hahn, M.; McLeod, D. G., Chronic orchialgia in the pain prone patient: The clinical perspective. *Journal of Urology*, 146, 1571-1574, December, 1991.

- Cox, Brian; Sneyd, Mary J.; Paul, Charlotte; Delahunt, Brett; Skegg, David C. G., Vasectomy and risk of prostate cancer. *JAMA*, 287: 23, 3110-3115, June 19, 2002.

- Crozier, Ruth; Bernstein, Gerald S., Health Status of American Men. *Journal of Clinical Epidemiology*, 46: 8, 697-706, 1993.

- Cruickshank, B.; Eidus, L.; Barkin, M., Regeneration of vas deferens after vasectomy. *Urology*, 30: 2, 137-142, August, 1987.

- Cui, S. Y., Treatment of epididymal stasis after vasoligation with audio-frequency therapy applied on the points. *Chinese Journal of Integrated Traditional and Western Medicine*, 6:2, 89, 1986.

- Curtis, G. L.; Ryan, W. L.; Sushil, S. L., Sperm-agglutinating and –immobilizing antibody formation following vasectomy prevented with dexamethasome in cynomolgus monkeys. *Fertility and Sterility*, 38: 1, 97-99, July, 1982.

- Dahl, J. B.; Kehlet, H.; Hansen, B. L.; Hjortso, N. C.; Erichsen, C. J.; Moiniche, S., (correspondence re. pre-emptive analgesia), *British Journal of Anaesthesia*, 70, 379, 1993.

- Davies, A. H.; Sharp, R. J.; Cranston, D.; Mitchell, R. G., The long-term outcome following "special clearance" after vasectomy., *British Journal of Urology*, 66: 2, 21-2, August 1990.

- Davis, B. E.; Noble, M. J.; Weigel, J. W.; Foret, J. D.; Mebust. W. K., Analysis and management of chronic testicular pain., *Journal of Urology*, 143: 5, 936-9, May, 1990.

- Davis, R. S., Intratesticular Spermatocele., *Urology*, 51: 5A, Supplement, 167-9, May, 1998.

- de Diego, Rodriguez E.; Correas, Gomez M. A.; Martin, Garcia B.; Hernandez, Rodriguez R.; Portillo, Martin J. A.; Gutierrez, Banos J. L.; del Valle, Schaan J. I.; Roca, Edreira A.; Villanueva, Pena A., Gutierrez, Garcia R., Founier's gangrene after vasectomy., *Archivos Espanoles De Urologia*, 53: 3, 275-8, April, 2000.

- DeGaris, R. M.; Pennefather, J. N., Prolonged supersensitivity to noradrenaline of smooth muscle of the epididymal half of the rat vas deferens denervated by vasectomy. *Journal of Autonomic Pharmacology*, 7: 3, 267-279, September, 1987.

- De Knijff, D. W.; Vrijhof, H. J.; Arends, J.; Janknegt, R. A., Persistence or reappearance of nonmotile sperm after vasectomy: does it have clinical consequences?, *Fertility and Sterility*, 67: 2, 332-5, February, 1997.

- De Krester, D. M.; Meinhardt, A.; Meehan, T.; Phillips, D. J.; O'Bryan, M. K.; Loveland, K. A., The roles of inhibin and related peptides in gonadal function., *Molecular and cellular Endocrinology*, 161: 1-2,43-6, March 30, 2000.

- Denniston, G. C., Vasectomy by electrocautery: Outcomes in a series of 2,500 patients. *Journal of Family Practice*, 21:1, 35-40, July, 1985.

- DeSchryver-Kecskemeti, Katherine; Balogh, Karoly; Neet, Kenneth E., Nerve growth factor and the concept of neural-epithelial interactions. *Archives of Pathological Laboratory Medicine*, 111, 833-835, September, 1987.

- Dias, P. L. R, The long-term effects of vasectomy on sexual behavior. *Acta Psychiatrica Scandinavica*, 67: 5, 333-338, May, 1983.

- Dias, P. L. R., The effects of vasectomy on testicular volume. *British Journal of Urology*, 55, 83-84, 1983.

- Digital Urology Journal, No Scalpel Vasectomy, [Online], http://www.duj.com/vasectomy.html, undated, downloaded 8/2/00.

- Discovery Health, The Testes and Scrotum/ Testicular Self-Exam, [Online], http://www.discoveryhealth.com/DH/ihtlH/WSDSCOOO/9105/9105.html, last updated April 20,2000.

- Discovery Health/Health Newsroom/Report, Chinese Researchers Successfully Test Male Birth Control Pill., [Online], http://www.discoveryhealth.com, August 1, 2000.

- Dixon, J. S.; Gilpin, C. J.; Gilpin, S. A.; Gosling, J.A.; Grant, J. F., The effects of vasectomy on the autonomic innervation of the human vas deferens. *Journal of Urology*, 137: 5, 1014-1016, May, 1987.

- Dym, Martin; Newton, Robert A.; Howards, Stuart S., Response of the human testis to vasectomy., *Journal of Andrology*, 3:1, 21-22, January/February, 1982.

- Edwards, I. S., Pain on ejaculation after vasectomy., *British Medical Journal*, 284, 1710, June 5, 1982.

- Ehn, B. E.; Liljestrand, J., A long-term follow-up of 108 vasectomized men. Good counseling routines are important., *Scandinavian Journal of Urology and Nephrology*, 29: 4, 477-81, December, 1995.

- Emard, J. F.; Drouin, G.; Thouez, J. P.; Ghadirian, P., Vasectomy and prostate cancer in Quebec, Canada. *Health and Place*, 7: 2, 131-139, June, 2001.

- Elicker, E. R.; Evans, A. T., Granulomatous orchitis., *Journal of Urology*, 113: 2, 199-200, February, 1975.

- Errey. B. B.; Edwards, I. S., Open-ended vasectomy: An Assessment., *Fertility and Sterility*, 45: 6, 843-846, June, 1986.

- Esen, U. I., Compensation for failed sterilization. *Hospital Medicine*, 63: 9, 533-534, September, 2002.

- Esho, Julius O.; Cass, Alexander S.; Ireland, Gerald W., Morbidity associated with vasectomy. *Journal of Urology*, 110, 413-415, October, 1973.

- Esk, Peter-Christian; Pabst, Reinhard, Improved results of vasovasostomy after sparing of nerves during vasectomy., *Fertility and Sterility*, 35: 3, 363-364, March, 1981.

- Fahrenbach, Hildegard B.; Alexander, Nancy J.; Senner, John W.; Fulgham, David L.; Coon, Lynn J., Effect of vasectomy on the retinal vasculature of men., *Journal of Andrology*, 1, 299-303, 1980.

- Farley, T. M.; Meirik, O.; Mehta, S.; Waites, G. M., The safety of vasectomy: recent concerns., *Bulletin of the World Health Organization*, 71: 3-4, 413-9, 1993.

- Feng, H. M.; Wen, R. Q.; Li, S. Q.; Wang, C.; Wang, Q. H.; Jiang, Y.; Li, Q. K., Proteins in fluid from the proximal vas deferens of normal fertile and vasectomized men., *International Journal of Andrology*, 18: 2, 63-6, April, 1995.

- Ferber, Andrew S.; Tietze, Christopher; Lewit, Sarah, Men with vasectomies: A study of medical, sexual, and psychosocial changes. *Psychosomatic Medicine*, 29: 4, 354-366, June-August, 1967.

- Fervenza, F. C.; Contreras, G. E.; Garratt, K. N.; Steckelberg, J. M., Staphylococcus lugdunesis endocartis: a complication of vasectomy?, *Mayo Clinic Proceedings*, 74: 12, 1227-30, December, 1999.

- Fisch, H.; Laor, E.; BarChama, N.; Witkin, S. S.; Tolia, B. M.; Reid, R. E.; Detection of testicular endocrine abnormalities and their correlation with serum antisperm antibodies in men following vasectomy., *Journal of Urology*, 141: 5, 1129-32, May, 1989.

- Flickinger, C. J.; Howards, S. S.; Herr, J. C., Effects of vasectomy on the epididymis., *Microscopy Research and Technique*, 30: 1, 82-100, January 1, 1995.

- Flores, A. J.; Lavernia, C. J.; Owens, P. W., Anatomy and physiology of peripheral nerve injury and repair., *American Journal of Orthopedics*, 29: 3, 167-73, March, 2000.

- Foley, Kathleen M., Opiods and chronic neuropathic pain. *New England Journal of Medicine*, 348: 13, 1279-1281, March 27, 2003.

- Fonseca, R.; Rajkumar, S. V.; White, W. L.; Tefferi, A.; Hoagland, H. C., Anemia after orchiectomy., *American Journal of Hematology*, 59: 3, 230-3, November, 1998.

- Fortunati, L. N.; Floerchinger-Franks, G., Men and family Planning: What is their future role? *Journal of the American Academy of Nurse Practitioners*. 13: 10, 473-479, October, 2001.

- Frances, M.; Gabor, G. T., The Medical Task Force, A comprehensive review of the sequelae of male sterilization. *Contraception*, 28:5, 455-473, November, 1983.

- Fuchs, E. F.; Alexander, N. J., Immunologic considerations before and after vasovasostomy. *Fertility and Sterility*, 40: 4, 497-499, October, 1983.

- Gehlbach, Dan; Hass, Gilbert Jr., Immunological Factor and Fertility, Center for Reproductive Health, 1000 N. Lincoln Blvd., Oklahoma City, OK 73104.

- Giovannucci, E.; Tosteson, T. D.; Speizer, F. E.; Vessey, M. P.; Colditz, G. A., A long-term study of mortality in men who have undergone vasectomy., *New England Journal of Medicine*, 326: 21, 1392-8, May 21, 1992.

- Giovannucci, E.; Ascherio, A.; Rimm, E. B.; Colditz, G. A.; Stampfer, M. J.; Willett, W. C., A prospective cohort study of vasectomy and prostate cancer in US men., *Journal of the American Medical Association*, 269: 7, 873-7, February 17, 1993.

- Giovannucci, E.; Tosteson, T. D.; Speizer, F. E.; Ascherio, A.; Vessey, M. P.; Colditz, G. A., A retrospective cohort study of vasectomy and prostate cancer in US men., *JAMA*, 269: 7, 878-82, February 17, 1993.

- Giovannucci, E., Insulin-like growth factor-I and binding protein-3 and risk of cancer., *Hormone Research*, 51 Supplement 3, 34-41, 1999.

- Goebel, P.; Ortmana, K., Risk factors in vasectomy-a comparison of satisfied vasectomized males with dissatisfied males seeking refertilization., *Urologe Ausgabe A*, 26: 3, 142-145, May, 1987.

- Goldstein, Marc; Gilbert, Bruce R.; Dicker, Adam P.; Dwosh, Jack; Gnecco, Claire, Microsurgical inguinal varicocelectomy with delivery of the testis: An artery and lymphatic sparing technique. *Journal of Urology*, 148: 6, 1808-1811, December, 1992.

- Gonadotropins: Luteinizing and Follicle Stimulating Hormones, anonymous, [Online], URL:arbl.cvmbs.colostate.edu/hbooks/pathphys…opit/lhfsh.html, dated December 1, 1998.

- Gower, Timothy, Healthy Man: The other prostate problem., [online] www.latimes.com/features/health/la-000003413jan14.column?coll=la-headlines-health-manual dated January 14, 2002.

- Graham, Sam D., Jr., Surgery of the testicle., <u>Surgical Management of Urologic Disease: An Anatomic Approach</u>, Droller, Michael J., editor, Mosby, St. Louis, 1992.

- Green, P. G.; Miano, F. J.; Strausbaugh, H.; Heller, P.; Janig, W.; Levine, J. D., Endocrine and vagal controls of sympathetically dependent neurogenic inflammation., *Annals of the New York Academy of Sciences*, 840, 282-288, May 1, 1998.

- Green, Tom, How I Beat Cancer, *US Weekly*, 70-3, April 24, 2000.

- Grimes, David A.; Peterson, Herbert B.; Rosenberg, Michael J., Fishburne, John I.; Rochat, Roger W.; Khan, Atiqur R.; Islam, Rafiqul, Sterilization-attributable deaths in Bangladesh. *International Journal of Gynaecology and Obstetrics*, 20, 149-154, 1982.

- Grimes, David A.; Satterthwaite, Adaline P.; Rochat, Roger W.; Akhter, Nargis, Deaths from contraceptive sterilization in Bangladesh: Rates, causes, and prevention., *Obstetrics and Gynecology*, 60: 5, 635-640, November, 1982.

- Guernsey, Diane, Live With Your Allergies, *Reader's Digest*, 162-7, April, 2000.

- Guess, Harry A., Invited commentary: Vasectomy and prostate cancer., *American Journal of Epidemiology*, 132: 6, 1062-1065, 1990.

- Gupta, I.; Dhawan, S.; Goel, G. D.; Saha, K., Low Fertility rate in vasovasotomized males and its possible immunological mechanism., *International Journal of Fertility*, 20: 3, 183-191, 1975.

- Haas, G. G.; Cines, D. B.; Schreiber, A. D., Immunologic infertility: identification of patients with antisperm antibody. *New England Journal of Medicine*, 303: 13, 722-727, September 25, 1980.

- Halder, N.; Cranston, D.; Turner, E; MacKenzie, I; Guillebaud, J, How reliable is vasectomy? Long-term follow-up of vasectomized men [letter]. *Lancet*, 356: 9223, 43-44, July 1, 2000.

- Hallan, R. I.; May, A. R., Vasectomy: How much is enough?, *British Journal of Urology*, 62:4. 377-379, October, 1988.

- Hamersma, R. J.; Anderegg, T.; Miller, C.; Rudolph, B, Psychological dynamics and self-perceptions of vasectomy candidates., *Perceptual and Motor Skills*, 40: 3, 1004-1006, June, 1975.

- Hamman, W., Neuropathic pain: A condition which is not always well appreciated. *British Journal of Anaesthesia*, 71:6, 779-780, December, 1993.

- Handelsman, D. J.; Conway, A. J.; Howe, C. J.; Turner, L.; Mackey, M. A., Establishing the minimum effective dose and additive effects of depot progestin in suppression of human spermatogenesis by a testosterone depot. *Journal of Clinical Endocrinology and Metabolism*, 81: 11, 4113-4121, 1996.

- Handelsman, D. J.; Farley, T. M.; Peregodov, A.; Waites, G. M., Factors in nonniform induction of azoospermia by testosterone enanthate in normal men. World Health Organization Task Force on Methods for the Regulation of Male Fertility., *Fertility and Sterility*, 63: 1, 125-133, January, 1995.

- Hargreave, T. B.; Hjort, T., Is low titre agglutination seen when testing male sera for antisperm antibodies an immunological phenomenon?, *Andrologia*, 15:1, 90-96, January-February, 1983.

- Harris, N. M.; Holmes, S. A. V., Requests for vasectomy: Counseling and consent., *Journal of the Royal Society of Medicine*, 94, 510-511, October, 2001.

- Hatcher, Robert A., Archived Questions and Answers: Why aren't men being warned about chronic post vasectomy pain before having the procedure performed? [online] www.managingcontraception.com downloaded 6/18/02.

- Hattikudur, N. S.; Shanta, S. R.; Shahani, S. K.; Shastri, P. R.; Thakker, P. V.; Bordekar, A. D., Immunological and clinical consequences of vasectomy., *Andrologia*, 14: 1, 15-22, January-February, 1982.

- Haws, J. M.; McKenzie, M.; Mehta, M.; Pollack, A. E., Increasing the availability of vasectomy in public-sector clinics., *Family Planning Perspectives*, 29: 4, 185-6 & 190, July-August, 1997.

- Haws, J. M.; Morgan, G. T.; Pollack, A. E.; Koonin, L. M.; Magnani, R. J.; Gargiullo, P. M., Clinical aspects of vasectomies performed in the United States in 1995., *Urology*, 52: 4, 685-91, October, 1998.

- Heidenreich, A.; Zumbe, J.; Martinez, F.; Grozinger, K.; Engelmann, U. H., Microsurgical testicular denervation as therapy option in chronic testalgia., *Urologe Ausgabe A*, 36: 2, 177-80, March 1997.

- Heidenreich, Alex; Olbert, Peter; Becker, T; Hofmann, R., Microsurgical testicular Denervation in patients with chronic testicular pain., *European Urology*, 39:1, supplement 5, 216, 2001.

- Heidenreich, Axel, Re: Microsurgical testicular denervation of the spermatic cord as primary surgical treatment of chronic orchialgia (letter)., *Journal of Urology*, 165, 2322-2333, 2001.

- Heidenreich, Axel; Olbert, Peter; Engelmann, Udo H., Management of chronic testalgia by microsurgical testicular denervation., *European Urology*, 41, 392-397, 2002.

- Hellma, H. W.; Samuel, T.; Rumke, P., Sperm autoantibodies as a consequence of vasectomy. II. Long-term follow-up studies., *Clinical and Experimental Immunology*, 38: 1, 31-36, October, 1979.

- Hendry, W.F., Bilateral aseptic necrosis of femoral heads following intermittent high-dose steroid therapy. *Fertility and Sterility*, 38: 1, 120, July, 1982.

- Hendry, W. F., Iatrogenic damage to the male reproductive function., *Journal of the Royal Society of Medicine*, 88: 10, 579P- 584P, October, 1995.

- Hendry, W. F., Testicular, epididymal and vassal injuries., *BJU International*, 86, 344-348, 2000.

- Hillis, S. D.; Marchbanks, P. A.; Tylor, L. R.; Peterson, H. B., Higher hysterectomy risk for sterilized than nonsterilized women: findings from the U.S. Collaborative Review of Sterilization. The U.S. Collaborative Review of Sterilization Working Group., *Obstetrics and Gynecology*, 91: 2, 241-6, February, 1998.

- Hofmeyr, G. J.; Rabson, A. R., Prevention of antisperm antibody response in vasectomized Swiss white mice by infusion of heterologous antisperm serum., *British Journal of Urology*, 56, 418-421, January, 1984.

- Holl-Allen, Robert, Counseling and consent in vasectomy., *Journal of the Royal Society of Medicine*, 95: 3, 165-166, March, 2002.

- Holman, C. D. J.; Wisniewski, Z. S.; Semmens, J. B.; Rouse, I. L.; Bass, A. J., Population-based outcomes after 28,246 in-hospital vasectomies and 1902 vasovasostomies in Wetsen Australia., *BJU International*, 86, 1043-1049, 2000.

- Hollman, P. C.; Katan, M. B., Health effects and bioavailability of dietary flavenols., *Free Radical Research*, 31 Supplement: S, 75-80, December 31, 1999.

- Horan, Anthony H, Are There Long-Term Consequences of Vasectomy., [Online], http://home.swbell.net.birons/vas.htm, downloaded March 5, 2000.

- Horenstein, D.; Houston, B. K., The effects of vasectomy on postoperative psychological adjustment and self-concept., *Journal of Psychology*, 89: 2nd half, 167-173, March, 1975.

- Howard, Geraldine, Who asks for vasectomy reversal and why?, *British Medical Journal* (Clinical Research Edition), 285: 6340, 490-492, August 14, 1982.

- Hsing, A. W.; Wang, R. T.; Gu, F. L.; Lee, M.; Wang, T.; Leng, T. J.; Spitz, M.; Blot, W. J., Vasectomy and prostate cancer risk in China., *Cancer Epidemiology, Biomarkers and Prevention*, 3: 4, 285-8, June, 1994.

- Hurtenbach, U.; Shearer, G. M., Germ cell-induced immune suppression in mice: Effect of inoculation of syngeneic spermatozoa on cell-mediated immune responses. *Journal of Experimental Medicine*; 155, 1719-1729, June, 1982.

- Hyperhealth V99.1, Luteinizing hormone.

- Hyperhealth V99.1, Testosterone – factors that enhance.

- Hyperhealth V99.1, Tribulus terrestris.

- Imai, K.; Yamanaka, H.; Mashimo, M.; Asano, M.; Yoshida, M., Testosterone replacement therapy for male hypogonadism with a radiation-polymerized testicular prosthesis., *International Journal of Urology*, 4: 2, 157-62, March 1997.

- Infinite Mind: Pain. [online] http://www.lcmedia.com/mind276.htm dated June 25, 2003.

- Isidor, A.; Aversa, A.; Fabbri, A., Erectile dysfunction. *Recenti Progressi In Medicina* (In Itialian), 90: 7-8, 396-402, July-August, 1999.

- James, W. H., Prostatic cancer, coital rates, vasectomy and testosterone., *Journal of Biosocial Science*, 26: 2, 269-72, April, 1994.

- Jarow, J. P.; Budin, R. E.; Dym, M.; Zirkin, B. R.; Noren, S.; Marshall, F., Quantitative pathologic changes in the human testis after vasectomy. A controlled study., *New England Journal of Medicine*, 313: 20, 1252-6, November 14, 1985.

- Jarow, J. P.; Goluboff, E. T.; Chang, T. S.; Marshall, F. F.; Relationship between antisperm antibodies and testicular histologic changes in humans after vasectomy., *Urology*, 43: 4, 521-4, April, 1994.

- Jarvis J. D.; Dubbins P. A., Changes in the epididymis after vasectomy: sonographic findings., *American Journal of Roentgenology*, 152: 3, 531-4, March, 1989.

- Jenkins, I. L.; Muir, V. Y.; Blacklock, N. J.; Turk, J. L.; Hanley, H. G., Consequences of vasectomy: An immunological and histological study related to subsequent fertility., *British Journal of Urology*, 51: 5, 406-410, October, 1979.

- Jequier, A. M., Vasectomy related infertility: a major and costly medical problem., *Human Reproduction*, 13: 7, 1757-9, July, 1998.

- Jerome, Richard; Breu, Giovanna, Mind over misery. *People*, 153-157, May 5, 2003.

- Johnson, A. L.; Howards, S. S., Intratubular hydrostatic pressure in testis and epididymis before and after vasectomy., *American Journal of Physiology*, 228: 2, 556-564, February, 1975.

- Jones, W. R.; Tischler, E.; Goulston, E., Psychological aspects of vasectomy: 1. Helping the patient decide., *Medical Journal of Australia*, 1:11, 521-522, March 17, 1973.

- Junnila, J.; Lassen, P., Testicular Masses., *American Family Physician*, 57: 4, 685-692, February, 1998.

- Kabat-Zinn, Jon, <u>Full Catastrophe Living</u>, Dell Publishing, 1540 Broadway, New York, 1990.

- Katz, J.; Kavanagh, B. P.; Clairoux, M. Sandler, A. N., Pre-emptive analgesia. *British Journal of Anaesthesia*, 70: 3, 378, March, 1993.

- Kaufman, Steven C.; Alexander, Nancy J., Vasectomy: Autoimmunity and safety. <u>Reproductive Immunology</u>, edited by R. A. Bronson, 1996.

- Keetch, David W.; Humphrey, Peter; Ratliff, Timothy L., Development of a mouse model for nonbacterial prostatitis., *Journal of Urology*, 152, 2247-250, July, 1994.

- Kelleher, Kathleen, Many real men have unreal fears about vasectomies. *Los Angeles Times*, Monday April 22, 2002.

- Khan, M. A.; Cranston, D., Recanalization of the vas following vasectomy., *British Journal of Urology*, 79:3, 484, March, 1997.

- Kendrick, J. S.; Gonzales, B.; Huber, D.H.; Grubb, G. S.; Rubin, G. L., Complications of vasectomies in the United States., *Journal of Family Practice*, 25: 3, 245-248, September, 1987.

- Kenogbon, J. I., Evidence-based counseling for vasectomy., *International Journal of Clinical Practice*, 54: 5, 317-21, June, 2000.

- Kerin, J. F.; Carignan, C. S.; Cher, D., The safety and effectiveness of a new hysteroscopic method for permanent birth control: results of the first Essure pbc clinical study., *Australian and New Zealand Journal of Obstetrics and Gynaecology*, 41: 4, 364-370, November, 2001.

- Kessler, Robert, Vasectomy and Vasovasostomy., *Surgical Clinics of North America*, 62: 6, 971-980, December, 1982.

- Khanna, Y. K.; Khanna, A.; Heda, K.;, Mathur, G.; Jhanji, R. N., pre-pubic vasectomy-a new approach., *Journal of Postgraduate Medicine*, 37: 2, 65-8 68A-68D, April, 1991.

- Kim, Edward D.; Lipshultz, Larry I., Evaluation and imaging of the infertile male. *Infertility and Reproductive Medicine Clinics of North America*, Philip E. Werthman, M.D., guest editor, 10: 3, 377-409, July, 1999.

- Kovi, Joseph; Agrata, Anthony; Benign neural invasion in vasitis nodosa. *JAMA*, 228: 12, 1519, June 17, 1974.

- Kronmal, R. A.; Krieger, J. N.; Coxon, V.; Wortley, P.; Thompson, L.; Sherrard, D. J., Vasectomy is associated with an increased risk for urolithiasis., *American Journal of Kidney Diseases*, 29: 2, 207-13, February, 1997.

- Labreque, M.; Bedard, L.; Laperriere, L., Efficacy an complications associated with vasectomies in two clinics in the Quebec region., *Canadian Family Physician*, 44, 1860-6, September 1998.

- Lacayo, Richard, Are You Man Enough?, *Time*, April 24, 2000, 58-68.

- Lacy, S. S.; Curtis, G. L.; Ryan, W. L., Prevention of autoimmunization to spermatozoa by passive antibody., *Urology*, 17:6, 566-569, June, 1981.

- Lahita, R. G.; Chiorazzi, N.; Reeves, W. H., editors, <u>Textbook of Autoimmune Diseases</u>. 484-489, Lippincott, Williams & Wilkins, Philadelphia, PA, 2000.

- Lamberg, A.; Rosenberg, J., Emergency care during ambulatory vasectomy., *Ugeskrift for Lager*, 158: 33, 4649-50, August 12, 1996.

- Lassen, P. M.; Thompson, I. M. Jr.; Helfrick, B., Serum prostate specific antigen concentration before and after vasectomy., *Military Medicine*, 161: 6, 356-357, June, 1996.

- Leavesley, J. H., Vasectomy: Psychological effects and pre-operative counseling [abstract]., *Australian Family Physician*, 5: 2, 142-150, March, 1976.

- Lee, Chung; Kozlowski, James K.; Grayhacj, John T., Etiology of benign prostatic hyperplasia., *Urologic Clinics of North America*, 22: 2, 237-246, May, 1995.

- Lee, Hee Yong, A 20-year experience with epididymovasostomy for pathologic epididymal obstruction. *Fertility and Sterility*, 47: 3, 487-491, March, 1987.

- Lee, S. K.; Wolfe, S. W., Peripheral nerve injury and repair., *Journal of the American Academy of Orthopaedic Surgeons*, 8: 4, 243-252, July-August, 2000.

- Levine, L. A.; Matkov, T. G.; Lubenow, T. R., Microsurgical denervation of the spermatic cord: a surgical alternative in the treatment of chronic orchialgia., *Journal of Urology*, 155: 3, 1005-7, March, 1996.

- Levine, L. A.; Matkov, T. G., Microsurgical denervation of the spermatic cord as primary surgical treatment of chronic orchialgia., *Journal of Urology*, 165, 1927-1929, June 2001.

- Levine, Peter A., <u>Waking the Tiger: Healing Trauma</u>. North Atlantic Books, Berkely, CA, 1997.

- Lewin, Lawrence M.; Shalev, Daniel Pace; Weissenberg, Ruth; Soffer, Yigal, Carnitine and acylcarnitines in semen from azoospermic patients., *Fertility and Sterility*, 36: 2, 214-218, August 1981.

- Li, Shunqiang; Goldstein, Mark; Zhu, Jinbo; Huber, Douglas, The no-scalpel vasectomy., *Journal of Urology*, 145, 341-344, February, 1991.

- Lindholm, Sally, Why Men Avoid the Doctor. *Vitality Digest*, 20-21, June/July, 2002.

- Linnet L, Clinical immunology of vasectomy and vasovasostomy., *Urology*, 22: 2, 101-112, August, 1983.

- Linnet, Lars; Hjort, Tage; Fogh-Andersen, Poul, Association between failure to impregnate after vasovasostomy and sperm agglutinins in semen., *Lancet*, 1:8212, 117-119, January 17, 1981.

- Linnet, L.; Suominen, J. J., A comparison of eight techniques for the evaluation of the auto-immune response to spermatozoa after vasectomy., *Journal of Reproductive Immunology*, 4: 3, 133-44, July, 1982.

- Loeser, John D., What is chronic pain?, *Theoretical Medicine*, 12: 3, 213-225, September, 1991.

- Loughlin, Kevin R., Microsurgical vasectomy reversal and varicocele ligation (letter)., *Urology*, 53: 1, 239-240, January, 1999.

- Ma, J.; Pollak, M. N.; Giovannucci, E.; Chan, J. M.; Tao, Y.; Hennekens, C. H.; Stampfer, M. J., Prospective study of colorectal cancer risk in men and plasma levels of insulin-like growth factor (IGF)-I and IGF-binding protein-3., *Journal of the National Cancer Institute*, 91: 7, 620-5, April 7, 1999.

- Maatman, T. J.; Aldrin, L.; Carothers, G. G., Patient non-compliance after vasectomy., *Fertility and Sterility*, 68: 3, 552-5, September, 1997.

- Magnani, R. J.; Haws, J. M.; Morgan, G. T.; Gargiullo, P. M.; Pollack, A. E.; Koonon, L. M., Vasectomy in the United States, 1991 and 1995., *American Journal of Public Health.*, 89: 1, 92-4, January, 1999.

- Marquette, Catherine M.; Koonin, Lisa M.; Antarsh, Libby; Gargiullo, Paul M.; Smith, Jack C., Vasectomy in the United States, 1991., *American Journal of Public Health*, 85: 5, 644-649, May, 1995.

- Massey, F. J.; Bernstein, G. S.; O'Fallon, W. M.; Schuman, L. M.; Coulson, A. H.; Crozier, M. A.; Mandel, J. S.; Benjamin, R. B.; Berendes, H. W.; Chang, P. C.; Detels, R.; Emslander, R. F.; Koreilitz, J.; Kurland, L. T.; Lepow, I. H.; McGregor, D. D.; Nakamura, R. N.; Quiroga, J.; Schmidt, S.; Spivey, G. H.; Sullivan, T., Vasectomy and Health: Results From a Large Cohort Study., *JAMA*, 252: 8, 1023-1029, August, 1984.

- Matthew Bender & Co., 2000, California Torts, Cause for Action for Negligence., Lexis Publishing.

- Mathews, J. D.; Skegg, D. C.; Vessey, M. P.; Konice, M.; Holborow, E. J.; Guillebraud, J., Weak autoantibody reactions to antigens other than sperm after vasectomy., *British Medical Journal*, 2: 6048, 1359-60, December 4, 1976.

- Mayor, S., French men invited to become "vasectomy tourists"., *British Medical Association*, 321: 7259, 470, August 19-26, 2000.

- Mazeh, D.; Merimsky, O.; Melamed, Y.; Inbar, M., Erotomania following an orchiectomy: a case report., *Journal of Sex and Marital Therapy*, 23: 2, 154-5, Summer, 1997.

- McConaghy, P.; Paxton, L. D.; Loughlin,. V, Chronic testicular pain following vasectomy., *British Journal of Urology*, 77, 328, 1996.

- McConaghy, P.; Reid, M.; Loughlin, V.; Huss, B. K., Pain after vasectomy., *Anesthesia*, 53: 1, 83-86, January, 1998.

- McCormack, Michael M.D.; Lapointe, Steven M.D., Physiologic consequences and complications of vasectomy., *Canadian Medical Association Journal*, 138:3, 223-225, February 1, 1988.

- McDonald, S. W., Cellular responses to vasectomy., *International Review of Cytology*, 199, 295-339, 2000.

- McDonald, S. W., Vasectomy review: sequelae in the human epididymis and ductus deferens., *Clinical Anatomy*, 9: 5, 337-42, 1996.

- McLachlan, R. I.; O'Donnell, L.; Stanton, P. G.; Balourdos, G.; Frydenberg, M.; de Kretster, D. M.; Robertson, D. M.; Effects of testosterone plus medroxyprogesterone acetate on semen quality, reproductive hormones, and germ cell populations in normal young men., *Journal of Clinical Endocrinology and Metabolism*, 87: 2, 546-556, February, 2002.

- McLachlan, R. I.; Wreford, N. G.; O'Donnell, L. O,; de Kretser, D. M.; Robertson, D. M., The endocrine regulation of spermatogenesis: independent roles for testosterone and FSH., *Journal of Endocrinology*, 148, 1-9, 1996.

- Mc Mahon, A. J.; Buckley, J.; Taylor, A.; Lloyd, S. N.; Deane, R. F.; Kirk, D., Chronic testicular pain following vasectomy., *British Journal of Urology*, 69: 2, 188-91, February, 1992.

- Meares, Edwin M., Serum antibody titers in urethritis and chronic bacterial prostatitis., *Urology*, X: 4, 305-309, October, 1977.

- Meares, Edwin M., Prostatitis., *Medical Clinics of North America*, 75: 2, 405-424, March, 1991.

- Menchini-Fabris, G. Fabrizio; Canale, Domenico; Izzo, Pier Luigi; Olivieri, Luigi; Bartelloni, Mauro, Free L-carnitine in human semen: Its variability in different andrologic pathologies., *Fertility and Sterility*, 42:2, 263-267, August 1984.

- Mendell, Jerry R.; Sahenk, Zarife, Painful sensory neuropathy., *New England Journal of Medicine*, 348: 13, 1243-1254, March 22, 2003.

- Meriggiola, M. C.; Bremmer, W. J.; Costantino, A.; Di Cintio, G.; Flamigni, C., Low dose of cyproterone acetate and testosterone enanthate for contraception in men., *Human Reproduction* 13: 5,1225-1229, May, 1998.

- Meriggiola, M. C.; Bremmer, W. J.; Constantino, A.; Pavani, A.; Capelli, M.; Flamigni, C., An oral regimen of cyproterone acetate and testosterone undecanoate for spermatogenic suppression in men., *Fertility and Sterility*, 68: 5, 844-850, November, 1997.

- Meriggiola, M. C.; Bremmer, W. J.; Paulsen, C. A.; Valdiserri, A.; Incorvaia, L.; Motta, R.; Pavani, A.; Capelli, M.; Flamigni,. C, A combined regimen of cyproterone acetate and testosterone enanthate as a potentially highly effective male contraceptive., *Journal of Clinical Endocrinology and Metabolism*, 81: 8, 3018-3023, August, 1996.

- Merz, Jon F., An Empirical Analysis of the Medical Informed Consent Doctrine: Search for a "Standard" of Disclosure. [online] http://www.flpc.edu/RISK/vol2/winter/merz.htm, downloaded 11/6/01.

- Mettlin, Curtis; Natarajan, Nachimuthu; Huben, Robert, Vasectomy and prostate cancer risk., *American Journal of Epidemiology*, 132: 6, 1056-1061, 1990.

- Miller, Dennis, Ranting Again, Doubleday, New York, 1998.

- Miller, Thomas W.; Kraus, Robert F., An overview of chronic pain., *Hospital and Community Psychiatry*, 41:4, 433-440, April, 1990.

- Miller, Warren B.; Shain, Rochelle N.; Pasta, David J., The pre- and poststerilization predictors of poststerilization regret in husbands and wives., *Journal of Nervous and Mental Disease*, 179: 10, 602-608, October, 1991.

- Mizoguchi, H.; Fukunaga, Y.; Kasagi, Y.; Ogata, J., Bilateral spermatocele developed after vasectomy: a case report., *Japanese Journal of Urology*, 85: 10, 1567-70, October, 1994.

- Mo, Z. N.; Huang, X.; Zhang, S. C.; Yang, J. R., Early and late long-term effects of vasectomy on serum testosterone, dihydrotestosterone, luteinizing hormone and follicle-stimulating hormone levels., *Journal of Urology*, 154: 6, 2065-9, December, 1995.

- Mosquera, L. F.; Urban, J., Laproscopic vasectomy., *Surgical Laparoscopy and Endoscopy*, 4: 6, 461-2, December, 1994.

- Moss, W. M., A comparison of open-end versus closed-end vasectomies: a report on 6220 cases., *Contraception*, 46: 6, 521-5, December 1992.

- MSNBC News Services, Sperm finding could lead to unisex contraceptive., [online], http://www.msnbc.com/news/640994.asp downloaded 6/19/02.

- Mullich, J., Proof of Pain., *Arthritis Today*, 17: 6, 35, November-December, 2003.

- Mumford, Stephen D., Vasectomy Counseling, San Francisco Press, Inc., 1997.

- Myers, Stanley A.; Mershon, Christopher E.; Fuchs, Eugene F., Vasectomy reversal for treatment of the post-vasectomy pain syndrome., *Journal of Urology*, 157, 518-520, February, 1997.

- Nader, Antoun; Candido, Kenneth D., Pelvic Pain., *Pain Practice*, 1: 2, 187-196, 2001.

- Nagler, Harris M.; Blick, Shawn D., Microsurgical reconstruction of the male reproductive tract., *Infertility and Reproductive Medicine Clinics of North America*, 10: 3, Philip Werthman, guest editor, 483-517, July, 1999.

- Nangia, Ajay K; Myles, Jonathan L; Thomas, Anthony J. Jr., Vasectomy reversal for the post-vasectomy pain syndrome: a clinical and histological evaluation., *Journal of Urology*, 164, 1939-1942, December, 2000.

- Nash, J. L.; Rich, J. D., The sexual aftereffects of vasectomy., *Fertility and Sterility*, 23:10, 715-8, October, 1972.

- National Institutes of Health; National Institute of Child Health and Human Development; National Cancer Institute; National Institute of Diabetes and Digestive and Kidney Diseases, Vasectomy and Prostate Cancer Conference, Final Statement- March 2,1993.

- National Institutes of Health; U.S. Department of Health and Human Services; National Institute of Child Health and Human Development, Facts About Vasectomy Safety., NIH Publication number 96-4094, April, 1996.

- Nirpathpongporn, A.; Huber, D. H.; Krieger, J. N., No-scalpel vasectomy at the King's birthday vasectomy festival., *Lancet*, 335: 8694, 894-895, April 14, 1990.

- Northrup, Christiane, M.D., <u>The Wisdom of Menopause: Creating Physical and Emotional Health and Healing During the Change</u>., Bantam Books, NewYork, 2001.Noonan, R. P., Comments on vasectomy closure techniques. *American Family Physician*, 61: 2, 306-307, January 15, 2000.

- O'Brien, T. S.; Cranston, D.; Ashwin, P.; Turner, E.; MacKenzi, I. Z.; Guillebaud. J., Temporary reappearance of sperm 12 months after vasectomy clearance., *British Journal of Urology*, 76: 3, 371-2, Sep., 1995.

- Olsson, Yngve, Professor, Department of Genetics and Pathology, Uppsala University, Sweden, "Chapter 11, Trauma (Nerve)", undated article on the Internet, <u>www.genpat.uu.se/persons/yo/Microenv/11.html</u>, downloaded August 31, 2000.

- Oversen, P.; Flyvbjerg, A.; Orskov, H., Insulin-like growth factor I (IGF-I) and IGF binding proteins in seminal plasma before and after vasectomy in normal men., *Fertility and Sterility*, 63: 4, 913-8, April, 1995.

- Pabst, R.; Martin, O.; Lippert. H., Is the low fertility rate after vasovasostomy caused by nerve resection during vasectomy?, *Fertility and Sterility*, 31: 3, 316-20, March, 1979.

- Padmore, D. E.; Norman, R. W.; Millard, O. .H, Analyses of indications for and outcomes of epididymectomy., *Journal of Urology*, 156: 1, 95-6, July, 1996.

- Pardanani, D. S.; Patil, N. G.; Pawar, H. N., Some Gross observations of the epididymis following vasectomy: a clinical study., *Fertility and Sterility*, 27: 3, 267-70, March, 1976.

- Patel, A.; Ramsay, J. W. A.; Whitfield, H. N., Fournier's gangrene of the scrotum following day case vasectomy. *Journal of the Royal Society of Medicine*, 1991.

- Patel, B.; Gujral, S.; Jefferson, K.; Evans, S. Persad, R., Seminal vesicle cysts and associated anomolies., *BJU International*, 90: 3, 265-271, August, 2002.

- Paxton, L. D.; Huss, B. K.; Loughlin, V.; Mirakhur, R. K., Intra-vas deferens bupivacaine for prevention of acute pain and chronic discomfort after vasectomy., *British Journal of Anesthesiology*, 74, 612-613, 1995.

- Peterson, Andrew C.; Lance, Raymond S.; Ruiz, Henry E., Outcomes of varicocele ligation done for pain., *Journal of Urology.* 159: 5, 1565-1567, May, 1998.

- Peterson, D. F.; Brown, A. M., Functional afferent innervation of testis., *Journal of Neurophyiology*, 36: 3, 425-433, May, 1973.

- Peterson, Herbert B.; Howards, Stuart S., Vasectomy and prostate cancer: the evidence to date., *Fertility and Sterility*, 70: 2, 201-203, August, 1998.

- Peterson, Herbert B.: Huber, Douglas H.; Belke, Arnold M., Vasectomy: an appraisal for the obstetrician-gynecologist., *Obstetrics and Gynecology*, 76: 3 Pt 2, 568-72, September, 1990.

- Petitti, Diana B.; Klein, Robert; Kipp, Harald; Kahn, William; Siegelaub, Abraham B.; Friedman, Gary D., A survey of personal habits, symptoms of illness, and histories of disease in men with and without vasectomies., *American Journal of Public Health*, 72: 5, 476-480, May, 1982.

- Platz, E. A.; Yeole, B. B.; Cho, E.; Jussawalla, D, J.; Giovannucci, E.; Ascherio, A., Vasectomy and prostate cancer: a case control study in India., *International Journal of Epidemiology*, 26: 5, 933-8, October, 1997.

- Pollack AE, Vasectomy and prostate cancer., *Advances in Contraception*, 9: 2, 181-6, June, 1993.

- Pollack, William, <u>Real Boys</u>, Henry Holt and Co., 1998.

- Potts, J. M.; Pasqualotto, F. F.; Nelson, D.; Thomas, A. J. Jr.; Agarwal, A., Patient characteristics associated with vasectomy reversal., *Journal of Urology*, 161: 6, 1835-9, June, 1999.

- Preston, JM, Vasectomy: common medicolegal pitfalls., *BJU International*, 86, 339-343, 2000.

- Prostate Forum Newsletter, P. O. Box 6696, Charlottesville, VA 22906-6696, Volume 2, Number 12, December 1997.

- Protatitis Website, Prostatitis: Two new articles on prostatitis., [Online], <u>www.prostatitis.org/ux2articles.html downloaded 1/15/02</u>.

- Prostatitis Website, Vasectomy Page, [Online], <u>http://www.prostatitis.org/vasectomy.html</u>, downloaded December 1, 1999.

- Pryor, J. P., Vasectomy: an effective form of contraception., *Human Reproduction*, 13: 7, 1758-1760, July, 1998.

- Radio National Health Report, Long-term Complications after a Vasectomy Operation, [Online], <u>http://www.abc.net.au/rn/talks/8.30/helthrpt/stories/s178.htm</u> dated July 7, 1997.

- Raffer, Jacob; Koyle, Martin A; Canfield, Craig W., Surgery of the spermatic cord., In <u>Surgical Management of Urologic Disease: An Anatomic Approach</u>, Droller, Michael J. editor, Mosby, St. Louis, 1992.

- Randall, P. E.; Ganguli, L.; Marcuson, R. W., Wound infection following vasectomy., *British Journal of Urology*, 55: 5, 564-567, October, 1983.

- Rasmussen, L. A.; Sorensen, E. W.; Sorensen, C.; Eldrup, J., Inguinal funicular block in vasectomy., *Ugeskrift for Laeger*, 156: 23, 3501-2, June 6, 1994.

- Raspa, R. F., Complications of vasectomy., *American Family Physician*, 48: 7,126-8, Nov. 15, 1993.

- Reda, Kenneth D., Open-ended Vasectomy: Improved Reversibility with Less Chance of Chronic Pain., [Online], <u>http://www.erols.com/kreda/index.html</u> downloaded November 15, 1999.

- Reynolds, J. L., Venting for post-vasectomy orchitis., *The Journal of Family Practice*, 44: 4, 329-330, April, 1997.

- Roberts, H. J., M.D., <u>Is Vasectomy Worth the Risk?</u>, Sunshine Sentinel Press, West Palm Beach, FL 33407, 1993.

- Rogers, Phil, Acupuncture in genitourinary and related conditions: 3c. Summary of points and protocols for "male disorders.", [Online], <u>http://homepage.tinet.ie/~progers/gu3c.htm downloaded 1/13/02</u>.

- Rose, Noel, Autoimmunity-the common thread., American Autoimmune Related Disease Association, Eastpointe, MI, undated.

- Rosenberg, J. C.; Lysz, K., Suppression of the immune system response by steroids., *Transplantation*, 29:5, 425-428, May, 1980.

- Rosenberg, L.; Palmer, J. R.; Zauber, A. G.; Warshauer, M. E.; Stolley, P. D.; Shapiro, S., Vasectomy and the risk of prostate cancer., *American Journal of Epidemiology*, 132: 6, 1051-5, discussion 1062-5, December, 1990.

- Rosenberg, L.; Schwingl, P. J.; Kaufman, D. W.; Helmrich, S. P.; Palmer, J. R.; Shapiro, S., The risk of myocardial infarction 10 or more years after vasectomy in men under 55 years of age., *American Journal of Epidemiology*, 123: 6, 1049-56, June, 1986.

- Ross, Marvin, Vasectomy: A Permanent Option, [Online], http://www.webM.D..com downloaded May 9, 1999.

- Rowbotham, Michael C.; Twilling, Lisa; Davies, Pamela S.; Riesner, Lori; Taylor, Kirk; Mohr, David, Oral opiod therapy for chronic peripheral and central neuropathic pain., *New England Journal of Medicine*, 348: 13, 1223-1232, March 27, 2003.

- Sakamoto, Y.; Matsumoto, T.; Mizuone, Y.; Haraoka, M.; Sakumoto, M.; Kumazawa, J., Testicular injury induces cell-mediated autoimmune response to testis., *Journal of Urology*, 153, 1316-1320, April, 1995.

- Sakamoto, Y.; Matsumoto, T.; Mizunoe, Y.; Kumazawa, J., Murine "sympathetic orchitis" induced by unilateral testicular injury and autoimmune response. Nippon Hinyokika Gakkai Zasshi, 86:12, 1751-1756, December, 1995.

- Sandlow, J. I.; Kreder, K. J., A change in practice: current urologic practice in response to reports concerning vasectomy and prostate cancer., *Fertility and Sterility*, 66: 2, 281-4, Aug., 1996.

- Sandlow, Jay I.; Westefeld; John S., Maples, Michael R.; Scheel, Karen R., Psychological correlates of vasectomy., *Fertility and Sterility*, 75: 3, 544-548, March 2001.

- Schlegel, Peter N.; Goldstein, Marc, Surgery of the vas deferens. In <u>Surgical Management of Urologic Disease: An Anatomic Approach</u>, Droller, Michael J. editor, Mosby, St Louis, 1992.

- Schmidt, Stanwood S., Technics and complications of elective vasectomy: The role of spermatic granuloma in spontaneous recanalization., *Fertility and Sterility*, 17: 4. 467-481, July-August, 1966.

- Schmidt SS, Spermatic granuloma: an often painful lesion., *Fertility and Sterility*, 31: 2, 178-81, February, 1979.

- Schmidt, Stanwood S., Vasectomy., *Urology Clinics of North America*, 14:1, 149-154, February, 1987.

- Schmidt, Stanwood S., Vasectomy., *JAMA*, 259:21, 3176, June 3, 1988.

- Schmidt, Stanwood S.; Minckler, Tate M., The vas after vasectomy: comparison of cauterization methods., *Urology*, 40: 5, 468-470, November, 1992.

- Schned, Alan; Selikowitz, Stuart, Morphologic changes in the epididymides removed for unremitting post-vasectomy pain., *Laboratory Investigations*, 50: 1, 51A-52A, 1984.

- Schned, Alan R. M.D.; Selikowitz, Stuart M. M.D., Epididymitis nodosa: an epididymal lesion analogous to vasitis nodosa., *Archives of Pathology and Laboratory Medicine*, 110, 61-64, January, 1986.

- Schuman, L. M.; Coulson, A. H.; Mandel, J. S.; Massey, F. J.; O'Fallon, W. M., Health status of American men-a study of post-vasectomy sequelae., *Journal of Clinical Epidemiology*, 46: 8, 697-958, August, 1993.

- Schwager, Edward J., Treatment of bacterial prostatitis., *American Family Physician*, 44: 6, 2137-2141, December, 1991.

- Schwartzman, Robert J.; McLellan, Toni L., Reflex sympathetic dystrophy: A review., *Archives of Neurology*, 44, 555-561, May, 1987.

- Schwingl PJ, Guess HA, Safety and effectiveness of vasectomy., *Fertility and Sterility*, 73: 5, 923-36, May, 2000.

- Sebben, Jack E., The hazards of electrosurgery., *Journal of the American Academy of Dermatology*, 16: 4, 869-871, April, 1987.

- Seidl, J.; Brotzman, G., The rate of hydrocele perforation during vasectomy. Is perforation dangerous?, *Journal of Family Practice*, 49: 6, 537-40, June, 2000.

- Selikowitz, Stuart M.; Schned, Alan R., A Late Post Vasectomy Syndrome., *The Journal of Urology*, 134, 494–7, September, 1985.

- Shafik, A., Electrovasogram in normal and vasectomized men and patients with obstructive azoospermia and absent vas deferens., *Archives of Andrology*, 36: 1, 67-79, January-February, 1996.

- Shafik, A., Electrovasography in normal and vasectomized men before and after reversal., *International Journal of Urology*, 19: 1, 33-8, February, 1996.

- Shahani, S. K.; Hattikudur, N. S., Immunological consequences of vasectomy., *Archives of Andrology*, 7: 2, 193-9, September, 1981.

- Shapiro, E. I.; Silber, S. J., Open-ended vasectomy, sperm granuloma, and post-vasectomy orchialgia., *Fertility and Sterility*, 32: 5, 546-50, November, 1979.

- Sharma, J.; Sadasukhi, T. C., Infectious complications of vasectomy: a study of 200 cases., *International Surgery*, 68: 1, 79-80, January-March, 1983.

- Shearer, G. M.; Hurtenbach, U., Is sperm immunosuppressive in male homosexuals and vasectomized men? *Immunology Today*, 3, 153, 1982.

- Sherlock, D. J.; Holl-Allen, R. T. J., Delayed spontaneous recanalization of the vas deferens., *British Journal of Surgery*, 71, 532-533, July, 1984.

- Shiraishi, K.; Takihara, H.; Naito, K., Influence of interstitial fibrosis on spermatogenesis after vasectomy and vasovasostomy., *Contraception*, 65: 3, 245-249, March 2002.

- Shoskes, D. A.; Zeitlin, S. I.; Rajfer, J., Quercetin in men with category III chronic prostatitis: A preliminary prospective, double blind, placebo-controlled trial., *Urology*, 54: 6, 960-3, December, 1999.

- Silber, Sherman J., Reversal of vasectomy and the treatment of male infertility., *Journal of Andrology*, 1, 261-268, November- December, 1980.

- Simon, H.; Etkin, M. J.; Godine, J. E.; Heller, D.; Kuter, I.; Shellito, P. C.; Stern, T. A.; Peckham, C., What Is Vasectomy?, [Online], http://webM.D..lycos.com/content/dmk/dmk_article_40087, September, 1998.

- Smith, J. C.; Cranston, D.; O'Brein, T.; Guillebaud, J.; Hindmarsh, J.; Turner. A. G., Fatherhood without apparent spermatozoa after vasectomy., *Lancet*, 344: 8914, 30, July 2, 1994.

- Smith, K. D.; Tcholakian, R. K.; Chowdhury, M.; Steinberger, E., An investigation of plasma hormone levels before and after vasectomy., *Fertility and Sterility*, 27: 2, 144-51, February, 1976.

- Soderdahl, Dougla W., Vasectomy: The most unkindest cut of all?, *Surgery, Gynecology and Obstetrics*, 155:5, 734-736, November, 1982.

- Sokal, D.; McMullen, S.; Gates, D.; Dominik, R., A comparison study of the no scalpel and standard incision approaches to vasectomy in 5 counties. The Male Sterilization Investigator Team., *Journal of Urology*, 162: 5, 1621-5, November, 1999.

- Sokol, Rebecca Z., Endocrinology and male infertility., *Infertility and Reproductive Medicine of North America*, 10: 3, 427-434, July, 1999.

- Stanford, J. L.; Wicklund, K. G.; McKnight, B,; Daling, J. R.; Brawer, M. K., Vasectomy and risk of prostate cancer., *Cancer Epidemiology, Biomarkers and Prevention*, 8: 10, 881-6, October, 1999.

- Starling, J. R.; Harms, B. A.; Schroeder, M. E.; Eichman, P. L., Diagnosis and treatment of genitofemoral and ilioinguinal entrapment neuralgia., *Surgery*, 102:4, 581-586, October, 1987.

- Starling, James R.; Harms, Bruce A., Diagnosis and treatment of genitofemoral and ilioinguinal neuralgia., *World Journal of Surgery*, 13:5, 586-591, September/October, 1989.

- Stulz, P.; Pfeiffer, K. M., Peripheral nerve injuries resulting from common surgical procedures in the lower portion of the abdomen., *Archives of Surgery*, 117: 3, 324-327, March, 1982.

- Stump, Bill, Are you ready for vasectomy?, *Men's Health,* December 2001, 112-115.

- Sweeney, P.; Tan, J.; Butler, M. R.; McDermott, T. E.; Grainger, R.; Thornhill, J. A., Epididymectomy in the management of intrascrotal disease: a critical reappraisal., *British Journal of Urology*, 81: 5, 753-5, May, 1998.

- Taguchi, Yosh M.D., <u>Private Parts: An Owner's Guide to the Male Anatomy</u>., McClelland & Stewart, Inc., The Canadian Publishers, Toronto, 1996.

- TCR Public Newsletter, Montrose General: Botched Vasectomy Victim Gets Record Award in Philadelphia. [Online] <u>http://bankrupt.com/CARPublic/</u> 991004.MBX, downloaded 11/6/2001.

- Testicular self-examination., (anonymous), *Postgraduate Medicine*, 105: 4, 241, April, 1999.

- Testosterone-Fertility.com, [online] www.testosterone-fertility.com, downloaded 9/30/03.

- Theodoskas, Jason M.D.; Feinberg, David T. M.D., <u>Don't Let Your HMO Kill You</u>, Routledge Publishing, 2000.

- Thompson, B.; MacGregor, J. E.; MacGillivray, I.; Garvie, W. H., Experience with sperm counts following vasectomy., *British Journal of Urology*, 68: 3, 230-3, September, 1991.

- Tripathy, S. P.; Ramachandran, C. R.; Ramachandran, P., Health consequences of vasectomy in India., *Bulletin of the World Health Organization*, 72: 5, 779-82, 1994.

- Tung, Kenneth S. K.; Teuscher, Cory; Goldberg, Ellen H.; Wild, Gaynor, Genetic control of antisperm autoantibody response in vasectomized guinea pigs., *Journal of Immunology*, 127:3, 835-839, September, 1981.

- Tung, Kenneth S. K., Department of Pathology, University of Virginia, Charlottesville, VA 22908; Teuscher, Cory, Department of Microbiology, Brigham Young University, Provo, UT 84602, Untitled research article regarding autoimmune orchitis and oophoritis dated August 5, 1994.

- Tung, Kenneth S. K.; Unanue, Emil R.; Dixon, Frank J., The immunopathology of experimental allergic orchitis., *American Journal of Pathology*, 60: 3, 313-327, September, 1970.

- Tung, Kenneth S. K.; Unanue, Emil R.; Dixon, Frank J., Pathogenesis of experimental allergic orchitis: The role of antibody., *Journal of Immunology*, 106: 6, 1463-1472, June, 1971.

- Turek, Paul J., Infections, immunology, and male infertility., *Infertility and Reproductive Medicine Clinics of North America*, 10: 3, 435-470, July, 1999.

- Tverskoy, Mark; Cozacov, Carlos Ayache; Bradley, Edwin L.; Kissin, Igor, Postoperative pain after inguinal herniorrhaphy with different types of anesthesia., *Anesthesia and Analgesia*, 70: 1, 29-35, January, 1990.

- Upadhyaya, M.; Hibbard, B. M,; Walker, S. M., Antisperm antibodies and male infertility., *British Journal of Urology*, 56, 531-536, 1984.

- Urology Forum, epididymectomy page., [Online], http//medhlp.netusa.net/forums/urology/messages/C30278-23.html downloaded July 4, 2000.

- Van Der Poel H. G.; Meuleman, E. J., Post-vasectomy pain, an underestimated side-effect., [Online], <u>http://www.uroweb.org/androweb/special/postvasectomy/body/shtml</u>, last updated June 17,1999.

- Vasectomymedical.com, No-scalpel vasectomy; post-vasectomy pain. [online] http://www.vasectomymedical.com/no-scalpel-vasectomy-pain.html updated 8/15/02.

- Verajankorva, E.; Martikainen, M.; Saraste, A,; Sundstrom, J.; Pollanen, P., Sperm antibodies in rat models of male hormonal contraception and vasectomy., *Reproduction, Fertility and Development*, 11: 1, 49-57, 1999.

- Verhulst, A. P.; Hoekstra, J. W., Paternity after bilateral vasectomy., *BJU International*, 83: 3, 280-2, February, 1999.

- Viddeleer, A. C.; Lycklama a Nijeholt, G. A., Lethal Fournier's gangrene following vasectomy., *Journal of Urology*, 147: 6, 1613-4, June, 1992.

- Walker, A. M.; Jick, H.; Hunter, J. R.; Danord, A.; Rothman, K. J., Hospitalization rates in vasectomized men., *JAMA*, 245: 22, 2315-7, June 12, 1981.

- Wallace, D. M. A.; Gunter, P. A.; Landon, G. V.; Pugh, R. C. B.; Hendry, W. F., Sympathetic orchiopathia- an experimental and clinical study., *British Journal of Urology*, 54, 765-768, 1982.

- Wallace, D. M. A.; Hendry, W. F.; Gunter, P. A.; Landon, G. V.; Pugh, R. C. B., Sympathetic orchiopathia., *Lancet*, 2: 8256, 1173, November 21, 1981.

- WebM.D., Chronic Pain. [online] http://my.webM.D..com/content/article/1680.50737 downloaded 10/31/02.

- WebM.D./World Health Organization (1990), Three-Step Analgesic Ladder., [online] at http://my.webM.D..com/content/dmk/dmk_article_3961306 downloaded 10/14/00.

- Weiske, WH, Vasectomy., *Andologia*, 33: 3, 125-134, May, 2001.

- Wen, R. Q.; Li, S. Q.; Wang, C. X.; Wang, Q. H.; Li, Q. K.; Feng, H. M.; Jiang, Y. J.; Huang, J. C., Analysis of spermatozoa from the proximal vas deferens of vasectomized men., *International Journal of Andrology*, 17: 4, 181-5, August, 1994.

- West, A. F.; Leung, H. Y.; Powell, P. H., Epididymectomy is an effective treatment for scrotal pain after vasectomy., *BJU International*, 85: 9, 1097-1099, June, 2000.

- Whyte, J.; Sarrat, R.; Cisneros, A. I.; Whyte, A.; Mazo, R.; Torres, A.; Lazaro, J., The vasectomized testis., *International Surgery*, 85: 2, 167-174, April-June, 2000.

- Wiest, W. M.; Janke, L. D., A methodological critique of research on psychological effects of vasectomy., *Psychosomatic Medicine*, 36: 5, 438-49, September-October, 1974.

- Wildschut, H. I.; Monincx, W., Vasectomy and the risk of prostate cancer., *Bulletin of the World Health Organization*, 72: 5, 777-8, 1994.

- Williams, David G., Virtuoso on a minor scale., *Alternatives for the Health-Conscious Individual*, 9: 16, 121-124, October, 2002.

- Williams, Dorie; Swicegood, Gray; Clark, Margaret P.; Bean, Frank D, Masculinity-femininity and the desire for sexual intercourse after vasectomy., *Social Psychology Quarterly*, 43: 3, 347-352, 1980.

- Wilson, Charles L., No-needle anesthetic for no-scalpel vasectomy., *American Family Physician*, 63:7, 1295, April 1,2001.

- Winters, S. J., Inhibin is released together with testosterone by the human testis., *Journal of Clinical Endocrinology and Metabolism*, 70: 2, 548-50, February, 1990.

- Winters, S. J., Current status of testosterone replacement therapy in men., *Archives of Family Medicine*, 8: 3, 257-63, May-June, 1999.

- Witkin, S. S.; Shahani, S. K.; Gupta, S.; Good, R. A.; Day, Noorbibi K., Demonstration of IgG Fe receptors on spermatozoa and their utilization for the detection of circulating immune complexes in human serum., *Clinical and Experimental Immunology*, 41: 3, 441-452, September, 1980.

- Witt, Michael A.; Heron, Sean; Lipshultz, Larry I., The post-vasectomy length of the testicular vassal remnant: A predictor of surgical outcome in microscopic vasectomy reversal., *Journal of Urology*, 151: 4, 892-894, April, 1994.

- Wolfers, David and Helen, Vasectomania., *Family Planning Perspectives*, 5: 4, 196-199, Fall, 1973.

- Wolfers, Helen, Psychological aspects of vasectomy., *British Medical Journal*, 4: 730, 297-300, October 31, 1970.

- Woolf, C. J.; Chong, M. S., Preemptive analgesia-treating postoperative pain by preventing the establishment of central sensitization., *Anesthesia and Analgesia*, 77: 2, 362-379, August, 1993.

- Wyburn, M. R., Sympathetic orchiopathia., *Lancet*, 2: 8260-61, 1417-1418, December 19-26, 1981.

- Yamamoto, M.; Hibi, H.; Katsuno, S.; Miyake,. K, Management of chronic orchialgia of unknown etiology., *International Journal of Urology*, 2: 1, 47-9, March, 1995.

- Yee, Andrew J.; Silver, Lee M., Contraceptive vaccine formulations with sperm proteins., *Reproductive Immunology*, chapter 33, 693-712, 1996.

- Zaninovich, Lou, <u>Vasectomy-before and after</u>., Infinity Publishing, Haverford, PA, <u>www.buybooksontheweb.com</u> 2002.

- Ziegler, Fredrick J.; Rodgers, David A.; Kriegman, Sali Ann, Effect of vasectomy on psychological functioning., *Psychosomatic Medicine*, 28: 1, 50-63, January/February 1966.

- Ziegler, Fredrick J.; Rodgers, David A.; Prentiss, Robert J., Psychosocial response to Vasectomy., *Archives of General Psychiatry*, 21, 46-54, July, 1969.

- Zhengwei, Y.; Wreford, N. G.; Royce, P.; de Kretser, D. M.; McLachlan, R. I., Stereological evaluation of human spermatogenesis after suppression by testosterone treatment: Heterogeneous pattern of spermatogenic impairment., *Journal of Clinical Endocrinology and Metabolism*, April 1998; 83: 4, 1284 –1291.

- Zorn, B. H.; Rauchenwald, M.; Steers, W. D., Periprostatic injection of local anesthesia for relief of chronic orchialgia., *Journal of Urology*, pt. 2, 151, 411A, abstract #735, 1994.

Index

ABC News, 18, 192, 223
abortion, 197
acupuncture, 37, 38, 41, 54, 55, 180, 195, 238
adrenal gland, 46, 150
aggressive surgical debridement, 76
AIDS, 92
allium, 184
analgesic, 41, 135, 242
anastomosis, 80
Androgel, 119, 120, 121, 124, 126, 180
andropause, 122, 123
androstenedione, 89
anesthesia, 13, 50, 54, 56, 67, 69, 130, 135, 136, 137, 138, 140, 144, 153, 166, 168, 179, 180, 208, 220, 241, 243
antibiotic, 53, 58, 61, 64, 76, 77
antibody titre, 178
anti-convulsant, 135, 179
anti-depressant, 19, 179
antigen, 92, 95, 96, 106, 128, 225, 233
anti-inflammatories, 179, 217
antioxidant, 62, 184
anti-seizure medication, 40, 103, 135, 179
antisperm antibodies, 92, 93, 95, 99, 103, 104, 105, 107, 110, 118, 147, 149, 169, 181, 212, 214, 215, 223, 225, 226, 229, 230, 231, 232
arteriosclerosis, 149
arteriovenous fistula, 198, 224
atherosclerosis, 79, 94, 95, 149, 212, 214, 223
atrophy, 24, 104
audio-frequency therapy, 180, 227
autoimmune, 3, 76, 92, 93, 94, 95, 96, 99, 100, 103, 104, 105, 106, 107, 108, 118, 122, 123, 125, 133, 134, 137, 144, 145, 147, 148, 149, 157, 160, 166, 169, 178, 181, 188, 193, 195, 201, 202, 212, 239, 241
autoimmune orchitis, 99, 100, 104, 106, 122, 147, 149
AVSC, 110
barrier, 103, 104, 110, 118, 165, 166, 215
bilateral, 29, 52, 76, 104, 168, 180, 216, 226, 242
biofeedback, 180
bioflavenoid, 62
biological mechanism, 98, 150
blood supply, 53, 58, 136, 178, 197
blood-testis barrier, 104
Botox, 153
breast carcinoma, 95
buccal, 126
bupivicaine, 168
cadmium, 184
carbocaine, 141
cardiac arrest, 144, 198
Dr. Malcolm Carruthers, 6, 27, 90, 94, 95, 100, 110, 115, 122, 123, 124, 133, 171, 174, 185, 197, 198, 213, 214, 218, 219, 226
castration, 5, 89, 90, 114, 115, 117, 118, 137, 144, 177, 195, 196, 199, 217
cauda epididymis, 133
causalgia, 137, 149
cauterization, 32, 33, 54, 239
CBS News, 157
Celebrex, 180
cellulitis, 75

cervical cap, 165
chirocaine, 141
chiropractic, 180
chiropractor, 41
chromosome, 82, 99
chronic post-vasectomy testicular pain, 47, 104, 146
chronic testicular pain, 16, 19, 20, 58, 79, 82, 110, 135, 136, 145, 147, 149, 177, 178, 196, 212, 213, 215, 216, 223, 224, 227, 231, 235
circumcision, 6
coital, 112, 232
Complex Regional Pain Syndrome, 137
complication, 6, 10, 52, 76, 86, 87, 106, 110, 111, 116, 144, 147, 168, 171, 173, 195, 196, 198, 212, 213, 215, 224, 228
condoms, 165, 167, 200
congestive epididymitis, 46, 144, 146, 196, 212
contraception, 3, 9, 12, 21, 82, 105, 106, 107, 108, 115, 148, 161, 163, 164, 165, 166, 167, 178, 192, 200, 201, 205, 212, 214, 235, 238, 242
contraceptive vaccine, 104, 106
contraindication, 25, 116
contralateral, 118
cord block, 38, 49, 50, 53, 55, 187
corticosteroids, 108, 123, 180
cost shifting, 130, 131
counseling, 38, 41, 75, 78, 110, 114, 115, 128, 173, 180, 187, 212, 213, 215, 216, 219, 228, 233
Couple to Couple League, 165
cremaster muscle, 28, 137, 178
Crohn's disease, 169
cross-reaction, 94
cryptorchidism, 167
Crystal Wand, 152
cysts, 10, 23, 46, 100, 107, 110, 125, 136, 145, 146, 149, 161, 168, 179, 201, 213, 237
death, 21, 22, 40, 76, 77, 89, 90, 115, 116, 135, 145, 165, 172, 195, 230
dehydroepiandrosterone, 89
denervation, 133, 136, 137, 178, 197, 223, 226, 231, 234
dexamethasone, 180
DHEA, 123
diabetes, 94, 110, 150, 236
diaphragm, 83, 113, 163, 165, 200
dietary measures, 184
digestive distress, 41
digital rectal exam, 63
dihydrotestosterone, 89, 236
disclose, 53, 145, 148, 170, 171, 173, 174, 185, 195
dissonance reduction, 113
dorsal, 135, 168, 217
Dr. Lou Zaninovich, 158
ejaculation, 28, 47, 56, 81, 111, 114, 115, 133, 147, 152, 164, 168, 176, 185, 195, 197, 215, 220, 226, 228
electric muscle stimulation, 180
electro-cautery, 30, 201
electroejaculation, 56
ELMA, 168
endogenous, 122
endometriosis, 118
epididymal cyst, 100, 125, 149
epididymal pain, 52, 212, 213

epididymectomy, 52, 53, 136, 137, 147, 177, 195, 196, 198, 216, 217, 219, 222, 237, 241
epididymis, 25, 28, 35, 45, 46, 47, 48, 52, 53, 58, 64, 80, 81, 93, 94, 104, 108, 118, 125, 133, 146, 147, 178, 181, 196, 205, 212, 213, 214, 215, 216, 217, 218, 220, 222, 229, 232, 235, 237
epididymitis, 6, 25, 35, 46, 48, 62, 64, 76, 110, 125, 144, 146, 149, 161, 167, 195, 196, 198, 201, 212, 215, 217, 218, 220, 239
epidural, 50, 55, 67, 68, 73, 168, 179
erectile dysfunction, 25, 123, 176, 178, 196, 224, 225
estradiol, 123
estrogen, 62
etiology, 98, 105, 216, 243
eugenic, 6
Experimental Autoimmune Orchitis, 104
experimental autoimmunization, 94
expert witness, 174
extravasation, 46, 214
fallopian tubes, 165
family planning, 8, 9, 12, 86
fertilization, 22, 81, 99, 166
fibromyalgia, 169
flecanide, 139
follicle-stimulating, 28, 89, 91, 103, 236
Fournier's gangrene, 76, 199, 237, 242
Free Androgen Index, 181
friable, 28, 47
gag order, 128
gangrene, 76, 149, 195, 198, 227
gatekeeper, 127
germ cells, 99
granuloma, 46, 47, 57, 72, 80, 85, 86, 94, 100, 107, 133, 146, 147, 149, 161, 179, 195, 197, 201, 212, 213, 215, 216, 217, 218, 225, 226, 239, 240
Graves' disease, 169
groin, 15, 16, 17, 19, 22, 25, 28, 32, 37, 38, 41, 42, 44, 49, 52, 63, 70, 79, 121, 124, 136, 137, 139, 144, 154, 168, 173, 176, 177, 178, 187, 189, 197, 205, 208, 218, 220
haploid, 92
Dr. Alex Heidenreich, 16, 178, 179, 197, 216, 231
hematoma, 47, 76, 86, 110, 149, 168, 198, 212
hemostat, 48, 54
hepatitis, 150
hernia, 17, 32, 63, 94, 167, 168, 189, 197
HLA, 169
HMO, 42, 127, 129, 131, 145, 158, 202, 205, 220, 222, 241
homeostasis, 90
homosexual, 93, 224, 240
hormonal, 3, 27, 76, 90, 91, 95, 114, 122, 123, 124, 145, 149, 166, 167, 168, 177, 212, 214, 242
hormone, 62, 89, 90, 91, 95, 103, 107, 117, 118, 119, 120, 123, 124, 125, 126, 136, 161, 163, 165, 166, 167, 169, 178, 179, 181, 201, 204, 232, 236, 240
HRT, 124
hydrocele, 23, 24, 25, 125, 133, 149, 167, 168, 178, 239
hydrocortisone, 100, 180
hypercholesterolaemia, 167
hypertension, 167
hypnotherapy, 180
hypoglycemia, 95, 150
hypogonadism, 91, 232
hysterectomy, 165, 206, 231
ICSI, 81, 99, 225
IgA, 93

IgG, 93, 243
IgM, 93
immune compliment, 94
immune system, 81, 91, 92, 93, 94, 96, 100, 103, 105, 107, 108, 145, 147, 148, 169, 180, 195, 201, 211, 238
immunobead assay, 104, 125, 169, 181
immunosurveillance, 95, 98
impotence, 40, 56, 114, 115, 135, 149, 195, 212
incision, 32, 48, 146, 173, 177, 207, 208, 226, 240
infection, 32, 34, 35, 46, 47, 53, 58, 64, 75, 76, 86, 92, 94, 100, 110, 149, 168, 189, 198, 199, 212, 215, 217, 218, 238
infertility, 23, 56, 81, 99, 100, 103, 104, 113, 115, 189, 225, 226, 230, 232, 240, 241
Infinite Mind, 18, 33, 232
inflammation, 25, 35, 38, 62, 64, 73, 86, 94, 100, 103, 104, 107, 110, 125, 137, 147, 149, 154, 169, 176, 187, 196, 201, 216, 217, 218, 230
informed consent, 157, 170, 171, 173, 174, 192, 213, 214
inguinal, 28, 32, 104, 136, 137, 167, 168, 192, 197, 203, 216, 229, 241
inguinal orchiectomy, 177
insurance, 12, 38, 42, 48, 66, 67, 115, 127, 128, 129, 130, 131, 144, 145, 148, 158, 161, 162, 174, 177, 192, 202, 205
intercourse, 32, 46, 47, 82, 85, 113, 114, 115, 164, 166, 176, 242
Internet, 10, 12, 32, 46, 52, 96, 107, 110, 144, 152, 156, 157, 167, 197, 198, 205, 237
interstitial fibrosis, 46, 48, 122, 240
intraepithelial vesicle, 99
intravenous lidocaine infusion, 138
in-vitro fertilization, 81
IUD, 113, 166, 206
joint pain, 94
Jon Kabat-Zinn, 41, 96, 180
Journal of the American Medical Association, 87, 96, 229
Journal of Urology, 6, 32, 52, 76, 91, 110, 212, 213, 214, 215, 223, 224, 225, 226, 227, 228, 229, 230, 231, 232, 233, 234, 235, 236, 237, 238, 239, 240, 241, 242, 243
kidney, 52, 94, 95, 103, 145, 149, 212, 214
kidney stone, 95
late post-vasectomy syndrome, 52, 213
L-Carnitine, 205
legal liability, 111, 162, 177
Leydig cells, 124
Li method, 17, 228, 234, 242
libido, 90, 112, 113, 118, 119, 121, 149, 160
lidocaine, 41, 50, 69, 70, 138, 139
ligation, 9, 113, 180, 195, 234, 237
litigation, 53, 86, 145, 173, 212, 214
liver, 150
local anesthetic, 50, 53, 54, 168, 207, 208
loss of consortium, 173
lumbar, 41
lung cancer, 95, 98, 149
Lupron, 118, 119
lupus, 92, 149, 169
luteinizing hormone, 28, 89, 90, 91, 236
lymph, 27, 28, 125, 133, 134, 137, 150, 178, 189, 201, 212, 229
macrophages, 99, 147
male menopause, 99, 115, 122
malpractice insurance, 172, 173, 174
marcaine, 50, 141
medical malpractice, 173, 174
meditation, 41, 46
melanoma, 95

membrane stabilizers, 135
MESA, 81
methyl testosterone, 123
methylprednisolone, 180
microsurgery, 53, 55, 62, 79, 80
migraine, 95, 150
mindfulness training, 41
mitral valve, 76
morbidity, 95, 146, 214
motile, 28, 81, 86, 144
motility, 93, 103, 205
MRI, 82, 100, 154
multiple immunologic responses, 94, 105
multiple myeloma, 95, 149
multiple sclerosis, 94, 95, 150, 169, 212
mumps, 110, 122, 167
myocardial infarction, 76, 95, 226, 238
myofascial release, 151, 153, 180
narcolepsy, 95, 150
narcotic, 13, 33, 60, 135, 139, 148
National Cancer Institute, 93, 224, 234, 236
National Institute of Health, 6, 28, 46, 89, 92, 94, 95, 96, 97,
    167
nausea, 15, 16, 34, 52, 70, 218
Nazi, 6
necrectomy, 76
neoplasm, 196
nerve block, 49, 136, 137, 139, 140, 179, 187
nerve damage, 117, 126, 133, 135, 136, 148, 154, 174, 177,
    187, 201, 202, 204, 220
nerve entrapment, 134, 212
neuralgia, 19, 149, 240, 241
neurectomy, 178
neurogenic inflammation, 154, 203
neurography, 154, 203
Neurontin, 40, 135, 139, 140
neuropathic pain, 33, 230
neuropathy, 136, 189, 202, 235
New England Journal of Medicine, 95, 184, 202, 229, 230, 232,
    235, 239
New Times, 157
nociceptive pain, 33, 168
No-Needle Anesthetic, 168
non-Hodgkin's lymphoma, 95, 149
no-scalpel vasectomy, 12, 31, 48, 54, 86, 146, 168, 169, 174,
    234, 242
OB-GYN, 9, 10
oestrone, 89
open-ended vasectomy, 47, 48, 49, 53, 54, 55, 80, 85, 146, 147,
    161, 168, 178, 195, 216, 238
opiate, 60
opiod, 135, 229, 239
oral contraceptive, 113, 185
orchialgia, 149, 195, 213, 215, 227, 231, 234, 240, 243
Orchidometer, 28
orchiectomy, 136, 137, 147, 216, 229, 235
orchitis, 53, 99, 103, 104, 106, 122, 196, 214, 225, 228, 238,
    239, 241
orthopedic consultation, 178
pain management, 18, 38, 42, 44, 46, 58, 111, 221, 222
paracrine, 122
pathogenesis, 82, 98
pelvic floor muscles, 151
pelvic floor release, 151, 152
pelvic plexus, 136

penis, 25, 49, 58, 136, 137, 173, 183, 184, 187, 216
perineum, 135
peripheral nerves, 132, 135, 137
personality disturbances, 149
Peyronie's disease, 25
phlebitis, 94, 149
photon therapy, 186, 187, 188, 189
physical therapy, 107, 144, 180, 221
Physicians Desk Reference, 48
pituitary gland, 28, 89, 90, 107, 118, 124, 222
Planned Parenthood, 9
polyphenols, 184
post-vasectomy pain syndrome, 48, 52, 53, 58, 60, 64, 82, 104,
    131, 132, 135, 137, 144, 146, 147, 149, 161, 173, 174, 185,
    187, 191, 195, 196, 197, 205, 212, 216, 222, 225, 236
post-vasectomy syndrome, 46, 52, 82, 213
pouch, 165
PPO, 129
Prednisone, 38, 39, 108, 123, 181
pregnenolone, 89
premature ejaculation, 56, 114
progesterone, 124, 125, 166, 180
progestin, 166, 230
prolactin, 123
Proscar, 184
prostate, 6, 10, 14, 25, 28, 62, 79, 89, 90, 94, 95, 96, 97, 98, 99,
    111, 118, 123, 124, 128, 135, 136, 148, 149, 151, 164, 166,
    176, 184, 185, 197, 199, 212, 214, 215, 220, 221, 224, 226,
    227, 228, 229, 230, 232, 233, 236, 237, 238, 239, 240, 242
prostate cancer, 25, 89, 96, 97, 98, 99, 124, 149, 164, 176, 184,
    212
prostatic fluid, 98
prostatitis, 25, 48, 62, 76, 96, 131, 149, 151, 176, 196, 197,
    220, 233, 235, 238, 239, 240
PSA, 124, 176, 184
psoriasis, 169
psychological, 96, 112, 113, 114, 115, 116, 117, 145, 177, 181,
    187, 225, 231, 242, 243
pulmonary embolism, 95, 149
PVPS. *See* post-vasectomy pain syndrome
Quercetin, 62, 180, 240
reanastomosis, 103
recanalization, 48, 85, 133, 148, 197, 239, 240
rectum, 14
reflex sympathetic dystrophy (RSD), 137, 173, 186, 187
rete testes, 104
rheumatoid arthritis, 92, 94, 149, 169, 212
rhythm method, 165
RISUG, 166
RONSI, 81
rupture, 45, 46, 47, 100, 133, 146, 147, 178, 201, 215
sacral plexus, 135
sacrum, 138
Saw Palmento, 184
scalpel, 10, 12, 31, 32, 48, 54, 55, 86, 137, 144, 145, 146, 168,
    178, 192, 201, 207, 217, 234, 237, 240, 242
scrotal abscess, 75
scrotal orchiectomy, 177
scrotal pain, 46, 82, 110, 111, 168, 173, 195, 196, 212, 213,
    215, 242
scrotum, 10, 12, 13, 14, 23, 24, 25, 28, 29, 30, 31, 32, 33, 43,
    47, 54, 58, 64, 69, 76, 83, 100, 124, 125, 135, 136, 137, 166,
    168, 173, 177, 184, 187, 198, 201, 207, 208, 237
sedation, 48, 67, 68, 70, 139, 141
selenium, 184

semen analysis, 77, 109, 181, 197, 212
seminal vesicle, 94, 221
seminiferous tubules, 48, 223
sexually transmitted diseases, 8, 165
shave, 12, 187
smooth muscle, 28, 227
special clamping device, 31
sperm, 10, 21, 27, 28, 30, 45, 46, 47, 48, 54, 56, 57, 58, 79, 80,
    81, 83, 85, 86, 87, 89, 90, 91, 92, 93, 94, 95, 96, 98, 100,
    103, 104, 105, 106, 107, 108, 110, 115, 118, 119, 122, 124,
    125, 126, 133, 137, 144, 146, 147, 148, 149, 161, 163, 164,
    165, 166, 169, 178, 180, 182, 183, 184, 192, 197, 201, 205,
    212, 213, 214, 215, 216, 217, 222, 223, 225, 227, 234, 235,
    237, 240, 241, 243
sperm antibodies, 92, 93, 94, 103, 148
sperm autoantibody, 93, 95
spermatic cord, 22, 28, 29, 32, 49, 52, 58, 64, 111, 133, 136,
    137, 147, 177, 179, 187, 195, 196, 197, 198, 204, 213, 215,
    223, 231, 234, 238
spermatids, 122
spermatocele, 110, 125, 149, 161, 201, 236
spermatozoa, 46, 80, 104, 147, 197, 216, 224, 232, 233, 234,
    240, 242, 243
spinal cord stimulator, 154
squamous cell carcinoma, 95
standard bilateral vasectomy, 29, 76
Standard of Care, 174
Staph infection, 75, 76, 100, 149, 197
sterilization, 5, 6, 8, 9, 21, 87, 90, 97, 110, 112, 113, 114, 116,
    149, 162, 165, 167, 192, 212, 223, 225, 228, 229, 230
steroid, 179, 180, 231
Steroli cells, 122
stitch, 32, 48, 55, 69
stress management, 41, 129, 180
suffering, 22, 76, 157, 161, 167, 168, 220, 221
Superior Hypogastric Nerve Block, 138
suture, 198
sympathetic opthalmia, 118
sympathetic orchiopathia, 104, 118, 177
Tantra, 182
TENS, 43, 44, 180
testalgia, 149, 231
testicle, 10, 22, 23, 24, 25, 27, 28, 47, 52, 53, 54, 58, 69, 75, 76,
    99, 104, 118, 126, 136, 147, 152, 157, 168, 177, 181, 182,
    189, 196, 197, 198, 199, 218, 219, 220, 229
testicles, 12, 15, 16, 17, 23, 25, 27, 28, 29, 35, 38, 41, 45, 46,
    47, 52, 58, 62, 67, 76, 79, 80, 82, 89, 93, 99, 100, 101, 104,
    106, 107, 108, 109, 111, 117, 119, 121, 122, 124, 125, 129,
    131, 135, 136, 143, 146, 149, 152, 153, 154, 157, 160, 163,
    173, 176, 177, 178, 181, 182, 183, 188, 192, 196, 197, 198,
    201, 203, 204, 208, 218, 219, 220, 222
testicular artery, 178, 197
testicular atrophy, 23, 125, 136, 166, 176, 178, 189, 196, 216
testicular biopsies, 122
testicular cancer, 22, 95, 149, 181, 212
testicular massage, 182
testicular pain, 16, 19, 20, 34, 41, 47, 53, 58, 79, 82, 104, 110,
    135, 136, 145, 147, 149, 177, 178, 182, 184, 189, 195, 196,
    197, 212, 213, 215, 216, 222, 223, 224, 226, 227, 231, 235
testicular self-exam, 11, 163, 169, 181
testicular sonography, 178
testicular torsion, 25
testicular ultrasound, 17, 35, 125

testis, 91, 93, 100, 104, 110, 118, 122, 133, 146, 147, 185, 192,
    195, 197, 212, 213, 214, 215, 218, 228, 229, 232, 237, 239,
    242, 243
testosterone, 23, 27, 28, 89, 90, 91, 96, 107, 108, 118, 119, 120,
    121, 122, 123, 124, 125, 126, 133, 137, 149, 166, 168, 179,
    181, 185, 188, 219, 222, 224, 225, 226, 230, 232, 235, 236,
    241, 243
testosterone implant, 126
testosterone therapy, 107, 108, 122, 124, 125, 180, 181, 206,
    222
thermal imaging, 188
thrombophlebitis, 94, 95, 212
thymectomy, 104
tolerogenic, 93
transrectal ultrasound, 178
traumatic neuroma, 73, 134, 174, 201
Tribulus Terrestris, 122
tricyclic antidepressant, 135
trigger-point injection, 153, 201
trophic nerves, 118
tubal ligation, 165, 206
tubular dilatation, 46, 122, 147
tumorigenesis, 95
U. S. Department of Health and Human Services, 6, 46, 92
unilateral, 52, 239
unmyelinated C-fibers, 135
urinalysis, 77
urologist, 5, 10, 11, 12, 15, 17, 22, 25, 34, 35, 38, 39, 40, 46,
    48, 51, 52, 53, 55, 56, 58, 62, 75, 77, 80, 85, 99, 107, 109,
    111, 117, 130, 135, 136, 137, 145, 154, 158, 161, 171, 172,
    173, 174, 187, 192, 199, 200, 205, 206, 219, 220, 222
USA Today, 157
uterus, 165
varicocele, 23, 167, 234, 237
vas deferens, 28, 31, 32, 45, 53, 79, 110, 133, 137, 146, 148,
    168, 181, 182, 213, 214, 215, 221, 225, 227, 228, 237, 239,
    240, 242
vasectomy failure, 86, 87
vasectomy reversal, 78, 79, 80, 82, 99, 103, 133, 147, 148, 192,
    195, 196, 197, 213, 217, 219, 222, 231, 234, 238, 243
vasitis nodosa, 86, 110, 147, 149, 161, 197, 215, 233, 239
vasoepididymostomy, 55, 80, 81, 178
vasovasostomy, 79, 80, 82, 133, 148, 178, 214, 215, 220, 223,
    224, 225, 226, 228, 229, 234, 237, 240
Vice-Grip Empathy Test, 16, 18
Wayne Dyer, 15
withdrawal method, 164
Wobenzym, 180
World Health Organization, 96, 98, 99, 107, 124, 125, 135,
    160, 180, 228, 230, 241, 242
yoga, 41, 42, 180
Dr. Lou Zaninovich, 158, 243
zero population growth, 191
zinc, 205
Zoladex, 118

Author Kevin Hauber makes his home with his family on the Central Coast of California. When he's not undergoing some kind of unsavory medical procedure because of his botched vasectomy, he works as mortgage loan officer giving away his company's money. The company even likes it that way. Kevin is the father of two lovely children and the lucky husband of a wonderful woman, all of whom have put up with a tremendous amount of grief due to his vasectomy medical experience. Hopefully, you won't have to endure the same kind of problems given what you find out in this book. With any luck, you will find out what you need to know in time.

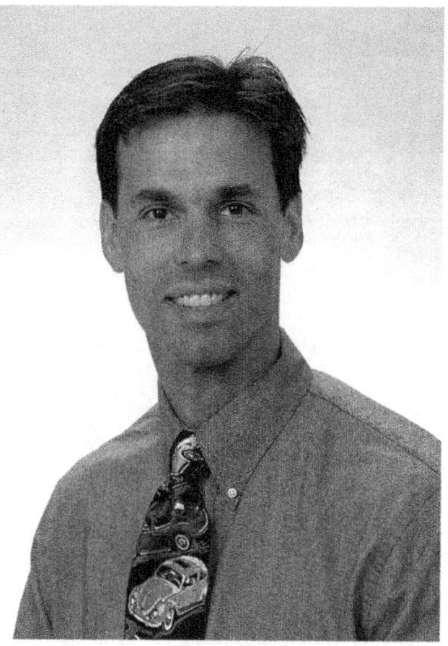

Kevin can be contacted by email at kevin@dontfixit.org or by phone at 805/459-8844.

You can read more about the experiences of Kevin and many others at: www.dontfixit.org

Made in the USA
Monee, IL
07 July 2026

56564655R00144